Obesity and Pregnancy

Books are to be returned on or before
the last date below.

7 – DAY LOAN

Obesity and Pregnancy

Edited by
Margaret Rees
Mahantesh Karoshi
Louis Keith

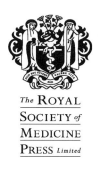

The ROYAL
SOCIETY *of*
MEDICINE
PRESS *Limited*

© 2008 Royal Society of Medicine Ltd

Published by the Royal Society of Medicine Press Ltd
1 Wimpole Street, London W1G 0AE, UK
Tel: +44 (0)20 7290 2921
Fax: +44 (0)20 7290 2929
E-mail: publishing@rsmpress.co.uk

British Library Cataloguing in Publication Data
A catalogue record for this book is available from the British Library

ISBN: 978-1-85315-761-5

Distribution in Europe and Rest of the World:
Marston Book Services Ltd
PO Box 269
Abingdon
Oxon OX14 4YN, UK
Tel: +44 (0)1235 465500
Fax: +44 (0)1235 465555
Email: direct.order@marston.co.uk

Distribution in USA and Canada:
Royal Society of Medicine Press Ltd
c/o BookMasters Inc
30 Amberwood Parkway
Ashland, OH 44805, USA
Tel: +1 800 247 6553/ +1 800 266 5564
Fax: +1 410 281 6883
Email: order@bookmasters.com

Distribution in Australia and New Zealand:
Elsevier Australia
30–52 Smidmore Street
Marrickville NSW 2204, Australia
Tel: +61 2 9517 8999
Fax: +61 2 9517 2249
Email: service@elsevier.com.au

Typeset by Saxon Graphics Ltd, Derby
Printed in the UK by MPG Books Limited

Contents

Contributors

Randall B Barnes MD
Associate Professor, Northwestern University, Chicago, USA

Rebecca Black MA MD MRCOG
Consultant Obstetrician, Women's Centre, John Radcliffe Hospital, Oxford, UK

Kirsten Duckitt MRCOG
Consultant Obstetrician and Gynecologist, Prince George Regional Hospital, Prince George, Canada

Ailsa E Gebbie MBChB FRCOG FFSRH
Consultant Gynaecologist, Family Planning and Well Woman Services, Edinburgh, UK

Lisa Gittens–Williams MD
Associate Professor of Obstetrics and Gynecology, UMDNJ, University Hospital, Newark, USA

Moshe Hod MD
Director, Division of Maternal Fetal Medicine, Helen Schneider Hospital for Women, Tel-Aviv University, Petah-Tiqva, Israel

Leslie Iffy MD
Professor of Obstetrics and Gynecology, UMDNJ, University Hospital, Newark, USA

Georgina Jones BA(Hons) MA DPhil
Senior Lecturer in Social Science, Health Services Research Section, University of Sheffield, Sheffield, UK

John G Kral MD PhD FACS
Professor of Surgery and Medicine, SUNY Downstate Medical Center, Brooklyn, New York, USA

Oded Langer MD PhD
Babcock Professor and Chairman, St Luke's-Roosevelt Hospital Center, University Hospital of Columbia University, New York, USA

David CW Lau MD PhD FRCPC
Professor of Medicine, Biochemistry and Molecular Biology, Julia McFarlane Diabetes Research Center; Chair, Diabetes and Endocrine Research Group, University of Calgary, Calgary, Canada

Erica E Marsh MD
Assistant Professor, Northwestern University, Chicago, USA

Orli Most MD
Atlantic Maternal Fetal Medicine, Morristown Memorial Hospital, Morristown, USA

LaTasha Nelson MD
Assistant Professor, Northwestern University, Chicago, USA

Manny Noakes PhD DipNut&Diet BSc
Associate Professor Program Leader – Diet and Lifestyle Interventions, CSIRO
Human Nutrition, Adelaide, Australia

Galia Oron MD
Senior Physician, Helen Schneider Hospital for Women, Tel-Aviv University,
Petah-Tiqva, Israel

Alan M Peaceman MD
Professor and Chief, Division of Maternal-Fetal Medicine, Northwestern
University, Chicago, USA

Daghni Rajasingam MBBS MD MRCOG
Consultant Obstetrician, Guy's and St Thomas' NHS Foundation Trust,
London, UK

Alice R Richman MPH
Doctoral Candidate, University of South Florida, Tampa, USA

Hannah Rickard MBBS MA
Specialty Trainee in Obstetrics and Gynaecology, Guy's and St Thomas' NHS
Foundation Trust, London, UK

Hamisu M Salihu MD PhD
Director, Center for Research and Evaluation, Lawton and Rhea Chiles Center
for Health Mothers and Babies, University of South Florida, Tampa, USA

Jane Scott PhD MPH Grad Dip Diet BSc
Associate Professor, Department of Nutrician and Dietetics, Finders University,
Adelaide, Australia

Eyal Sheiner MD PhD
Consultant Obstetrician, Soroka University Medical Center, Ben Gurion
University of the Negev, Beer-Sheva, Israel

Adi Y Weintraub MD
Resident, Soroka University Medical Center, Ben Gurion University of the
Negev, Beer-Sheva, Israel

Melanie J Woolnough BMedSci MB ChB FRCA
Anaesthetic SpR, Royal Hallamshire Hospital, Sheffield, UK

Steven M Yentis BSc MBBS FRCA MD MA
Anaesthetic Consultant, Chelsea and Westminster Hospital, London, UK

Yariv Yogev MD
Senior Physician, Helen Schneider Hospital for Women, Tel-Aviv University,
Petah-Tiqva, Israel

Preface

Unlike other areas of medicine where statistics are meticulously kept by governments and global organizations, there are no accurate data to describe the number of the world's inhabitants who are overweight, obese, or morbidly obese. Despite this knowledge deficit, it should come as no surprise to readers that the medical community is facing an epidemic. Obesity is present in many of the developed countries and can also be observed in some urban areas of developing nations. The cause of this epidemic, simply stated, is overeating, but the overriding concern is more complex. Social factors, such as growing affluence since the 1950s, increasing reliance on pre-prepared meals, and the popularity of fast foods and sweetened drinks, have all contributed to the problem. Though there has been no official Olympiad in this area of life, some observers suggest that the UK and US are in constant competition for the title of 'Obesity Capital of the World'.

Without doubt, the obesity epidemic has had adverse effects on both men and women, but in the case of women, some of its worse complications occur with those who are severely obese and pregnant. Obviously, this combination has been seen in the past, but it has increased so dramatically in its frequency that research has yet to catch up. Studies may discuss one or another aspect of caring for the obese pregnant patient, but until now, there has been no attempt to draw all such material together to try and present a comprehensive appraisal of the problem.

We are pleased to have the opportunity to review this topic here, and have invited some of the world's experts on this subject to share their knowledge and experience, and ensure that the material discussed is evidence-based. We have initially presented some 'core issues' that relate to obesity in both sexes, while then going on to discuss obesity in the pregnant patient, concluding with information on care of the obese parturient (e.g. difficulties of surgery and anaesthesia).

We hope that our efforts will be of value to all health care professionals who deal with this problem on a day-to-day basis, and that the book provides them with adequate suggestions to augment their care plans and counselling processes.

Margaret Rees
Reader in Reproductive Medicine and Honorary Consultant in Medical Gynaecology, John Radcliffe Hospital, Oxford, UK; Visiting Professor, University of Glasgow, Glasgow, UK

Mahantesh Karoshi
Specialist Registrar, Department of Obstetrics and Gynaecology, Frimley Park Foundation Hospital NHS Trust, Frimley, UK

Louis Keith
Professor Emeritus and Former Head, Department of Obstetrics and Gynecology, Northwestern University Medical School, Chicago, USA

SECTION 1

Core Issues

1 Epidemiology and long-term health consequences of obesity

Hamisu M Salihu, Alice R Richman

Introduction

Obesity is a complex and multifactorial disease of epic proportions, developing from a combination of behavioral, genetic, and environmental factors and resulting in a global burden of chronic disease, death, and disability. Obesity is most often measured through an assessment of excessive body fat as compared with height by the body mass index (BMI), which is calculated by dividing a person's weight in kilograms by the square of their height in meters (BMI = kg/m^2).[1,2] A summary of the typical obesity classifications, based on BMI values, is provided in Table 1.1. Although BMI is most often used to measure obesity, it does have limitations. For example, BMI may overestimate body fat in extremely muscular individuals or may underestimate body fat in individuals, such as the elderly, who may have little muscle mass. Therefore, interpretations of BMI within a clinical setting must take into account lean mass (muscularity) to avoid incorrect assessments of body fat.[3]

Another, albeit less frequently used, method of classification of obesity categorizes obese individuals according to body fat distribution into peripheral, truncal (central), and generalized obesity. Central obesity is defined as waist circumference or waist/hip ratio (WHR) above the 95th percentile, peripheral obesity is defined as WHR below the 5th percentile, and generalized obesity describes a person whose waist circumference lies between the 5th and the 95th percentiles.[4]

BMI measurements are most accurate as weight and height of a person and are measured by a healthcare professional in contrast to self-reports, which tend to be inexact. Despite potential inaccuracy, research data often utilize self-reported estimates, which tend to overreport height and underreport weight.[5-11] Perhaps as a result of culturally dictated ideas of desirable body image, women tend to underestimate their weight more than men, and men tend to overestimate their height more than women.[5-11] As age increases, both sexes tend to overestimate their height, an error that may be related to an unawareness of postural shrinkage secondary to osteoporotic spinal fractures.[5-11] It is likely, therefore, that reported BMI values represent underestimates, and the association between BMI and morbidity and mortality outcomes could in fact be conservative estimations at best.

TABLE 1.1 Classifications of BMI

	BMI (kg/m^2)	**Risk of comorbidities**
Underweight	<18.5	Low – but other problems
Normal weight	18.5–24.9	Average
Overweight	25–29.9	Increased
Obesity (class 1)	30–34.9	Moderate
Obesity (class 2)	35–39.9	Severe
Extreme obesity (class 3)	≥40	Very severe

Adapted with permission from WHO, 2000.[2]

Epidemiology of obesity

Obesity is a global epidemic in both developed and developing countries, with approximately 1 billion overweight and at least 300 million obese adults worldwide.[12] The World Health Organization (WHO) projects that the number of obese individuals will increase to 700 million by the year 2010.[12]

The prevalence of obesity varies greatly by geographical location, from as low as 5% in China, Japan, the Philippines, and some African nations to over 75% in such places as urban Samoa.[12] Even in China, where low rates are prevalent, obesity rates are 20% in some urban areas.[12]

In the USA, only four states had obesity rates less than 20% in 2006, while 22 had obesity rates equal to or greater than 25%.[13] Such rates exceed the 15% of Canadians, 21% of Germans, and 5% of Norwegians who are obese.[2] Variations also exist in Middle Eastern countries (e.g., 29% of Bahrainians vs 10% of Iranians) and in Africa as well.[14]

Trends in obesity

The extent of the obesity epidemic is such that it is replacing more long-established public-health concerns such as undernutrition and infectious disease in terms of public health priorities.[2] Figure 1.1 shows overall trends in obesity in the USA from 1960 to 2004, using data collected by the National Health and Nutrition Examination Survey (NHANES) program. NHANES is a cross-sectional, nationally representative survey that collects and disseminates estimates of several health indicators for the US population. This figure demonstrates a rise in obesity rates over time, climbing nearly 2.5 times in the period 1960–2004, doubling in just two decades from 1980 to 2000, with extreme obesity growing in 2004 to almost six times what it was in 1960.

Though counterintuitive, increases in obesity rates are often faster in developing countries than in developed ones.[12] The WHO classifies obesity prevalence data into six regions: (1) Africa, (2) the Americas, (3) south-east Asia, (4) Europe, (5) the eastern Mediterranean, and (6) the western Pacific. All six regions, including both developing and developed nations, experienced an increase in obesity prevalence rates over the 5-year period 1987–92.[2] Figure 1.2 shows a comparison of obesity rates among both developed and developing nations.

Childhood obesity is also more prevalent and on the rise.[15–17] Since parental obesity is the strongest predictor of childhood obesity, it is no surprise that childhood obesity is growing. Globally, approximately 22 million children under the age of 5 are overweight.[12] In the USA, childhood obesity rates have tripled since 1980. Child obesity rates in Switzerland are almost five times what they were in 1960,[15] and rates have more than doubled from 1974 to 2003 in England.[16] Similarly, in Spain, adolescent obesity rates more than doubled from 1985 to 2002.[17]

Risk factors

A combination of behavioral, environmental, and genetic factors places a person at risk of obesity. In terms of behavior, a person's sustained choices in eating (energy intake) and physical activity (energy expenditure) balance over time determine obesity onset.[20] Energy surplus is thought to occur when the number of calories consumed exceeds the number of calories used or burned by the body.

Home or workplace environments that encourage physical activity (e.g., the availability of parks, playfields) contribute to reduced storage of body fat. For

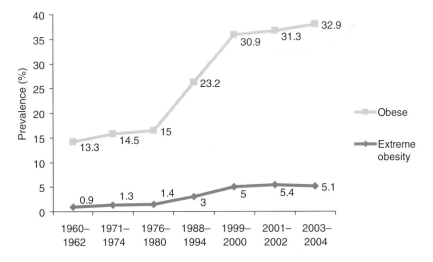

FIGURE 1.1 Prevalence and trends of obesity among adults aged 20–74 years in the USA, 1960–2004. Obesity, BMI ≥ 30; extreme obesity, BMI ≥ 40. Significant increasing trend ($P < 0.05$). The x-axis is not reflected to scale, meaning that the times between survey years are not equivalent. Adapted with permission from Ogden et al;[5] data from National Health and Nutrition Examination Survey (NHANES).[18]

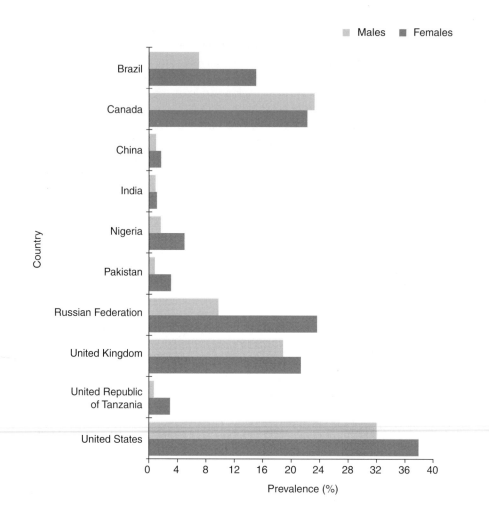

FIGURE 1.2 Obesity rates of both developed and developing nations by gender in 2002. Reproduced with permission from Ono et al.[19]

children, the home and school are particularly important in terms of excess weight acquisition. School-related factors include the types of food available during school hours, physical activity programs, available facilities for physical activity, and school policy,[21] wherein a child's freedom to be outside before or after regular school hours reflects of the safety of the neighborhood.[22–25]

Standard demographic variables such as age, race, gender, and socioeconomic status (SES) also represent risk factors for obesity. Older adults are more likely to be obese than younger ones, although this trend ceases after 80 years of age.[26] In a population-based survey among US adults, 26.8% of adults aged 20–39 years were obese compared with to 34.8% of adults aged 40–59 and 35.2% of adults aged 60–79. Family SES affects the physical activity outlets available in the community.[27–30] Wealthy communities tend to have parks and recreation areas in proximity to residential locations, and this encourages group participation in physical activities. The farther a family is from a park or activity site, the more unlikely they are to frequent it.

Large racial and ethnic disparities exist in obesity prevalence, especially among women. In the USA, minority women have higher rates of obesity than non-minority women, 53% of non-Hispanic black women and 48% of Mexican–American women being obese compared with 36% of non-Hispanic white women (Figure 1.3). Interestingly, this racial/ethnic disparity is not observed among US men, although racial and ethnic disparities to the disadvantage of minority groups are pronounced in both boys and girls and adolescents. For example, Mexican–American boys are significantly more overweight than non-Hispanic white and non-Hispanic black boys. Among girls, non-Hispanic black girls are the group at highest risk of overweight.[31] The same gender differences are also noted in Europe.[5]

Like most public health issues, obesity is linked to SES. In 2005, Ball and Crawford performed a systematic review of 34 papers worldwide and found that, in general, people with lower SES are at increased risk of weight gain.[32] It is thought that the association between poverty and obesity is due to the wide availability of low-cost foods that are high in calories and fat, people in the lower-income group being unable to afford healthy food, which tends to be more expensive.[33] Of equal importance, poor neighborhoods often are surrounded by fast-food restaurants and small convenience stores, making healthy food options particularly difficult to find.[33–38] Globally, as the gross national product (GNP) increases, the burden of obesity shifts to populations with lower SES. This shift particularly affects women with lower SES, who become obese earlier than men of equivalent SES.[39]

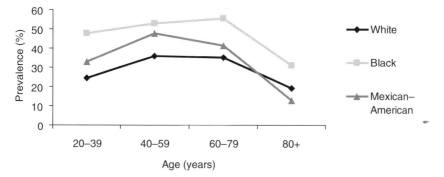

FIGURE 1.3 Prevalence of obesity among adults aged 20+ by race/ethnicity in the USA, 1999–2004. Obesity, BMI ≥ 30; significant at $P < 0.05$. Adapted from Ogden et al;[5] data from National Health and Nutrition Examination Survey (NHANES).[1]

Most of the genetic evidence for obesity comes from twin, family-member, and adoptee studies of resemblance and differences.[40] One twin study demonstrated that identical twins have a similar BMI, even when raised in different environments.[41] Another twin study showed that twin binge-eating disorders are due to shared genetic factors.[42] Many family studies have demonstrated a positive correlation between parental and child obesity, and some purport that parental obesity is the strongest predictor of childhood obesity.[43-45]

The role of obesity-related genes has also been investigated, as discussed further in Chapter 4. Although identifying genes that can be linked to common forms of obesity is a slow process, some studies have linked certain genes to obesity by demonstrating that they are present at higher frequencies among obese individuals.[40] Other studies have shown that certain mutations identified on the genome are associated with being overweight.[46-48] In particular, mutations in the single-gene, melanocortin 4-receptor gene have been linked to around 5% of obesity cases in identified populations, and this receptor gene is thought to mediate feeding behavior.[40]

In 2003, Loos and Bouchard performed a large review of the literature and found genetics to be responsible for about 30–70% of human adiposity, estimating the risk of obesity to be 2–3 times higher for those with a family history of obesity.[49] The same authors quantified four levels of genetic determination of obesity: (1) genetic obesity (1–5% of cases, not dependent on environment), (2) strong genetic predisposition (obese when living in obesigenic environment and overweight in non-obesigenic environment), (3) slight genetic predisposition (overweight in obesigenic environment and normal weight in non-obesigenic environment), and (4) genetically resistant (normal weight in obesigenic environment). An obesigenic environment is defined as an environment that encourages obesity and aids in the expression of genetic influences to gain weight.[49] In addition to these genomic studies, a handful of population-based studies have identified a gene with an unknown function (FTO, fat mass and obesity-associated gene) that may be responsible for 22% of obesity cases.[50] At this time, more research is needed in this area before genomic strategies can be incorporated into public health interventions.

Consequences of obesity: morbidity

The negative health consequences associated with obesity and the exponential growth of the disorder are such that the word 'alarming' is sedate compared with the need to address the problem urgently. Unfortunately, the enumeration of morbidities, disabilities, and quality-of-life issues below is hardly exhaustive:[51-59]

– cardiovascular diseases (e.g., coronary heart disease, hypertension, dyslipidemia, and stroke)
– many types of cancer: endometrial, cervical, ovarian, prostate, breast, colon, etc.
– type 2 diabetes mellitus
– end-stage kidney disease

- fatty liver disease
- osteoarthritis
- pulmonary embolism
- deep vein thrombosis
- polycystic ovary syndrome
- hyperuricemia and gout
- gallstones
- reproductive disorders
- low back pain
- breathlessness
- sleep apnea
- psychological and social problems
- complications in pregnancy
- complications in surgery
- social and psychological problems.

Only the most pressing issues will be addressed in some detail. The association between diabetes and obesity for adults is possibly the strongest relationship observed.[5] Several large, prospective studies found that overweight and obesity (BMI >25) account for roughly 65–80% of all new type 2 diabetes.[59] Eighty percent of people with diabetes are overweight or obese.[54] One study found that people with pre-obesity (BMI 25–30) are 3.5–4.6 times as likely to have diabetes as normal weight individuals (BMI 18.5–24.9).[60] Further, the relative risk increases as BMI increases, so that both men and women with BMIs of 35 are 20 times as likely to develop type 2 diabetes than individuals of normal weight.[60] Racial and ethnic disparities are present in this area as well, such minorities having a higher risk of acquiring obesity-related diabetes than non-Hispanic whites. The same level of disparity exists for minority children compared with their non-Hispanic white counterparts.[5]

Obesity is a risk factor for cardiovascular disease (CVD), specifically through its relationship to hypertension and high cholesterol. Obese individuals are 1.5–2.5 times as likely to have CVD (myocardial infarction and stroke) as persons of normal weight.[59] Persons who are overweight or obese (BMI >25) have a higher incidence of heart disease including heart attack, congestive heart failure, sudden cardiac death, angina or chest pain, and abnormal heart rhythm.[54] They are also twice as likely to have high blood pressure as those of normal weight, and obese people are more likely to maintain elevated levels of triglycerides and low concentrations of high-density lipoprotein (HDL)-cholesterol.[54,55,61] Like type 2 diabetes, racial and ethnic disparities are present in the relationship between obesity and CVD, with non-Hispanic whites having more risk of CVD than non-Hispanic blacks at a certain BMI, while people of Asian descent bear the greatest risk of obesity-associated CVD. These differences are perhaps due to variation in body fat distribution across population subgroups.[5,61,62]

Obesity also acts as a risk factor for many types of cancer, including endometrial, colon, gallbladder, prostate, kidney, and postmenopausal breast cancer.[54] A large prospective study of over 900 000 US adults found that obese men have over a 50% increased risk of dying from liver and gallbladder cancers, and non-Hodgkin's lymphoma, and obese women have a more than 50% increased risk of dying from gallbladder, breast, uterine, and kidney cancers.[63] The same study found that extremely obese women (BMI $\geq$ 40) have a more than 4–6 times increased risk of dying from kidney and uterine cancer than normal-weight women. As BMI increases past 35, so does the number of cancer sites.[63]

Lastly, obese individuals run a greater risk of adverse social circumstances and psychological problems than do non-obese individuals.[64] In terms of social bias, obese individuals are discriminated against in numerous settings:[65] (1) in the workplace, where overweight women receive lower wages, are denied higher-level positions, and receive fewer promotions,[66] and where employers and coworkers view overweight men and women as lazier, less competent, and less self-disciplined than non-overweight employees;[67] (2) in the healthcare industry by healthcare professionals; and (3) in the application process for college admission and employment.[65] The social stigma of obesity is not confined exclusively to adults, because overweight and obese children and adolescents also experience an increased risk of social and psychological problems, particularly self-esteem and behavioral problems.[68]

Consequences of obesity: mortality

Most obesity literature shows an association between this condition and an increased risk of mortality, although the exact nature of the relationship remains unclear.[5,69] Many studies support a curvilinear relationship, whereby risk of death is increased for both high and low BMI.[70–86] However, controversy exists over the finding that low BMI is related to mortality, because most study populations fail to exclude smokers and individuals with other comorbidities.[77,79,81,85,87,88] Given this circumstance, the Centers for Disease Control and Prevention (CDC) estimates that approximately 365 000 lives are lost from obesity and related comorbidities annually in the USA, placing obesity second only to smoking as the leading cause of death in the USA.[89]

CVD is the main cause of obesity-related mortality.[90] One review examined 26 other studies and found that obesity was related to all-cause mortality (relative risk [RR] =1.22), to coronary heart disease (RR = 1.57), and to CVD mortality (RR = 1.48).[91] Figure 1.4 displays the relative risk of death from all causes by BMI, race, and sex. A curvilinear relationship is depicted, and there is minimal variation until the higher BMIs, wherein white women and men acquire higher RR of death than black women and men. For higher BMIs, white men have a greater RR for all causes of death than white women. Unfortunately, data are missing for black men with BMI >35, and so no comparisons to black women can be made.

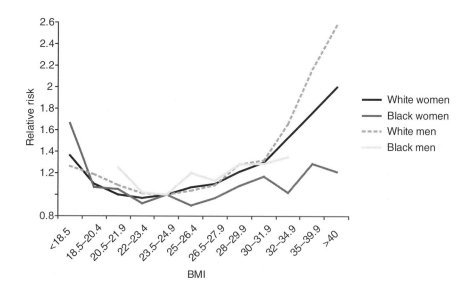

FIGURE 1.4 Relative risk of death from all causes by BMI, races and sex. Subjects had never smoked and did not have a history of disease. Adapted with permission from Calle et al.[69]

Obesity and reproductive health outcomes

As global obesity rates rise in both developed and developing nations, so also does the prevalence of obese pregnant women. Overweight and obesity affect girls before they reach puberty, and studies have shown that obesity is associated with early menarche; this linkage is even stronger among black and Hispanic girls.[92] Early maturation may have considerable implications for social, behavioral, and educational development and also may be predictive of future obesity, breast cancer, and mental health problems (see Chapter 3).[93,94]

Overweight and obesity are associated with several adverse reproductive health outcomes, including infertility,[95] gestational diabetes,[96] pregnancy-induced hypertension and pre-eclampsia,[97] birth defects, large-for-gestational-age (LGA) infants or macrosomia,[98] increased risk of cesarean delivery,[99–101] prolonged labor,[102] postpartum anemia,[103–105] and perinatal and maternal mortality.[54,106]

The relationship between gradations of obesity and in utero fetal demise was recently clearly demonstrated in a large, population-based study covering more than 1.5 million deliveries in the USA.[107] In doing so, the authors categorized obese mothers into the three typical obesity subclasses; namely, class I (BMI = 30.0–34.9), class II (BMI = 35.0–39.9), and class III (extreme obesity) (BMI ≥ 40). Overall, obese mothers were 40% more likely to experience stillbirth than non-obese gravidas (hazards ratio = 1.4; 95% CI = 1.3–1.5). These authors also noted that the risk of stillbirth increased in a dose-related fashion with ascending obesity class ($P < 0.01$). Perhaps the most striking and unique finding of this study was the pronounced risk of stillbirth among black mothers compared with their white counterparts. It is equally intriguing that the black disadvantage in stillbirth widened significantly with increase in BMI, with the greatest black–white difference observed among extremely obese mothers. These findings are unique in that they may provide a new point of view in the study of racial disparities, not only in the USA but also in other countries where obesity is a problem.

A number of hypotheses have been advanced to explain the adverse fetal outcomes associated with maternal obesity. It is well established that obese women are at elevated risk of gestational diabetes and hypertensive disorders.[108] However, even in the absence of these complications, the risk of heightened adverse birth outcomes among obese women still persists.[109,110] Obese mothers are less likely than thinner women to perceive fetal kicks, so that in diminished fetal movements preceding fetal demise, thinner women are more likely to perceive a change and seek prompt medical care.[108] Obese gravidas tend to have hyperlipidemia, which suppresses prostacyclin secretion while enhancing peroxidase production.[111] This imbalance favors vasoconstriction and platelet aggregation, processes that impede the maternal–fetal circulation, thus hampering normal fetal growth and development. Compared with non-obese mothers, obese pregnant women experience more extended periods of snoring during sleep with more frequent apnea hypoxia incidents, leading to prolonged episodes of oxygen desaturation.[112] This also could reduce blood flow to the fetus, leading to fetal compromise and greater likelihood of in utero fetal demise.

Conclusions

An attempt has been made to offer a global epidemiologic picture of the current pandemic of obesity and its consequences. There is little doubt that the prevalence of obesity is rising globally, and the increased prevalence has been observed among both developed and developing nations. Obesity is a risk factor for mortality and is a major determinant of CVD, stroke, many forms of cancer, and type 2 diabetes, in addition to psychosocial and behavioral disorders. Although some individuals are predisposed to obesity through genetic and biologic factors, much of obesity is due to societal, environmental, and behavioral influences. The good news is that obesity is a modifiable risk factor, and health policymakers and care providers have a golden opportunity to take action to avert a bleak future for growing numbers of the world's population.

References

1. Mei Z, Grummer-Strawn LM, Pietrobelli A, et al. Validity of body mass index compared with other body-composition screening indexes for the assessment of body fatness in children and adolescents. *Am J Clin Nutr* 2002;**75**:978–85.
2. World Health Organization. *Obesity: preventing and managing the global epidemic. Report of a WHO Consultation*. Geneva: World Health Organization, 2000 (WHO

Technical Report Series, no. 894). Available at: www.who.int/nutrition/publications/obesity/en/index.html.

3. National Institutes of Health, National Heart, Lung, and Blood Institute, NHBLI Obesity Education Initiative and North American Association for the study of Obesity. *The practical guide. Identification, evaluation, and treatment of overweight and obesity in adults*. NIH Publication no. 00–4084, 2000. Available at: www.nhlbi.nih.gov.

4. See R, Abdullah SM, McGuire DK, et al. The association of differing measures of overweight and obesity with prevalent atherosclerosis: Dallas Heart Study. *J Am Coll Cardiol* 2007;**50**:752–9.

5. Ogden CL, Yanovski SZ, Carroll MD, Flegal KM. The epidemiology of obesity. *Gastroenterology* 2007;**132**:2087–3102.

6. Kuczmarski MF, Kuczmarski RJ, Najjar M. Effects of age on validity of self-reported height, weight, and body mass index: findings from the Third National Health and Nutrition Examination Survey, 1988–1994. *J Am Diet Assoc* 2001;**101**:28–34.

7. Niedhammer I, Bugel I, Bonenfant S, et al. Validity of self-reported weight and height in the French GAZEL cohort. *Int J Obes* 2000;**24**:1111–18.

8. Flood V, Webb K, Lazarus R, Pang G. Use of self-report to monitor overweight and obesity in populations: some issues for consideration. *Aust N Z J Public Health* 1999;**24**:96–99.

9. Nieto-Garcia FJ, Bush TL, Keyl PM. Body mass definitions of obesity: sensitivity and specificity using self-reported weight and height. *Epidemiology* 1990;**1**:146–52.

10. Rowland M. Self-reported weight and height. *Am J Clin Nutr* 1990;**52**:1125–33.

11. Perry GS, Byers TE, Mokdad AH, et al. The validity of self-reports of past body weights by U.S. adults. *Epidemiology* 1995;**6**:61–6.

12. World Health Organization. Information sheets on obesity and overweight. Available at: www.who.int/dietphysicalactivity/publications/facts/obesity/en/; www.who.int/mediacentre/factsheets/fs311/en/index.html.

13. Centers for Disease Control and Prevention. State-specific prevalence of obesity among adults – United States, 2005. *MMWR Weekly*, 15 September, 2006;**55**: 985–88.

14. Prentice AM. The emerging epidemic of obesity in developing countries. *Int J Epidemiol* 2006;**35**:93–9.

15. Zimmermann MB, Gübeli C, Püntener C, Molinari L. Overweight and obesity in 6–12 year old children in Switzerland. *Swiss Med Wkly* 2004;**134**:523–8.

16. Stamatakis E, Primatesta P, Chinn S, et al. Overweight and obesity trends from 1974 to 2003 in English children: what is the role of the socioeconomic factors? *Arch Dis Child* 2005;**90**:999–1004.

17. Moreno LA, Mesana MI, Fleta J, et al. Overweight, obesity and body fat composition in Spanish adolescents. The AVENA Study. *Ann Nutr Metab* 2005;**49**:71–6.

18. National Health Examination Survey (1963–1965; 1966–1970); National Health and Nutrition Examination Survey (I, 1971–1974; II, 1976–1980;

III, 1988–1994; 1999–2000; 2001–2002; 2003–2004). Available at: www.cdc. gov/nchs/about/major/nhanes/datalink.htm.

19. Ono T, Guthold R, Strong K. WHO Global comparable Estimates, 2005. Available at: www.who.int/infobase/report.aspx.

20. Centers for Disease Control and Prevention. Contributing factors. Overweight and obesity: An overview. Available at: www.cdc.gov/nccdphp/dnpa/obesity/ contributing_factors.htm.

21. Alio AP, Salihu HM, Berrings TJ, et al. Obesity research and the forgotten African American child. *Ethn Dis* 2006;**16**:569–75.

22. Timperio A, Crawford D, Telford A, Salmon J. Perceptions about the local neighborhood and walking and cycling among children. *Prev Med* 2004;**38**: 39–47.

23. Saelens BE, Sallis JF, Black JB, Chen D. Neighborhood-based differences in physical activity: an environment scale evaluation. *Am J Public Health* 2003;**93**:1552–8.

24. Gordon-Larsen P, McMurray RG, Popkin BM. Determinants of adolescent physical activity and inactivity patterns. *Pediatrics* 2000;**105**:E83–E91.

25. Timperio A, Salmon J, Crawford D. Perceptions of local neighbourhood environments and their relationship to childhood overweight and obesity. *Int J Obes* 2005;**29**:170–5.

26. MacDonald KG Jr. Overview of the epidemiology of obesity and the early history of procedures to remedy morbid obesity. *Arch Surg* 2003;**138**: 357–60.

27. Estabrooks PA, Lee RE, Gyurcsik NC. Resources for physical activity: do availability and accessibility differ by neighborhood socioeconomic status? *Ann Behav Med* 2003;**25**:100–4.

28. Giles-Corti B, Donovan RJ. Socioeconomic status differences in recreational physical activity levels and real and perceived access to supportive physical environment. *Prev Med* 2002;**35**:601–11.

29. Brownson RC, Baker EA, Housemann RA, et al. Environmental and policy determinants of physical activity in the United States. *Am J Public Health* 2001;**91**:1995–2003.

30. Gordon-Larson P, Griffiths P, Bentley ME, et al. Barriers to physical activity: quantitative data on caregiver–daughter perceptions and practices. *Am J Prev Med* 2004;**27**:218–23.

31. National Health and Nutrition Examination Survey, 1999–2004. Available at: www.cdc.gov/nchs/nhanes.htm.

32. Ball K, Crawford D. Socioeconomic status and weight change in adults: A review. *Soc Sci Med* 2005;**60**:1987–2010.

33. Drewnowski A, Specter SE. Poverty and obesity: the role of energy density and energy costs. *Am J Clin Nutr* 2004;**79**:6–16.

34. Haas JS, Lee LB, Kaplan CP, et al. The association of race, socioeconomic status, and health insurance status with prevalence of overweight among adolescents. *Am J Public Health* 2003;**93**:2105–10.

35. French SA, Harnack L, Jeffery RW. Fast food restaurant use among women in the Pound of Prevention study: dietary, behavioral and demographic correlates. *Int J Obes* 2000;**24**:1353–9.

36. Jeffery RW, French SA. Epidemic obesity in the United States: are fast foods and television viewing contributing? *Am J Public Health* 1998;**88**:277–80.

37. Reidpath DD, Burns C, Garrard J, et al. An ecological study of the relationship between social and environmental determinants of obesity. *Health Place* 2002;**8**:141–5.

38. Morland K, Wing S, Roux AD, Poole C. Neighborhood characteristics associated with the location of food stores and food service places. *Am J Prev Med* 2002;**22**:23–9.

39. Monteiro CA, Moura EC, Conde WL, Popkin BM. Socioeconomic status and obesity in adult populations of developing countries: a review. *Bull WHO* 2004;**82**:940–6.

40. Centers for Disease Control and Prevention. National Office of Public Health Genomics. Obesity and genetics: a public health perspective. Available at: www.cdc.gov/genomics/training/perspectives/obesity.htm.

41. Stunkard AJ, Harris JR, Pedersen NL, McClearn GE. The body-mass index of twins who have been reared apart. *N Engl J Med* 1990;**322**:1483–7.

42. Tholin S, Rasmussen F, Tynelius P, Karlsson J. Genetic and environmental influences on eating behavior: the Swedish Young Male Twins Study. *Am J Clin Nutr* 2005;**81**:564–9.

43. Whitaker RC, Wright JA, Pepe MS, et al. Predicting obesity in young adulthood from childhood and parental obesity. *N Engl J Med* 1997;**337**:869–73.

44. Maffeis C, Talamini G, Tato L. Influence of diet, physical activity and parents' obesity on children's adiposity: a four-year longitudinal study. *Int J Obes Relat Metab Disord* 1998;**22**:758–64.

45. Wardle J, Guthrie C, Sanderson S, et al. Food and activity preferences in children of lean and obese parents. *Int J Obes Relat Metab Disord* 2001;**25**:971–7.

46. Farooqi IS, Keogh JM, Yeo GSH, et al. Clinical spectrum of obesity and mutations in the melanocortin 4 receptor gene. *N Engl J Med* 2003;**348**:1085–95.

47. Hinney A, Bettecken T, Brumm H, et al. Prevalence, spectrum and functional characterization of melanocortin-4 receptor gene variations in a representative population-based sample and obese adults from Germany. *J Clin Endocrinol Metab* 2006;**91**:1761–9.

48. Dempfle A, Hinney A, Heinzel-Gutenbrunner M, et al. Large quantitative effect of melanocortin-4 receptor gene mutations on body mass index. *J Med Genet* 2004;**41**:795–800.

49. Loos RJ, Bouchard C. Obesity – is it a genetic disorder? *J Intern Med* 2003;**254**:401–25.

50. Department of Health and Human Services, Centers for Disease Control and Prevention. Overweight and obesity: health consequences. Available at: www.cdc.gov/nccdphp/dnpa/obesity/consequences.htm.

51. Stein CJ, Colditz GA. The epidemic of obesity. *J Clin Endocrinol Metab* 2004; **89**:2522–5.

52. Mokdad AH, Serdula MK, Dietz WH, et al. The continuing epidemic of obesity in the United States. *JAMA* 2000;**284**:1650–1.

53. Must A, Spadano J, Coakley EH, et al. The disease burden associated with overweight and obesity. *JAMA* 1999;**282**:1523–9.

54. United States Department of Health and Human Services. Overweight and obesity: health consequences. Available at: www.surgeongeneral.gov/topics/obesity/calltoaction/fact_consequences.htm.

55. World Health Organization. The challenge of obesity in the WHO European Region and the strategies for response (e-book). Available at: www.euro.who.int/document/E89858.pdf.

56. Moghaddam AA, Woodward M, Huxley R. Obesity and risk of colorectal cancer: a meta-analysis of 31 studies with 70,000 events. *Cancer Epidemiol Biomarkers Prev* 2007;**16**:2533–47.

57. Stein PD, Beemath A, Olson RE. Obesity as a risk factor in venous thromboembolism. *Am J Med* 2005;**118**:978–80.

58. de Lusignan S, Hague N, van Vlymen J, et al. A study of cardiovascular risk in overweight and obese people in England. *Eur J Gen Pract* 2006;**12**:19–29.

59. Seidell JC. Time trends in obesity: an epidemiological perspective. *Horm Metab Res* 1997;**29**:155–8.

60. Field AE, Coakley EH, Must A, et al. Impact of overweight on the risk of developing common chronic diseases during a 10-year period. *Arch Intern Med* 2001;**161**:1581–6.

61. Helling TS, Gurram K. Nonalcoholic fatty liver disease, nonalcoholic steatohepatitis, and bariatric surgery: a review. *Surg Obes Relat Dis* 2006;**2**:213–20.

62. Howard BV, Criqui MH, Curb JD, et al. J. Risk factor clustering in the insulin resistance syndrome and its relationship to cardiovascular disease in postmenopausal white, black, Hispanic, and Asian/Pacific Islander women. *Metabolism* 2003;**52**:362–71.

63. Calle EE, Rodriguez C, Walker-Thurmond K, Thun MJ. Overweight, obesity, and mortality from cancer in a prospectively studied cohort of U.S. adults. *N Engl J Med* 2003;**348**:1625–38.

64. James DC. Factors influencing food choices, dietary intake, and nutrition-related attitudes among African Americans: application of a culturally sensitive model. *Ethn Health* 2004;**9**:349–67.

65. Hopper SV. The influence of ethnicity on the health of older women. *Clin Geriatr Med* 1993;**9**:231–59.

66. Ness R, Laskarzewski P, Price RA. Inheritance of extreme overweight in black families. *Hum Biol* 1991;**63**:39–52.

67. Colilla S, Rotimi C, Cooper R, et al. Genetic inheritance of body mass index in African-American and African families. *Genet Epidemiol* 2000;**18**:360–76.
68. Department of Health and Human Services, Center for Disease Control and Prevention. Defining overweight and obesity. Available at: www.cdc.gov/nccdphp/dnpa/obesity/defining.htm.
69. Calle EE, Thun MJ, Petrelli JM, et al. Body-mass index and mortality in a prospective cohort of U.S. adults. *N Engl J Med* 1999;**341**:1097–2105.
70. Allison DB, Gallagher D, Heo M, et al. Body mass index and all-cause mortality among people age 70 and over: the Longitudinal Study of Aging. *Int J Obes Relat Metab Disord* 1997;**21**:424–31.
71. Cornoni-Huntley JC, Harris TB, Everett DF, et al. An overview of body weight of older persons, including the impact on mortality. *J Clin Epidemiol* 1991;**44**:743–53.
72. Diehr P, Bild DE, Harris TB, et al. Body mass index and mortality in nonsmoking older adults: the Cardiovascular Health Study. *Am J Public Health* 1998;**88**:623–9.
73. Durazo-Arvizu R, Cooper RS, Luke A, et al. Relative weight and mortality in U.S. blacks and whites: findings from representative national population samples. *Ann Epidemiol* 1997;**7**:383–95.
74. Folsom AR, Kaye SA, Sellers TA, et al. Body fat distribution and 5-year risk of death in older women. *JAMA* 1993;**269**:483–7.
75. Garfinkel L. Overweight and mortality. *Cancer* 1986;**58**:1826–9.
76. Harris T, Cook EF, Garrison R, et al. Body mass index and mortality among nonsmoking older persons. *JAMA* 1988;**259**:1520–4.
77. Lee IM, Manson JE, Hennekens CH, Paffenbarger RS Jr. Body weight and mortality: a 27-year follow-up of middle-aged men. *JAMA* 1993;**270**:2823–8.
78. Lew EA, Garfinkel L. Variations in mortality by weight among 750,000 men and women. *J Chronic Dis* 1979;**32**:563–76.
79. Lindsted K, Tonstad S, Kuzma JW. Body mass index and patterns of mortality among Seventh-Day Adventist men. *Int J Obes* 1991;**15**:397–406.
80. Lindsted KD, Singh PN. Body mass and 26-year risk of mortality among women who never smoked: findings from the Adventist Mortality Study. *Am J Epidemiol* 1997;**146**:1–11.
81. Manson JE, Willett WC, Stampfer MJ, et al. Body weight and mortality among women. *N Engl J Med* 1995;**333**:677–85.
82. Losonczy KG, Harris TB, Cornoni-Huntley J, et al. Does weight loss from middle age to old age explain the inverse weight mortality relation in old age? *Am J Epidemiol* 1995;**141**:312–21.
83. Singh PN, Lindsted KD. Body mass and 26-year risk of mortality from specific diseases among women who never smoked. *Epidemiology* 1998;**9**:246–54.
84. Stevens J, Cai J, Pamuk ER, et al. The effect of age on the association between body-mass index and mortality. *N Engl J Med* 1998;**338**:1–7.
85. Troiano RP, Frongillo EA Jr, Sobal J, Levitsky DA. The relationship between body weight and mortality: a quantitative analysis of combined information from existing studies. *Int J Obes Relat Metab Disord* 1996;**20**:63–75.

86. Bray, G. *Contemporary Diagnosis and Management of Obesity*. Newtown, PA: Handbooks in Health Care, 2003.
87. Manson JE, Stampfer MJ, Hennekens CH, Willett WC. Body weight and longevity: a reassessment. *JAMA* 1987;**257**:353–8.
88. Willett WC, Stampfer M, Manson J, Vanltallie T. New weight guidelines for Americans: justified or injudicious? *Am J Clin Nutr* 1991;**53**:1102–3.
89. Mokdad AH, Marks JS, Stroup DF, Gerberding JL. Actual causes of death in the United States, 2000. *JAMA* 2004;**291**:1238–45.
90. Dorn JM, Schisterman EF, Winkelstein W Jr, Trevisan M. Body mass index and mortality in a general population sample of men and women. The Buffalo Health Study. *Am J Epidemiol* 1997;**146**:919–31.
91. McGee DL, Diverse Populations Collaboration. Body mass index and mortality: a meta-analysis based on person-level data from twenty-six observational studies. *Ann Epidemiol* 2005;**15**:87–97.
92. Kral JG. Preventing and treating obesity in girls and young women to curb the epidemic. *Obes Res* 2004;**12**:1539–46.
93. Johansson T, Ritzén EM. Very long-term follow-up of girls with early and late menarche. *Endocr Dev* 2005;**8**:126–36.
94. Group ECW. Hormones and breast cancer. *Hum Reprod Update* 2004;**10**: 281–93.
95. Zaadstra BM, Seidell JC, Van Noord PA, et al. Fat and female fecundity: prospective study of effect of body fat distribution on conception rates. *BMJ* 1993;**306**:484–7.
96. Solomon CG, Willett WC, Carey VJ, et al. A prospective study of pregravid determinants of gestational diabetes mellitus. *JAMA* 1997;**278**:1078–83.
97. Thadhani R, Stampfer MJ, Hunter DJ, et al. High body mass index and hypercholesterolemia: risk of hypertensive disorders of pregnancy. *Obstet Gynecol* 1999;**94**:543–50.
98. Larsen CE, Serdula MK, Sullivan KM. Macrosomia: influence of maternal overweight among a low-income population. *Am J Obstet Gynecol* 1990;**162**: 490–4.
99. Cnattingius S, Bergstrom R, Lipworth L, Kramer MS. Prepregnancy weight and the risk of adverse pregnancy outcomes. *N Engl J Med* 1998;**338**: 147–52.
100. Rosenberg TJ, Garbers S, Chavkin W, Chiasson MA. Prepregnancy weight and adverse perinatal outcomes in an ethnically diverse population. *Obstet Gynecol* 2003;**102**:1022–7.
101. Vahratian A, Siega-Riz AM, Zhang J, et al. Maternal pre-pregnancy overweight and obesity and the risk of primary cesarean delivery in nulliparous women. *Ann Epidemiol* 2005;**15**:467–74.
102. Vahratian A, Zhang J, Troendle J, et al. Maternal pre-pregnancy overweight and obesity and the pattern of labor progression in term nulliparous women. *Obstet Gynecol* 2004;**104**:943–51.
103. Bodnar LM, Siega-Riz AM, Cogswell M. High pregnancy body mass index increases the risk of postpartum anemia. *Obes Res* 2004;**12**:941–8.

104. Bodnar LM, Siega-Riz AM, Miller WC, et al. Who should be screened for postpartum anemia? An evaluation of current recommendations. *Am J Epidemiol* 2002;**156**:903–12.

105. Bodnar LM, Scanlon KS, Freedman DS, et al. High prevalence of postpartum anemia among low-income women in the United States. *Am J Obstet Gynecol* 2001;**185**:438–43.

106. Galtier-Dereure F, Boegner C, Bringer J. Obesity and pregnancy: complications and cost. *Am J Clin Nutr* 2000;**71**(Suppl 5):1242S–8S.

107. Salihu HM, Dunlop A-L, Alio AP, et al. Extreme obesity and risk of stillbirth among black and white gravidas. *Obstet Gynecol* 2007;**110**:552–7.

108. Fretts RC. Etiology and prevention of stillbirth. *Am J Obstet Gynecol* 2005;**193**:1923–35.

109. Kristensen J, Vestergaard M, Wisborg K, et al. Pre-pregnancy weight and the risk of stillbirth and neonatal death. *BJOG* 2005;**112**:403–8.

110. Cnattingius S, Bergstrom R, Lipworth L, Kramer MS. Prepregnancy weight and the risk of adverse pregnancy outcomes. *N Engl J Med* 1998;**338**: 147–52.

111. Stone JL, Lockwood CJ, Berkowitz GS, et al. Risk factors for severe preeclampsia. *Obstet Gynecol* 1994;**83**:357–61.

112. Maasilta P, Bachour A, Teramo K, et al. Sleep-related disordered breathing during pregnancy in obese women. *Chest* 2001;**120**:1448–54.

2 Pregravid obesity and excessive weight gain: implications on pregnancy

Galia Oron, Yariv Yogev and Moshe Hod

Introduction

Overweight and obesity are defined as abnormal or excessive fat accumulation that may impair health. As a rule, women have more body fat than men, and it is widely agreed that men with more than 30% body fat and women with more than 25% body fat are obese.

The World Health Organization (WHO) and the US National Institutes of Health define 'underweight' as a body mass index (BMI) of 18.5 or less, 'normal weight' as a BMI of 18.5–24.9, 'overweight' as a BMI of 25–29.9, and 'obesity' as a BMI of 30 or greater. Obesity is further characterized by BMI into class I (30–34.9), class II (35–39.9), and class III (< 40).[1]

There is a substantial increase in the prevalence of obesity in the population of reproductive-aged women. Although increased pregravid obesity is in and of itself a significant risk factor for adverse maternal and neonatal outcomes, additional weight gain during pregnancy compounds this risk for both the mother and her offspring. This chapter addresses issues concerning pregravid obesity and weight gain during pregnancy and their implication for reproduction and pregnancy outcome.

Global trends

The prevalence of obesity is increasing at an alarming rate on a global basis. The worldwide prevalence of obesity (BMI $\geq$ 30) is 15–20%, and obesity and its comorbid consequences account for 2–7% of the total global healthcare costs. The WHO's latest reports indicate that in 2007 approximately 1 billion adults (aged 15 and older) were overweight and at least 300 million adults were obese. This international agency also projects that, by 2015, approximately 2.3 billion adults will be overweight and more than 700 million will be obese.[2] Results from the latest (2003–4) US National Health and Nutrition Examination Survey (NHANES) indicate that 66.3% of adults are overweight (BMI $\geq$ 25) and 32.2% are obese (BMI $\geq$ 30). The prevalence of overweight and obesity among adults aged 20–74 years in the USA increased from 47.0% (in the 1976–80 survey) to 66.3% (in the 2003–4 survey). Over the same period, the prevalence of obesity has doubled among women from 16.5% to 33.2%[3,4] (Table 2.1).

TABLE 2.1 Age-adjusted prevalence of overweight and obesity among US adults aged 20–74 years (in %). NHANES reports[3,4]

	1976–80	1988–94	1999–2000	2001–2	2003–4
Overweight and obese (BMI ≥ 25)	47%	55.9%	64.5%	65.7%	66.3%
Obese (BMI ≥ 30)	15%	23.2%	30.9%	31.3%	32.2%

Obesity and pregnancy

As the prevalence of obesity is increasing, so is the number of women of reproductive age who are overweight and obese. The average BMI is increasing among all age categories, and women enter pregnancy at higher weights. Women are also more likely to retain gestational weight with each pregnancy.

Approximately one-third of women of reproductive age in the USA are obese, with no appreciable increase from 1999.[4–6] The prevalence of obesity is greatest among African–American women (48.8%), compared with Mexican–American (38.9%) and non-Hispanic white women (31.3%).[4]

Fertility

Several studies have shown an increased risk of anovulatory infertility in obese women (odds ratio [OR] of 2–3) by the mechanism of hyperandrogenism and polycystic ovary syndrome, which share several pathophysiologic characteristics, including insulin resistance.[7–11] Although some controversy still exists regarding the effect of obesity in patients who have in vitro fertilization (IVF), three large, population-based, retrospective studies have shown lower pregnancy rates in obese patients. Linsten et al[12] reported the results of 8457 IVF patients, showing significantly lower birth rate in women with a BMI of ≥27 (OR 0.67, 95% confidence interval [CI] 0.48–0.94). Fedorcsak et al[13] reviewed 5019 IVF cycles and found a significantly lower cumulative live birth rate in the obese group – 41.4% – than in normal-weight women – 50.3% (95% CI 32.1–50.7). Wang et al[14] reported the results of 3586 patients and established a significant linear reduction in fecundity from the moderately obese to the very obese ($P < 0.001$). Body fat distribution in women of reproductive age seems to have more impact on fertility than age or obesity itself; a 0.1 unit increase in waist–hip ratio led to a 30% decrease in probability of conception per cycle (hazard ratio [HR] 0.7, 95% CI 0.5–0.8).[9]

Miscarriage

Although the relationship between obesity and first-trimester miscarriage has been investigated extensively, the results are far from conclusive and require further research. Whereas several studies suggest that obesity may increase the risk of miscarriage[15–19] due to adverse influences on the embryo, the endometrium, or both,[20] others found no association between miscarriage and obesity.[21-24] These studies lack consistency, however, mainly because of the use of different obesity classification systems that disregard the WHO definitions.

Perinatal and neonatal complications

Obesity increases all pregnancy complications, as shown in Table 2.2. The risk of pregnancy complications increases in a linear fashion with increased BMI. In a prospective, multicenter study of more than 16 000 patients, Weiss et al[26] found that classes I and II obesity were associated with an increased risk of complications during pregnancy, including gestational diabetes (OR 2.6 and 4, respectively), fetal macrosomia (OR 1.7 and 1.9, respectively), gestational hypertension (OR 2.5 and 3.2, respectively), and pre-eclampsia (OR 1.6 and 3.3, respectively). The effect of obesity on the obstetric and perinatal outcome is most probably confounded by several pre-existing, undiagnosed comorbidities such as type 2 diabetes and hypertension.

TABLE 2.2 Obstetric perinatal and neonatal complications associated with obesity

Obstetric	Perinatal and neonatal
Gestational diabetes (OR = 2.6–4)[26]	Neural tube defect (OR = 1.8)[78]
Hypertension (OR = 2.5–3.2)[26,36]	Spina bifida (OR = 2.6)[78]
Pre-eclampsia (OR = 1.6–3.3)[26,36]	Omphalocele (OR = 3.3)[80]
Dyslipidemia	Macrosomia (OR = 1.2–2.1)[34,36]
Back pain	Head trauma
	Shoulder dystocia
Preterm delivery (OR = 2)[36]	Brachial plexus lesion
(HR for PPROM = 1.5)[63]	Fracture of the clavicle
More induced deliveries (HR = 1.2–1.8)[36,63]	Stillbirth (HR = 1.4–2.9) 35[49,51]
Prolonged delivery	Hemorrhage after delivery
Vulvar or perineal tears	(OR = 1.5)[36]
Cesarean section and its	
complications (OR = 1.4–3.9)[64,68]	
Thromboembolism	

HR, heart ratio; OR, odds ratio; PPROM, preterm premature rupture of membranes.

Gestational diabetes mellitus (GDM)

About 3–7% of women develop GDM during pregnancy. Although many factors are related to this risk, including ethnicity, previous occurrence of GDM, age, parity, family history of diabetes, and degree of hyperglycemia in pregnancy,[27-32] obesity is an independent risk factor for developing GDM, causing an increased risk of about 20%.[27,28] Even overweight women have 1.8–6.5 times greater risk of GDM.[29,33] A population-based cohort study of 96 801 singleton births found that not only obese women (BMI > 30.0) but also overweight women (BMI =

25.0–29.9) have a markedly increased risk of GDM (OR 5.0 and 2.4, respectively).[34] Of equal importance, women diagnosed with GDM have a considerably higher risk of developing type 2 diabetes mellitus later in life. In a case–control study, including 28 women diagnosed with GDM in 1984–5, and a control group of 53 women who gave birth in the same time period, Linné et al performed a 2-h oral glucose tolerance test 15 years later.[35] Ten women (35%) in the GDM group were diagnosed with type 2 diabetes mellitus but none in the control group ($P <$ 0.001). Mean BMI in the diabetic group was 27.4 and in the nondiabetic GDM group, 24.6 ($P < 0.05$).

Macrosomia

Morbid obesity (BMI > 35) increases the risk of birth weights under 4000 g (OR 2.1 (95% CI 1.3–3.2)).[36] Ehrenberg et al[37] reviewed the results of 12 950 pregnancies and found that both obesity and pregestational diabetes are independently associated with increased risk of macrosomia. After adjusting for confounding risk factors, these authors found that, compared with normal BMI women, obese women were at elevated risk of large-for-gestational-age (LGA) newborns at delivery (16.8% vs 10.5%; $P < 0.0001$), as were overweight women (12.3% vs 10.5%; $P = 0.01$). Baeten et al[34] found that the risk of delivering a macrosomic infant was increased (albeit not in a dose-related fashion) with each level of increasing BMI, independently of the diagnosis of diabetes: BMI > 30: OR 2.1 (95% CI 1.9–2.4); BMI 25–29.9: OR 1.5 (95% CI 1.4–1.6); BMI 20–24.9: OR 1.2 (95% CI 1.2–1.3). Because the prevalence and frequency of overweight and obesity in women are nearly 10 times that of diabetes (45% vs 4.5%), abnormal maternal body habitus appears to be the strongest influence on the prevalence of macrosomia.

Gestational hypertension and pre-eclampsia

Arterial blood pressure, hemoconcentration, and cardiac function are all altered by the hemodynamic changes brought about by obesity. The prevalence of hypertensive disorder and pre-eclampsia is higher in obese women.[38–40] Previous studies found pregnancy-associated obesity to be a risk factor for gestational hypertension, independently of diabetes, age,[41,42] and parity (OR 1.7, 95% CI 1.2–6.2).[40] Stone et al[43] found that the only risk factors associated with the development of severe pre-eclampsia were severe obesity in all patients (OR 3.5, 95% CI 1.6–7.4) and a history of pre-eclampsia in multiparous patients (OR 7.2, 95% CI 2.7–18.7). In a large, population-based, cohort study of 96 801 singleton births to nulliparous women, prepregnancy obese as well as overweight women had a markedly increased risk of pre-eclampsia (OR 3.3 and 2, respectively) and eclampsia (OR 3 and 2, respectively) compared with women with prepregnancy BMI < 20.0.[34]

Sibai et al[38] found that prepregnancy relative weight was strongly predictive of the risk of pre-eclampsia ($P < 0.01$), with the highest incidence among women whose relative weight was ≥ 140 lb (63 kg) (11.3%). A meta-analysis showed that the risk of pre-eclampsia doubled with each 5–7 kg/m^2 increase in prepregnancy BMI. This relation persisted in studies that excluded women with chronic hypertension, diabetes mellitus, multiple gestations, and other confounders.[44]

A retrospective cohort study of 24 241 women of whom 5308 (21.9%) were overweight, 1858 (7.7%) were obese, and 157 (0.6%) were morbidly obese (BMI ≥ 40) found a three times higher risk of pre-eclampsia in obese and a seven times higher risk in morbidly obese primigravid women.[36] Morbid obesity (BMI > 40) was associated with a substantially increased risk of pre-eclampsia (OR 4.82, 95% CI 4.04–5.74).[45]

Stillbirth and fetal death

Stillbirth remains a serious reproductive failure, with a frequency of 2–5 per 1000 births, and constitutes more than half of all perinatal deaths.[46,47] Prepregnancy BMI and fetal death were examined in the Danish National Birth Cohort among 54 505 pregnant women. They reported a fivefold increase in risk of stillbirth in obese women. Prepregnancy obesity correlated with an increased risk of both late spontaneous abortion and stillbirth, expressed as follows – before week 14: HR 0.8 (95% CI 0.5–1.4); weeks 14–19: HR 1.6 (95% CI 1.0–2.5); weeks 20–27: HR 1.9 (95% CI 1.1–3.3); weeks 28–36: HR 2.1 (95% CI 1.0–4.4); weeks 37–39: HR 3.5 (95% CI 1.9–6.4); and week 40: HR 4.6 (95% CI 1.6–13.4). Overweight women also experienced a higher risk after 28 weeks, and especially after 40 weeks' gestation HR 2.9 (95% CI 1.1–7.7).[48] In a large, British, register-based study, overweight and obesity were only modestly related to intrauterine death (OR 1.1 [95% CI 0.9–1.2] and OR 1.4 [95% CI 1.1–1.7]), respectively, after adjustment for obesity-related diseases in pregnancy.[48] In a large, Swedish, population-based cohort of 167 750 women, the OR for late fetal death was increased among nulliparous women with overweight and obesity (OR 3.2 [95% CI 1.6–6.2] and OR 4.3 [95% CI 2.0–9.3], respectively). Among parous women, only obese women had a significant increase in the risk of late fetal death: OR 2.0 (95% CI 1.2–3.3).[9]

In a large cohort of 134 527 obese women, Salihu et al[51] found that, overall, obese mothers were about 40% more likely to experience stillbirth than nonobese women (adjusted HR 1.4 [95% CI 1.3–1.5]). The risk of stillbirth increased in a dose-dependent fashion with increase in BMI: class I (BMI 30–34.9), HR 1.3 (95% CI 1.2–1.4); class II (BMI 35–39.9), HR 1.4 (95% CI 1.3–1.6); and extreme obesity (BMI 40), HR 1.9 (95% CI 1.6–2.1) (*P* for trend < 0.01). Furthermore, obese black mothers experienced more stillbirths than their white counterparts (adjusted HR 1.9, 95% CI 1.7–2.1 compared with adjusted HR 1.4, 95% CI 1.3–1.5). The black disadvantage in stillbirth widened with increase in BMI, with the greatest difference observed among extremely obese black mothers (adjusted HR 2.3, 95% CI 1.8–2.9).

Preterm delivery

Most investigators report both low prepregnancy weight and poor weight gain in low-BMI women as risk factors for preterm birth.[52–59] Ehrenberg et al[60] found that women with pregravid BMI of <19.8 were at a slightly increased risk of preterm labor: relative risk (RR) 1.22 (95% CI 1.02–1.46). Moreover, low maternal weight at delivery (BMI < 19.8) was associated with substantial risk of preterm labor and delivery (RR 2.5 [95% CI 1.02–6.33] and RR 2.45 [95% CI 1.4–4.4], respectively) and lower gestational age at delivery (36.8 vs 38.3 weeks; $P < 0.05$). These authors concluded that low weight and BMI at conception or delivery, as well as poor weight gain during pregnancy, were associated with prematurity and low birth weight. Schieve et al[61] reported that weight gain of less than 0.5 lb/week (0.23 kg) at 14–28 weeks of pregnancy was associated with increased risk of preterm delivery, particularly if women were underweight or of average weight before pregnancy (OR 6.7 and 1.6 for underweight and overweight women, respectively).

Regarding obese women, reports are inconclusive. Current evidence suggests that obesity may be associated with induced preterm delivery, but not spontaneous preterm birth. Smith et al[62] reported that, among nulliparous women, the risk of spontaneous preterm labor decreased with increasing BMI, whereas the risk of requiring an elective preterm delivery increased. Morbidly obese nulliparous women were at increased risk of all-cause preterm delivery. In contrast, obesity and elective preterm delivery were only weakly associated among multiparous women. Bhattacharya et al[36] also reported that the frequency of induced labor increased with increasing BMI, the risk being lowest in underweight women (BMI ≤ 19.9) (OR 0.8 [95% CI 0.8–0.9]) and highest in the morbidly obese (BMI > 35) (OR 1.8 [95% CI 1.3–2.5]). In a large retrospective cohort study including 62 167 women within the Danish National Birth Cohort, the crude risks of PPROM (preterm premature rupture of the membranes) and of induced preterm deliveries were higher in obese women than in normal-weight women, especially before 34 completed weeks of gestation (HR 1.5 [95% CI 1.2–1.9] and HR 1.2 [95% CI 1.0–1.6], respectively).[63]

Cesarean section

Studies report a nearly twofold increased risk of cesarean delivery in women who are obese even after controlling for other factors. Why obesity increases the risk of cesarean section, with even greater risk among morbidly obese women, needs further study. The increased risk of cesarean delivery in obese women should not be taken lightly. Apart from the immediate operative risk, the increased cesarean rate in overweight and obese women is also associated with increased postoperative complications such as wound infection/breakdown, excessive blood loss, deep venous thrombophlebitis, and postpartum endometritis.

In a large retrospective study that included 26 682 nulliparous women with singleton, term deliveries, the incidence of cesarean delivery increased with increased prepregnancy BMI from 14.3% for lean women (BMI < 19.8) to 42.6% for morbidly obese women (BMI ≥ 35). Among women without complications, the estimated adjusted RR was 1.4 (95% CI 1.0–1.8) among overweight women, 1.5 (95% CI 1.1–2.1) among obese women, and 3.1 (95% CI 2.3–4.8) among morbidly obese women.[64] Similar results were reported by Vahratian,[65] showing an unadjusted RR of 1.4 for cesarean delivery among overweight and obese women. After controlling for maternal height, education, weight gain during pregnancy, and labor induction, the adjusted RR for cesarean delivery among overweight women was 1.2 (95% CI 0.8–1.8) and among obese women 1.5 (95% CI 1.05–2.0).

Weiss et al[66] reported the rate of cesarean section among nulliparous women to be 20.7% for normal-weight women, 33.8% for obese women (BMI 30–34.9), and 47.4% for morbidly obese patients (BMI ≥ 35). Similar results were reported by Holger et al,[67] with the increased risk of cesarean section rising with increasing BMI, from 25.1% (BMI ≥ 30) to 30.2% (BMI > 35), and even to 43.1% in morbidly obese women (BMI ≥ 40), mainly because of repeat cesarean sections. Another study conducted among 1881 low-risk women reported an overall cesarean rate of 5.1%, but the rate rose to 7.7% for obese women (BMI > 29) compared with 4.1% for women with normal BMI. After adjustment for weight gain, short stature, advanced maternal age, parity, and intrapartum complications, the OR for obesity was 3.99 (95% CI 2.0–7.9; $P < 0.001$).[68] Cnattingius et al[69] found that the effect of prepregnant BMI on cesarean delivery rate was influenced by maternal height. Tall, lean women had the lowest cesarean rate (5%), followed by tall, obese women (11%), whereas short, obese women had the highest rate (36%). Brost et al[70] found that each unit increase in prepregnancy BMI or a third-trimester weight gain resulted in an increase in the odds of cesarean delivery of 7.0% and 7.8%, respectively. Witter et al[71] supported these findings and reported a statistically significantly increased risk of cesarean section associated with weight gain during pregnancy. The attributed risk of cesarean section of gaining more than 16 kg was 6.9%.

Obesity was also associated with increased risk of operative delivery: 33.8% in the obese and 47.4% in the morbidly obese group versus 20.7% in controls.[72]

Postpartum anemia

Bodnar et al suggested that high prepregnancy BMI predicts postpartum anemia, reporting that the adjusted RR increased as BMI increased from 24 to 38. Women with a BMI of 28 had nearly 1.8 times the risk of postpartum anemia of women with a BMI of 20 (95% CI 1.3–2.5), and obese women with a BMI of 36 had nearly 2.8 times this risk (95% CI 1.7–4.7).[73,75] These findings were recently supported by a large retrospective cohort study that found obese women more likely to sustain postpartum hemorrhage (OR 1.5, 95% CI 1.3–1.7).[36] Postpartum anemia in obese women is no doubt caused by several potential contributing factors, all of which are more prevalent among obese women; they include iron deficiency, a higher rate of cesarean section and operative delivery, a higher incidence of macrosomia (causing increased blood loss during delivery), and a lower rate of breastfeeding[76] (protecting against anemia by lengthening the postpartum amenorrhea).

Perinatal mortality

Perinatal mortality is increased among overweight and obese women. Cogswell et al[77] reported that perinatal mortality is 50% higher among infants born to overweight women and 200–430% higher among infants born to obese women. Obesity increases the perinatal mortality from 1.4 per 1000 in normal-weight women to 5.7 per 1000 in obese women.[72]

Birth defects

Apart from the increase in failure to detect birth defects in obese women due to difficult interpretation of serum markers (changes in the volume of distribution) and suboptimal visualization of fetal anatomy by ultrasound examination, several studies report a factual increase in birth defects among obese women. Waller et al[78] in 1994 first suggested that offspring of obese women were at increased risk of neural tube defects (OR 1.8, 95% CI 1.1–3.0), especially spina bifida (OR 2.6, 95% CI 1.5– 4.5). These results have been confirmed in subsequent studies and have also implicated maternal obesity in increased risk of heart defect (OR 1.18, 95% CI 1.09–1.27)[79] and omphalocele (OR 3.3, 95% CI 1.0–10.3).[80] Because these types of congenital anomalies are often seen with pregestational diabetes, some investigators suggest that many of these obese women may have had undiagnosed type 2 diabetes.[79] Neural tube defects are associated with folic acid deficiencies, yet it is inconclusive whether such a deficiency is a contributing factor to the increased risk of a neural tube defect in obese women. Mojtabai[81] suggested that women with a BMI greater than 30 would need to increase their folate consumption by 350 μg/day to achieve the same folate levels as women with a BMI less than 20. In contrast, Ray et al[82] in a Canadian population estimated whether the risk of neural tube defects was lower after flour was fortified with folic acid; surprisingly, they found the opposite. Before fortification of flour, increased maternal weight was associated with a modestly increased risk of neural tube defects (OR 1.4, 95% CI 1.0–1.8); after flour fortification, the risk actually increased (OR 2.8, 95% CI 1.2–6.6).

Infant and childhood implications

The implications of maternal obesity far surpass intrauterine life, extending into infancy and even adulthood with severe health repercussions. Maternal obesity has long been linked with the delivery of a macrosomic infant. Now there is abundant evidence linking macrosomia to increased overweight and obesity in adolescents as well as adults.[83–85] Perhaps more alarming is a recent, retrospective, cohort study by Whitaker[86] in over 8400 children in the USA in the early 1990s, which reported the prevalence of childhood obesity to be 2.4–2.7 times higher in offspring of obese women in the first trimester than in children whose mothers' BMI was in the normal range at this early stage of pregnancy. These findings remained consistent even after controlling for additional risk factors, including birth weight, parity, weight gain, and smoking during pregnancy (RR 2.0, 95% CI 1.7–2.3).

The epidemic of obesity and subsequent risk of diabetes and components of the metabolic syndrome clearly may begin in utero with fetal overgrowth and adiposity. Fully 50–90% of adolescents with type 2 diabetes have a BMI greater than 27,[87] and 25% of obese children 4–10 years of age have impaired glucose tolerance.[88]

Maternal long-term implications

Some women's pregnancies are associated with excessive weight gain.[89–91] Mean weight retention after pregnancy ranges between 0.4 and 3.8 kg.[92–95] Weight retention after pregnancy has been attributed to various causative factors, including smoking cessation, changes in activity leading to a more sedentary lifestyle, and socioeconomic factors such as low income. However, increased weight gain during pregnancy remains the strongest factor for weight retention after pregnancy.[96–98] Linné et al reported that women with a weight gain of 16 kg or more during pregnancy were 2.5 times more likely to be a high weight retainer 1 year postpartum.[99]

Recommended weight gain during pregnancy

Weight gain in pregnancy is considered to be the difference between a woman's weight at the last antenatal visit and her pregravid weight or her weight at first antenatal visit. The increment in weight gain during pregnancy takes into account the 4–5 kg in average 'net maternal weight gain' from the fetus (3.5 kg), placenta (0.5 kg), and amniotic fluid (0.5–1.0 kg).

Recommendations for optimal weight gain (20 lb or 9.1 kg) during pregnancy are inherited from the time when rickets was prevalent in Europe, and were initially intended to help decrease the risk of fetal macrosomia and complicated deliveries.[100] They were formulated as the Prochownick diet at a time when cesarean delivery was a formidable operation that carried a great risk of mortality. When cesarean sections became more routine as a result of improved medical conditions and operative care, weight recommendations became more liberal. In 1990, the Institute of Medicine (IOM) published guidelines for recommended weight gain during pregnancy based on prepregnancy weight.[101] This report was written at a time when concern was focused on the low-birth-weight infant. Since that time, the focus has shifted to the greater concern of increasing rates of obesity. The suggested weight gains are a gain of 11.2–15.9 kg for women with normal BMI, 6.8–11.2 kg for overweight women, and at least 6.8 kg for obese women (Table 2.3).

Based on the increasing evidence that overweight and obese women exceed the recommended weight gain during pregnancy together with the increasing prevalence of obesity in the population, the IOM currently is reviewing the recommendations for weight gain in pregnancy. Rode et al[102] tested the IOM recommendations by analyzing data from 2248 women with singleton, term pregnancies. These investigators established that the rate of birth of a macrosomic infant increased with an increasing weight gain in underweight and normal-weight women, but the association was less apparent in overweight and obese women. Underweight women seemed to benefit from gaining more weight than recommended by the IOM, because the OR of birth weight less than 3000 g was

TABLE 2.3 Institute of Medicine (IOM) recommendations for weight gain in pregnancy[101] versus the Swedish Medical Birth Register.[104] Optimal weight gain recommendations

Initial body mass index	IOM recommended gestational weight gain (lb/kg)	Swedish Medical Birth Register optimal weight gain recommendation (lb/kg)
< 20 (low)	28–40/12.5–18	9–22/4–10
20–24.9 (normal)	25–35/11.5–16	5–22/2–10
25–29.9 (high)	15–25/7–11.5	<20/9
30 (obese)	At least 15/6	<13/6

0.3 (95% CI 0.1–0.9) and the OR was 1.7 for birth weight greater than or equal to 4000 g (95% CI 0.8–3.6). The normal-weight women had an increased risk of birth weight less than 3000 g (OR 2.4, 95% CI 1.5–3.7) if weight gain was below the recommended range, and the OR of birth weight greater than or equal to 4000 g was 1.9 (95% CI 1.5–2.5) when the women gained more than recommended. They concluded that the upper IOM recommended limit for underweight women may have to be increased.

In 2006, the IOM convened a conference on this subject and published its workshop report, 'Influence of Pregnancy Weight on Maternal Child Health'. The goal of the workshop was to report on the available data relating to the recent trends in maternal obesity and weight gain on the health of the mothers and children. In the time between 1993 and 2003, the percentage of women gaining more than the IOM recommendations increased from 37% to 46%; this was accompanied by a decrease from 30% to 23% of women gaining less than the IOM weight gain recommendations. The report also noted the increasing trends in maternal complications, such as pre-eclampsia, gestational diabetes, and cesarean delivery, associated with maternal pregravid obesity and increased weight gain in pregnancy.[103]

A large, population-based, cohort study from the Swedish Medical Birth Register conducted on 298 648 singleton pregnancies recommended a slightly stricter weight gain during pregnancy in all prepregnancy BMI categories, in order to decrease the risk of adverse obstetric and neonatal outcomes[104] (Table 2.3).

Low weight gain during pregnancy

Low weight gain during pregnancy is associated with increased risk of preterm delivery and low birth weight. The magnitude of risk varies according to prepregnancy BMI. The risk is primarily evident in underweight (OR 6.7, 95% CI 1.1–40.6) and average-weight (OR 3.6, 95% CI 1.6–8.0) women, and less evident in overweight (OR 1.6, 95% CI 0.7–3.5) women.[105–110] Prospective cohort studies evaluating the effect of the Leningrad siege and the Dutch 'hunger winter' of World War II established the intrauterine influence of extreme maternal caloric deprivation with both short- and long-term consequences.

Studies of the Dutch hunger winter showed that the average birth weight for babies conceived or born during that winter was around 300 g lower than that previously established.[111] The siege of Leningrad was associated with an average fall in birth weight of 500–600 g (for term babies born in 1942). Of those born in the first half of 1942, half weighed less than 2500 g.[112] Low birth weight was found to correspond to an average increase in blood pressure of 1–2 mmHg in adult life,[113] a 15% increased risk of mortality from ischemic heart disease,[114] and a 35% increased risk of hemorrhagic stroke.[115] Exposure to famine in late or midgestation caused reduced glucose tolerance, whereas exposure to famine in early gestation caused a more atherogenic lipid profile, higher fibrinogen concentrations, reduced plasma concentrations of factor VII, a higher BMI, and a higher risk of coronary heart disease. These findings have led to the 'fetal origins' (Barker) hypothesis, which proposes that the fetus adapts to a limited supply of nutrients. In doing so, it permanently alters its physiology and metabolism, possibly increasing its risk of chronic disease later in life.[116–122]

High weigh gain during pregnancy

Excessive gestational weight gain can lead to increased risk of gestational diabetes, failed induction and postpartum infection,[123] pre-eclampsia,[124,125] cephalopelvic disproportion or failure to progress,[126,127] instrumental delivery,[124,126] preterm delivery,[127] cesarean delivery,[123,127,130,131] macrosomia,[124,125,128,130,132] low 5-min Apgar score,[132] and weight retention after pregnancy.[133–135]

Excessive weight gain during pregnancy also increases the risk of fetal death[136] and preterm labor and delivery.[129,136–138] Oken showed that increased weight gain increases the risk of having an overweight child at the age of 3 (OR 4.35 [95% CI 1.7–11.2]).[140] High weight gain during pregnancy, exceeding the current recommendations and leading to overweight or obesity, is associated with all the risks previously mentioned as associated with obesity during pregnancy.

Weight gain during multiple gestation pregnancy

Maternal weight gain recommendations during multiple gestation pregnancies can be based on pregravid BMI as with singletons. Weight gain during critical periods of gestation significantly influences twin birth weight; these critical periods vary by maternal pregravid weight status. Weight gain before 20 weeks had the largest effect on infants of underweight women, whereas weight gain after 28 weeks significantly affected the infant birth weights of normal-weight and overweight women.[141,142] A threshold weekly weight gain, from 20 weeks' gestation to delivery, of at least 1.75 lb/week (0.79 kg/week) in underweight women and at least 1.50 lb/week (0.68 kg/week) in normal-weight women was associated with the birth of both twins weighing at least 2500 g.[141]

The published recommendations for optimal maternal weight gain according to maternal pregravid BMI during critical periods of gestation are as follows:

- *Underweight women* – 1.25–1.75 lb/week (0.57–0.79 kg/week) until 20 weeks, 1.50–1.75 lb/week (0.68–0.79 kg/week) at 20–28 weeks, and 1.25 lb/week (0.57 kg/week) from 28 weeks to delivery
- *Normal-weight women* – 1–1.5 lb/week (0.45–0.68 kg/week) until 20 weeks, 1.25–1.75 lb/week (0.57–0.79 kg/week) at 20–28 weeks, and 1.0 lb/week (0.45 kg/week) from 28 weeks to delivery
- *Overweight women* – 1–1.25 lb/week (0.45–0.57 kg/week) until 20 weeks, 1–1.5 lb/week (0.45–0.68 kg/week) at 20–28 weeks, and 1 lb/week (0.45 kg/week) from 28 weeks to delivery
- *Obese women* – 0.75–1 lb/week (0.34–0.45 kg/week) to 20 weeks, 0.75–1.25 lb/week (0.34–0.57 kg/week) at 20–28 weeks, and 0.75 lb/week (0.34 kg/week) from 28 weeks to delivery.[143]

A constant maternal weight gain throughout gestation and not only an absolute weigh gain, even if gained during critical periods of gestation, was found to be important for maintaining a twin weight discordance of less than 25%.[144]

High-order multiple gestations

In a large, retrospective, observational study including 1166 triplet pregnancies with a normal (19.8–26) pregravid BMI, 208 of them (18%) had an adequate weight gain defined as over 680 g/week. In this study, adequate weight gain was not associated with a lower incidence of adverse outcome (defined as small-for-gestational-age infants and total triplet birth weight under 4500 g).[145]

In a recent retrospective study evaluating 56 triplet gestations, the total maternal weight gain was associated with increasing mean birth weight and higher gestational age at delivery. Pregnancy complications (such as GDM and gestational hypertension) were associated with prepregnancy BMI. The authors concluded that, for triplet gestation, a normal prepregnancy BMI and a total gestational weight gain of at least 15.9–20.5 kg (35–45 lb) is associated with fewer pregnancy complications.[146]

Key points
- Approximately one-third of women of reproductive age in the USA are obese.
- Maternal obesity is associated with a spectrum of reproductive problems, including infertility, and pregnancy and delivery complications in addition to the common general health repercussions.
- Obesity during pregnancy has been associated with a two- to fourfold increased risk of pregnancy-induced hypertension, gestational diabetes, fetal macrosomia, birth defects, cesarean and operative delivery, and postpartum anemia.
- Low weight gain during pregnancy is associated with increased risk of preterm delivery and low birth weight.
- Sustaining a healthy lifestyle by increased physical activity and healthy dieting leading to weight reduction before pregnancy is definitely the goal

in order to decrease the medical and obstetric risks associated with overweight and obesity during pregnancy.

References

1. World Health Organization. Obesity: preventing and managing a global epidemic. *World Health Organ Tech Rep Ser* 2000;**894**:1–4.
2. WHO Global Strategy on Diet, Physical Activity and Health 2003. Obesity and overweight. Available at: www.who.int/dietphysicalactivity/publications/facts/obesity/en/. World Health Organization. Information sheets an obesity and overweight. Available at: www.who.int/dietphysicalactivity/publications/facts/obesity/en.
3. Flegal KM, Carroll MD, Johnson CL, Ogden CL. Prevalence and trends in obesity among US adults, 1999–2000. *JAMA* 2002;**288**:1723–7.
4. Hedley AA, Ogden CL, Johnson CL, et al. Prevalence of overweight and obesity among US children, adolescents, and adults, 1999–2002. *JAMA* 2004;**291**:2847–50.
5. Ogden CL, Carroll MD, Curtin LR, et al. Prevalence of overweight and obesity in the United States, 1999–2004. *JAMA* 2006;**295**:1549–55.
6. Manson JE, Willet WC, Stampfer MJ, et al. Body weight and mortality among women. *N Engl J Med* 1995;**333**:677–85.
7. Green BB, Weiss NS, Daling JR. Risk of ovulatory infertility in relation to body weight. *Fertil Steril* 1988;**50**:721–6.
8. Grodstein F, Goldman MB, Cramer DW. Body mass index and ovulatory infertility. *Epidemiology* 1994;**5**:247–50.
9. Zaadstra BM, Seidell JC, Van Noord PA, et al. Fat and female fecundity: prospective study of effect of body fat distribution on conception rates. *BMJ* 1993;**306**:484–7.
10. Metwally M, Li TC, Ledger WL. The impact of obesity on female reproductive function. *Obesity Rev* 2007;**8**:515–23.
11. Frisch RE. Body fat, menarche and ovulation. *Baillière's Clin Obstet Gynaecol* 1990;**4**:419–39.
12. Lintsen AM, Pasker-de Jong PC, de Boer EJ, et al. Effects of subfertility, cause, smoking and body weight on the success rate of IVF. *Hum Reprod* 2005;**20**:1867–75.
13. Fedorcsak P, Dale PO, Storeng R, et al. Impact of overweight and underweight on assisted reproduction treatment. *Hum Reprod* 2004;**19**:2523–8.
14. Wang JX, Davies M, Norman RJ. Body mass and probability of pregnancy during assisted reproduction treatment: retrospective study. *BMJ* 2000;**321**:1320–1.
15. Hamilton-Fairley D, Kiddy D, Watson H, et al. Association of moderate obesity with a poor pregnancy outcome in women with polycystic ovary syndrome treated with low dose gonadotrophin. *Br J Obstet Gynaecol* 1992;**99**:128–31.
16. Wan GJX, Davies MJ, Norman RJ. Obesity increases the risk of spontaneous abortion during infertility treatment. *Obes Res* 2002;**10**:551–4.

17. Bussen S, Sutterlin M, Steck T. Endocrine abnormalities during the follicular phase in women with recurrent spontaneous abortion. *Hum Reprod* 1999;**14**:18–20.
18. Lashen H, Fear K, Sturdee DW. Obesity is associated with increased risk of first trimester and recurrent miscarriage: matched case-control study. *Hum Reprod* 2004;**19**:1644–6.
19. Fedorcsak P, Dale PO, Storeng R, et al. The impact of obesity and insulin resistance on the outcome of IVF or ICSI in women with polycystic ovarian syndrome. *Hum Reprod* 2001;**16**:1086–91.
20. Bellver J, Rossal LP, Bosch E, Zuniga A. Obesity and the risk of spontaneous abortion after oocyte donation. *Fertil Steril* 2003;**79**:1136–40.
21. Douglas CC, Gower BA, Darnell BE, et al. Role of diet in the treatment of polycystic ovary syndrome. *Fertil Steril* 2006;**85**:679–88.
22. Loveland JB, McClamrock HD, Malinow AM, Sharara FI. Increased body mass index has a deleterious effect on in vitro fertilization outcome. *J Assist Reprod Genet* 2001;**18**:382–6.
23. Lashen H, Ledger W, Bernal AL, Barlow D. Extremes of body mass do not adversely affect the outcome of superovulation and in-vitro fertilization. *Hum Reprod* 1999;**14**:712–15.
24. Winter E, Wang J, Davies MJ, Norman R. Early pregnancy loss following assisted reproductive technology treatment. *Hum Reprod* 2002;**17**:3220–3.
25. Roth D, Grazi RV, Lobel SM. Extremes of body mass index do not affect first-trimester pregnancy outcome in patients with infertility. *Am J Obstet Gynecol* 2003;**188**:1169–70.
26. Weiss JL, Malone FD, Eming D, et al. Obstetric complications and cesarean delivery rate: a population-based screening study. FASTER Research Consortium. *Am J Obstet Gynecol* 2004;**190**:1091–7.
27. Gabbe S. Gestational diabetes mellitus. *N Engl J Med* 1986;**315**:1025–6.
28. Guttorm E. Practical screening for diabetes mellitus in pregnant women. *Acta Endocrinol (Copenh)* 1974;**75**:11–24.
29. Abrams B, Parker J. Overweight and pregnancy complications. *Int J Obes* 1988;**12**:293–303.
30. Catalano P, Roman N, Tyzbir E, et al. Weight gain in women with gestational diabetes. *Obstet Gynecol* 1993;**81**:523–8.
31. Metzger B, Coustan D. Summary and recommendations of the fourth international workshop-conference on gestational diabetes mellitus. *Diabetes Care* 1998;**21**:B161–7.
32. Sepe S, Connell F, Geiss L, Teutsch S. Gestational diabetes: incidence, maternal characteristics and perinatal outcome. *Diabetes* 1985;**34**:13–16.
33. Perlow JH, Morgan MA, Montgomery D, et al. Perinatal outcome in pregnancy complicated by massive obesity. *Am J Obstet Gynecol* 1992;**167**:958–62.
34. Baeten JM, Bukusi EA, Lambe M. Pregnancy complications and outcomes among overweight and obese nulliparous women. *Am J Public Health* 2001;**91**:436–40.

35. Linné Y, Barkeling B, Rössner S. Natural course of gestational diabetes mellitus: long term follow up of women in the SPAWN study. *Br J Obstet Gynaecol* 2002;**109**:1127–31.

36. Bhattacharya S, Campbell DM, Liston WA, et al. Effect of body mass index on pregnancy outcomes in nulliparous women delivering singleton babies. *BMC Public Health* 2007;**7**:168.

37. Ehrenberg HM, Mercer BM, Catalano PM. The influence of obesity and diabetes on the prevalence of macrosomia. *Am J Obstet Gynecol* 2004;**191**: 964–8.

38. Sibai BM, Gordon T, Thom E, Caritis SN. Risk factors for pre-eclampsia in healthy nulliparous women: a prospective multicenter study. National Institute of Child Health and Human Development Network of Maternal-Fetal Medicine Units. *Am J Obstet Gynecol* 1995;**172**:642–8.

39. Easterling TR, Benedetti TJ, Schmucker BC, Millard SP. Maternal hemodynamics in normal and pre-eclamptic pregnancies: a longitudinal study. *Obstet Gynecol* 1990;**76**:1061–9.

40. Eskenazi B, Fenster L, Sidney S. A multivariate analysis of risk factors for preeclampsia. *JAMA* 1991;**266**:237–41.

41. Gross T, Sokol RJ, King KC. Obesity in pregnancy: risks and outcome. *Obstet Gynecol* 1980;**56**:446–50.

42. Galtier-Dereure F, Boegner C, Bringer J. Obesity and pregnancy: complications and cost. *Am J Clin Nutr* 2000;**71**(Suppl 5):1242S–8S.

43. Stone JL, Lockwood CJ, Berkowitz GS, et al. Risk factors for severe preeclampsia. *Obstet Gynecol* 1994;**83**:357–61.

44. O'Brien TE, Ray JG, Chan WS. Maternal body mass index and the risk of preeclampsia: a systematic review. *Epidemiology* 2003;**14**:368–74.

45. Cedergren MI. Maternal morbid obesity and the risk of adverse pregnancy outcome. *Obstet Gynecol* 2004;**103**:219–24.

46. Kalter H. Five-decade international trends in the relation of perinatal mortality and congenital malformations: stillbirth and neonatal death compared. *Int J Epidemiol* 1991;**20**:173–9.

47. Odlind V, Haglund B, Pakkanen M, et al. Deliveries, mothers and newborn infants in Sweden, 1973–2000. Trends in obstetrics as reported to the Swedish Medical Birth Register. *Acta Obstet Gynecol Scand* 2003;**82**:516–28.

48. Nohr EA, Bech BH, Davies MJ, et al. Prepregnancy obesity and fetal death. *Obstet Gynecol* 2005;**106**:250–9.

49. Sebire NJ, Jolly M, Harris JP, et al. Maternal obesity and pregnancy outcome: a study of 287,213 pregnancies in London. *Int J Obes Relat Metab Disord* 2001;**25**:1175–82.

50. Cnattingius S, Bergström R, Lipworth L, Kramer MS. Prepregnancy weight and the risk of adverse pregnancy outcomes. *N Engl J Med* 1998;**338**:147–52.

51. Salihu HM, Dunlop A, Hedayatzadeh M, et al. Extreme obesity and risk of stillbirth among black and white gravidas. *Obstet Gynecol* 2007;**110**:552–7.

52. Schieve LA, Cogswell ME, Scanlon KS. Maternal weight gain and preterm delivery: differential effects by body mass index. *Epidemiology* 1999;**10**:141–7.

53. Kramer MS, Coates AL, Michoud MC, et al. Maternal anthropometry and idiopathic preterm labor. *Obstet Gynecol* 1995;**86**:744–8.

54. Siega-Riz AM, Adair LS, Hobel CJ. Institute of Medicine maternal weight gain recommendations and pregnancy outcome in a predominantly Hispanic population. *Obstet Gynecol* 1994;**84**:565–73.

55. Spinillo A, Capuzzo E, Piazzi G, et al. Risk for spontaneous preterm delivery by combined body mass index and gestational weight gain patterns. *Acta Obstet Gynecol Scand* 1998;**77**:32–6.

56. Hickey CA, Cliver SP, McNeal SF, et al. Prenatal weight gain patterns and spontaneous preterm birth among nonobese black and white women. *Obstet Gynecol* 1995;**85**:909–14.

57. Hediger ML, Scholl TO, Belsky DH, et al. Patterns of weight gain in adolescent pregnancy: effects on birth weight and preterm delivery. *Obstet Gynecol* 1989;**74**:6–12.

58. Scholl TO, Hediger ML, Salmon RW, et al. Influence of prepregnant body mass and weight gain for gestation on spontaneous preterm delivery and duration of gestation during adolescent pregnancy. *Am J Hum Biol* 1989;**1**:657–64.

59. Abrams B, Newman V, Key T, Parker J. Maternal weight gain and preterm delivery. *Obstet Gynecol* 1989;**74**:577–83.

60. Ehrenberg HM, Dierker L, Milluzzi CRN, Mercer BM. Low maternal weight, failure to thrive in pregnancy, and adverse pregnancy outcomes. *Am J Obstet Gynecol* 2003;**189**:1726–30.

61. Schieve LA, Cogswell ME, Scanlon KS, et al. Prepregnancy body mass index and pregnancy weight gain: associations with preterm delivery. NMIHS Collaborative Study Group. *Obstet Gynecol* 2000;**96**:194–200.

62. Smith GCS, Shah I, Pell JP, et al. Maternal obesity in early pregnancy and risk of spontaneous and elective preterm deliveries: a retrospective cohort study. *Am J Public Health* 2007;**97**:157–62.

63. Nohr EA, Bech BH, Vaeth M, et al. Obesity, gestational weight gain and preterm birth: a study within the Danish National Birth Cohort. *Paediatr Perinat Epidemiol* 2007;**21**:5–14.

64. Dietz PM, Callaghan WM, Morrow B, Cogswell ME. Population-based assessment of the risk of primary cesarean delivery due to excess prepregnancy weight among nulliparous women delivering term infants. *Matern Child Health J* 2005;**9**:237–44.

65. Vahratian A, Siega-Riz AM, Zhang J, et al. Maternal pre-pregnancy overweight and obesity and the risk of primary cesarean delivery in nulliparous women. *Ann Epidemiol* 2005;**15**:467–74.

66. Weiss JL, Malone FD, Emig D, et al. Obesity, obstetric complications and cesarean delivery rate: a population based screening study. *Am J Obstet Gynecol* 2004;**190**:1091–7.

67. Holger S, Scheithauer S, Dornhofer N, et al. Obesity as an obstetric risk factor: does it matter in a perinatal center? *Obesity* 2006;**14**:770–3.

68. Kaiser PS, Kirby RS. Obesity as a risk factor for cesarean in a low-risk population. *Obstet Gynecol* 2001;**97**:39–43.

69. Cnattingius R, Cnattingius S, Notzon FC. Obstacles to reducing cesarean rates in a low-cesarean setting: the effect of maternal age, height, and weight. *Obstet Gynecol* 1998;**92**:501– 6.

70. Brost BC, Goldenberg RL, Mercer BM, et al. The Preterm Prediction Study: association of cesarean section with increases in maternal weight and body mass index. *Am J Obstet Gynecol* 1997;**177**:333–41.

71. Witter FR, Caufield LE, Stoltzfus RJ. Influence of maternal anthropometric status and birth weight on the risk of cesarean delivery. *Obstet Gynecol* 1995;**85**:947–51.

72. Yu CK, Teoh TG, Robinson S. Obesity in pregnancy. *Br J Obstet Gynaecol* 2006;**113**: 1117–25.

73. Bodnar LM, Siega-Riz AM, Miller WC, et al. Who should be screened for postpartum anemia? An evaluation of current recommendations. *Am J Epidemiol* 2002;**156**:903–12.

74. Bodnar LM, Scanlon KS, Freedman DS, et al. High prevalence of postpartum anemia among low-income women in the United States. *Am J Obstet Gynecol* 2001;**185**:438–43.

75. Bodnar LM, Siega-Riz AM, Miller WC, Cogswell ME. High prepregnancy BMI increases the risk of postpartum anemia. *Obes Res* 2004;**12**:941–8.

76. Donath SM, Amir LH. Does maternal obesity adversely affect breastfeeding initiation and duration? *Breastfeed Rev* 2000;**8**:29–33.

77. Cogswell ME, Perry GS, Schieve LA, Dietz WH. Obesity in women of childbearing age: risks, prevention, and treatment. *Primary Care Update Obstet Gynecol* 2001;**8**:89–105.

78. Waller DK, Mills JL, Simpson JL, et al. Are obese women at higher risk for producing malformed offspring? *Am J Obstet Gynecol* 1994;**170**:541–8.

79. Cedergren MI, Kallen BA. Maternal obesity and infant heart defects. *Obes Res* 2003;**11**:1065–71.

80. Watkins ML, Rasmussen SA, Honeru MA, et al. Maternal obesity and risk for birth defects. *Pediatrics* 2003;**111**:1152–8.

81. Mojtabai R. Body mass index and serum folate in childbearing women. *Eur J Epidemiol* 2004;**19**:1029–36.

82. Ray JG, Wyatt PR, Vermeulen MJ, et al. Greater maternal weight and the ongoing risk of neural tube defects after folic acid flour fortification. *Obstet Gynecol* 2005;**105**:261–5.

83. Garn SM, Clark DC. Trends in fatness and the origins of obesity. *Pediatrics* 1976;**57**:443–56.

84. Garn SM, Cole PE, Bailey SM. Living together as a factor in family line resemblances. *Hum Biol* 1979;**51**:565–87.

85. Martorell R, Stein AD, Schroeder DG. Early nutrition and adiposity. *J Nutr* 2001;**131**:874S–80S.

85. Whitaker RC. Predicting preschooler obesity at birth: the role of maternal obesity in early pregnancy. *Pediatrics* 2004;**114**:e29–36.

86. Mokdad AH, Ford ES, Bowman BA, et al. Diabetes trends in the U.S. 1990–1998. *Diabetes Care* 2000;**23**:1278–83.

88. Sinha R, Fisch G, Teague B, et al. Prevalence of impaired glucose tolerance among children and adolescents with marked obesity. *N Engl J Med* 2002;**346**:802–10.

89. Mullins A. Overweight in pregnancy. *Lancet* 1960;**i**:146–7.

90. Greene J. Clinical study of the etiology of obesity. *Ann Intern Med* 1939;**12**: 1797–803.

91. Sheldon J. Maternal obesity. *Lancet* 1949;**ii**:869–73.

92. Abrams B, Laros R. Prepregnancy weight, weight gain, and birth weight. *Am J Obstet Gynecol* 1986;**154**:503–9.

93. Cederlöf R, Kaij L. The effect of childbearing on body weight: a twin control study. *Acta Psychiatr Scand Suppl* 1970;**219**:47–9.

94. Forster J, Bloom E, Sorensen G, et al Reproductive history and body mass index in black and white women. *Prev Med* 1986;**15**:685–91.

95. Smith DE, Lewis CE, Caveny JL, et al. Longitudinal changes in adiposity associated with pregnancy. The CARDIA Study. Coronary Artery Risk Development in Young Adults Study. *JAMA* 1994;**271**:1747–51.

96. Öhlin A, Rössner S. Maternal body weight development after pregnancy. *Int J Obes Relat Metab Disord* 1990;**14**:159–73.

97. Walker LO. Predictors of weight gain at 6 and 18 months after childbirth: a pilot study. J *Obstet Gynecol Neonatal Nurs* 1996;**25**:39–48.

98. Greene GW, Smiciklas-Wright H, Scholl TO, Karp RJ. Postpartum weight change: how much of the weight gained in pregnancy will be lost after delivery? *Obstet Gynecol* 1988;**71**:701–7.

99. Linné Y, Neovius M. Identification of women at risk of adverse weight development following pregnancy. *Int J Obes* 2006;**30**:1234–39.

100. Dieckman W. *The Toxemias of Pregnancy*. St Louis, MO: Mosby, 1952.

101. Subcommittee on Nutritional Status and Weight Gain During Pregnancy, Subcommittee on Dietary Intake and Nutrient Supplements During Pregnancy, Committee on Nutritional Status During Pregnancy and Lactation Food and Nutrient Board, et al. *Nutrition During Pregnancy*. Washington DC: National Academy Press, 1990.

102. Rode L, Hegaard HK, Kjaergaard H, Moller LF. Association between maternal weight gain and birth weight. *Obstet Gynecol* 2007;**109**:1309–15.

103. Committee on the Impact of Pregnancy Weight on Maternal and Child Health, National Research Council. *Influence of Pregnancy Weight on Maternal and Child Health: Workshop Report*. Washington, DC: National Academies Press, 2007.

104. Cedergren MI. Optimal gestational weight gain for body mass index categories. *Obstet Gynecol* 2007;**110**:759–64.

105. Schieve L, Cogswell ME, Scanlon KS. Prepregnancy body mass index and pregnancy weight gain: associations with preterm delivery. NMIHS Collaborative Study Group. *Obstet Gynecol* 2000;**96**:194–200.

106. Schieve LA, Cogswell ME, Scanlon KS. Maternal weight gain and preterm delivery: differential effects by body mass index. *Epidemiology* 1999;**10**:141–7.

107. Spinillo A, Capuzzo E, Piazzi G, et al. Risk for spontaneous preterm delivery by combined body mass index and gestational weight gain patterns. *Acta Obstet Gynecol Scand* 1998;**77**:32–6.

108. Abrams B, Newman V, Key T, Parker J. Maternal weight gain and preterm delivery. *Obstet Gynecol* 1989;**74**:577–83.

109. Carmichael SL, Abrams B. A critical review of the relationship between gestational weight gain and preterm delivery. *Obstet Gynecol* 1997;**89**:865–73.

110. Carmichael SL, Abrams B, Selvin S. The association of pattern of maternal weight gain with length of gestation and risk of spontaneous preterm delivery. *Pediatr Perinat Epidemiol* 1997;**11**:392–406.

111. Stein Z, Susser M, Saengler G, Marolla F. *Famine and Human Development. The Dutch hunger winter of 1944–1945.* London: Oxford University Press, 1975.

112. Sparen P, Vagero D, Shestor DB, Plavinskaja S, et al. Long term mortality after severe starvation during the siege of Leningrad: prospective cohort study. *BMJ* 2004;**328**:11.

113. Leon D, Koupilová I. Birth weight, blood pressure and hypertension. Epidemiological studies. In: Barker DJ, ed. *Fetal Origins of Cardiovascular and Lung Disease.* New York: Marcel Dekker, 2001.

114. Leon DA, Lithell HO, Vagero D, et al. Reduced fetal growth rate and increased risk of death from ischaemic heart disease: cohort study of 15 000 Swedish men and women born 1915–29. *BMJ* 1998;**317**:241–5.

115. Hyppönen E, Leon DA, Kenward MG, Lithell H. Prenatal growth and risk of occlusive and haemorrhagic stroke in Swedish men and women born 1915–29: historical cohort study. *BMJ* 2001;**323**:1033–4.

116. Roseboom TJ, van der Meulen JH, Osmond C, Barker DJ. Coronary heart disease after prenatal exposure to the Dutch famine, 1944–45. *Heart* 2000;**84**:595–8.

117. Roseboom TJ, van der Meulen JH, Ravelli AC, van Montfrans GA. Blood pressure in adults after prenatal exposure to famine. *J Hypertens* 1999;**17**:325–30.

118. Ravelli AC, van Der Meulen JH, Osmond C, Barker DJ. Obesity at the age of 50 y in men and women exposed to famine prenatally. *Am J Clin Nutr* 1999;**70**:811–16.

119. Roseboom TJ, van der Meulen JH, Osmond C, Barker DJ. Plasma lipid profiles in adults after prenatal exposure to the Dutch famine. *Am J Clin Nutr* 2000;**72**:1101–6.

120. Roseboom TJ, van der Meulen JH, Osmond C, Barker DJ. Adult survival after prenatal exposure to the Dutch famine 1944–45. *Paediatr Perinat Epidemiol* 2001;**15**:220–5.

121. Roseboom TJ, van der Meulen JH, Ravelli AC, Osmond C. Effects of prenatal exposure to the Dutch famine on adult disease in later life: an overview. *Mol Cell Endocrinol* 2001;**4**:293–8.

122. Sparen P, Vagero D, Shestov DB, et al. Long term mortality after severe starvation during the siege of Leningrad: prospective cohort study. *BMJ* 2004;**328**:1.

123. Kabiru W, Raynor BD. Obstetric outcomes associated with increase in BMI category during pregnancy. *Am J Obstet Gynecol* 2004;**191**:928–32.

124. Johnson JW, Longmate JA, Frentzen B. Excessive maternal weight and pregnancy outcome. *Am J Obstet Gynecol* 1992;**167**:353–70.

125. Cedergren M. Effects of gestational weight gain and body mass index on obstetric outcome in Sweden. *Int J Gynaecol Obstet* 2006;**93**:269–74.

126. Chen G, Uryasev S, Young TK. On prediction of the cesarean delivery risk in a large private practice. *Am J Obstet Gynecol* 2004;**191**:617–24.

127. Young TK, Woodmansee B. Factors that are associated with cesarean delivery in a large private practice: the importance of prepregnancy body mass index and weight gain. *Am J Obstet Gynecol* 2002;**187**:312–18.

128. Thorsdottir I, Torfadottir JE, Birgisdottir BE, Geirsson RT. Weight gain in women of normal weight before pregnancy: complications in pregnancy or delivery and birth outcome. *Obstet Gynecol* 2002;**9**:799–806.

129. Dietz P, Callaghan W, Cogswell M, et al. Combined effects of prepregnancy body mass index and weight gain during pregnancy on the risk of preterm delivery. *Epidemiology* 2006;**17**:170–7.

130. Stotland NE, Hopkins LM, Caughey AB. Gestational weight gain, macrosomia, and risk of cesarean birth in nondiabetic nulliparas. *Obstet Gynecol* 2004;**104**:671–7.

131. Shepard MJ, Hellenbrand KG, Bracken MB. Proportional weight gain and complications of pregnancy, labor, and delivery in healthy women of normal prepregnant stature. *Am J Obstet Gynecol* 1987;**157**:217.

132. Stotland NE, Cheng YW, Hopkins LM, Caughey AB. Gestational weight gain and adverse neonatal outcome among term infants. *Obstet Gynecol* 2006;**108**:635–43.

133. Kac G, Benicio MH, Velasquez-Melendez G, et al. Gestational weight gain and prepregnancy weight influence postpartum weight retention in a cohort of Brazilian women. *J Nutr* 2004;**134**:661–6.

134. Scholl TO, Hediger ML, Schall JI, et al. Gestational weight gain, pregnancy outcome, and postpartum weight retention. *Obstet Gynecol* 1995;**86**:423–7.

135. Thorsdottir I, Birgisdottir BE. Different weight gain in women of normal weight before pregnancy: postpartum weight and birth weight. *Obstet Gynecol* 1998;**92**:377–83.

136. Villamor E, Dreyfuss ML, Baylin A, et al. Weight loss during pregnancy is associated with adverse pregnancy outcomes among HIV-1 infected women. *J Nutr* 2004;**134**:1424–31.

137. Ehrenberg HM, Dierker L, Milluzzi C, Mercer BM. Low maternal weight, failure to thrive in pregnancy, and adverse pregnancy outcomes. *Am J Obstet Gynecol* 2003;**189**:1726–30.

138. Schieve LA, Cogswell ME, Scanlon KS, et al. Prepregnancy body mass index and pregnancy weight gain: associations with preterm delivery. NMIHS Collaborative Study Group. *Obstet Gynecol* 2000;**96**:194–200.

139. Jacobsson B, Ladfors L, Milsom I. Advanced maternal age and adverse perinatal outcome. *Obstet Gynecol* 2004;**104**:727–33.

140. Oken E, Taveras EM, Kleinman KP, et al. Gestational weight gain and child adiposity at age 3 years. *Am J Obstet Gynecol* 2007;**196**:322 e1–8.
141. Lantz ME, Chez RA, Rodriguez A, et al. Maternal weight gain patterns and birth weight outcome in twin gestation. *Obstet Gynecol* 1996;**87**:551–6.
142. Luke B, Gillespie B, Min SJ, et al. Critical periods of maternal weight gain: effect on twin birth weight. *Am J Obstet Gynecol* 1997;**177**:1055–62.
143. Luke B, Hediger ML, Nugent C, Newman RB. Body mass index-specific weight gains associated with optimal birth weights in twin pregnancies. *J Reprod Med* 2003;**48**:217–24.
144. Lee KJ, Hur J, Yoo J. Twin weight discordance and maternal weight gain in twin pregnancies. *Int J Gynaecol Obstet* 2007;**96**:176–80.
145. Flidel-Rimon O, Rhea DJ, Shinwell ES, Keith LG. Early weight gain does not decrease the incidence of low birth weight and small for gestational age triplets in mothers with normal pre-gestational body mass index. *J Perinat Med* 2006;**34**:404–8.
146. Eddib A, Penvose-Yi J, Shelton JA, Yeh J. Triplet gestation outcomes in relation to maternal prepregnancy body mass index and weight gain. *J Matern Fetal Neonatal Med* 2007;**20**:515–19.

3 The psychology of obesity in women and pregnancy

Georgina Jones

Introduction

In the not so recent past, the relationship between weight gain and pregnancy focused primarily upon inadequate maternal weight gain.[1] The consequences of inadequate weight gain for fetal growth traditionally were thought to be such that pregnant women were advised to 'eat for two' and avoid slimming.[2] However, recently, the impact of excessive weight gain and obesity during pregnancy has shifted the focus.

Obesity (a body mass index [BMI] exceeding 30 kg/m^2) has now become a major public health concern in western societies because of the risk to health and the cost to health services that are commonly associated with the condition (see Chapters 1 and 2). The physical consequences of obesity, in particular cardiovascular diseases (coronary heart disease, hypertension, and ischaemic stroke), diabetes mellitus, and some cancers represent the impetus for most public health campaigns and weight loss interventions. Indeed, obese persons are expected to have more unhealthy life years than normal-weight individuals.[3]

In pregnancy, epidemiological studies show that maternal obesity is associated with infertility, miscarriage, poor pregnancy outcome, impaired fetal well-being, and gestational diabetes.[4] There is also a tendency for obese women to have larger babies, and, although the evidence is not conclusive, there is increased risk of caesarean section in overweight women.[5,6] The negative consequences of obesity for the delivery and provision of obstetric services in the UK, for example, has also been reported by health professionals in relation to the levels of care required, costs and resource issues, risks to the health of the child and the mother, and weight-related existing or developing morbidities.[7]

The aims of this chapter are to explore some of the psychological issues surrounding obesity in pregnancy because a growing body of literature has recently identified obesity as a significant predictor of poor psychological well-being and negative health-related quality of life (HRQoL), particularly in women.[8] Of equal importance, pregnancy and the postpartum period have been identified as vulnerable and at times confusing periods in women's lives when they gain and retain excessive weight (see Chapters 8 and 10).

For example, it is paradoxical that, although obesity is undesirable during pregnancy, weight gain is medically important to ensure healthy fetal development,[9] and childbearing has been attributed to adult weight gain in many obese women.[10] In a retrospective analysis of 128 women attending an obesity unit in Sweden, Rossner and Ohlin[11] found that 73% of their severely obese patients had retained over 10 kg in association with pregnancy. Numerous additional studies have examined factors associated with excessive weight gain during pregnancy; most find that a high prepregnancy BMI is associated with excessive gains in weight.[12,13] Indeed, one study found that 100% of women who were overweight or obese before their pregnancy gained weight in excess of the recommended guidelines.[14]

In particular, this chapter discusses:

- What are the mental health/psychological issues related to obesity?
- What are the consequences of obesity for body image and lifestyle?
- Why do women continue to eat excessively during pregnancy?
- Does obesity affect the desire for pregnancy?
- What are the implications for weight loss programmes in women who have retained weight?
- Is obesity considered to be an addiction?

What are the mental health/psychological issues?

Numerous studies have investigated the relationship between psychological well-being (in particular mood, anxiety, and depression) during pregnancy and the postnatal period. Pregnancy is often associated with depression, both antenatally and postnatally, and pregnancy and childbirth can have a profound and debilitating effect on mothers.[15] A great number of women feel exhausted after the birth of their baby, and are tearful and depressed in relation to this. The term 'postnatal illness' has been used to characterize a number of mental health conditions. Although a continuum may be present, three main degrees of unhappiness or depression have been identified. The mildest form, the 'baby blues', is said to affect 39–85% of women.[16] During the first days after the birth of their baby, women may feel more emotional than usual, irritable, anxious, and weepy, and have a low mood. Next, postnatal depression can begin soon after childbirth, and, finally, although far less common, puerperal psychosis is a severe mental illness affecting 1 in 1000 women in the first few months after delivery.

Given these circumstances, it is logical to ask to what extent obesity affects the mental health and psychological well-being of women, both antenatally and postnatally. Overall, the data on this relationship are scant. Despite the paucity of research, however, a negative effect of weight on both parameters appears evident. Antenatally, Amador et al[17] assessed the HRQoL of obese, pregnant Mexican women. Using the generic Short Form-12 quality-of-life (QoL) questionnaire (SF-12), these investigators compared the HRQoL of 110 obese and 110 non-obese pregnant women at the first pregnancy visit and again at 36–37 weeks' gestation. Classifications of BMI were based upon the Norma Oficial

Mexicana, whereby women with a BMI of 18.5–24.9 kg/m^2 were classified as non-obese and those over 27 kg/m^2 as obese. Overall, the obese women had a worse HRQoL. At the beginning of the pregnancy ($P = 0.01$) and during the third trimester ($P = 0.03$), obese pregnant women had significantly lower Mental Component Summary (MCS) scores. However, in both groups, MCS scores increased (thereby indicating better HRQoL) by the third trimester ($P = 0.001$). In contrast, no significant differences were noted between the groups at the beginning of gestation. However, scores significantly declined in both groups between the first- and third-trimester follow-up visit, more so in obese than non-obese women ($P = 0.04$).

These observations suggest that prepregnancy BMI is a significant factor in determining psychological well-being during pregnancy. Indeed, some postnatal research supports this finding. For example, Carter et al,[18] in their analysis of 64 American women, found that at 4 and 14 months post partum an interrelationship of symptoms of depression, anxiety and BMI was present. However, only 17 of the women had a BMI over 27, and there was insufficient power to analyse the data stratified by BMI.

The most comprehensive study investigating the relationship between postpartum depression and prepregnancy BMI was published recently.[19] In a retrospective analysis of the 2000–1 Utah data from the Pregnancy Risk Assessment Monitoring System, investigators found a potential association between prepregnancy BMI and self-reported depression. Prepregnancy BMI was calculated by self-reported height and weight. Overall, normal-weight women (BMI 19.8–25.9 kg/m^2) reported significantly fewer depressive symptoms (22.8%) than obese women (30.8%) (BMI > 29 kg/m^2). After controlling for income and marital status, a prepregnancy BMI over 29 was significantly associated with depressive symptoms (adjusted odds ratio [OR] 1.53, 95% confidence interval [CI] 1.15–2.02). Compared with the percentage of prepregnancy normal-weight women (1.53%), overweight (BMI 26–29.0 kg/m^2) (2.99%) and obese women (3.10%) reported a statistically significant, twofold increase in depressive symptoms requiring assistance. However, it is important to highlight that in this study women characterized as underweight (BMI < 19.8 kg/m^2) also reported more depressive symptoms than the normal and overweight groups of women.

The authors also found an increase in reported emotional and traumatic stress during pregnancy in overweight and obese women compared with normal-weight women.[19] However, again it is worth mentioning that women who were underweight also reported more stress than the normal group and more traumatic stress than the obese women.

Although high prepregnancy BMI appears to play a role in affecting the psychological well-being of antenatal and postnatal women, the issue is more complex, as research has found that, even in women within the normal BMI range, issues concerning their weight and negative health behaviours are still evident. For example, Dipietro et al[20] carried out a cross-sectional study of 130 women (mean age 31.3 years) (mean BMI = 24.9) in the USA at 36 weeks' gestation in normal, low-risk pregnancy in order to assess their attitude to weight gain. Overall, they found that 21% described weight-restrictive behaviours (including not eating before an obstetric visit, altering weight gain from month to month, and trying not to look pregnant early in the pregnancy), and these women were more likely to be anxious and stressed ($P < 0.01$), as well as depressed and angry ($P < 0.001$). They also reported feeling less uplifted about their pregnancy ($P < 0.05$). Those women who felt self-conscious about their weight felt more hassled about their pregnancy and greater anger, and had more support from their partners ($P < 0.05$). Prepregnancy BMI was unrelated.

The extent to which psychological well-being is affected by weight gain during pregnancy may differ between ethnicities. Cameron et al[21] looked at the relationship between depression and weight gain during pregnancy. Although this study was limited by sample size, the authors found that in 96 white, inner-city, American women, third-trimester depressive symptomatology was predicted by lower self-esteem and greater deviation from the medical recommendations of ideal weight, as measured on the Rosenberg Self-Esteem Scale and a shortened, 14-item version of the Beck Depression Inventory. For the sample of 36 African–American women also included in the analyses, only lower self-esteem predicted increased depressive symptomatology scores.

The observation that overweight and obese women of European–American descent are at increased risk of psychological distress has also been described in non-pregnant, middle-class samples of women.[21] One explanation may be that white European women are more vulnerable to the negative psychological impact of weight as a result of different expectations and norms in terms of acceptable body shapes and sizes compared with other cultures. Indeed, in obese, postmenopausal women, White et al[22] found that white women reported a worse HRQoL even though they had a significantly lower BMI than the African–American women in the study. Although the observations cited above are of interest, clearly more research is needed in specific relation to maternal obesity, ethnicity, and psychological well-being.

What are the consequences of obesity on body image?

Obesity and the body shape related to it generally are associated with negative attitudes, and the negative 'fat is bad' stereotype is evident from early childhood. For example, children as young as 6 years old characterize silhouettes of an overweight child as 'dirty', 'lazy', 'ugly', and 'stupid',[23] and these negative perceptions of obese people continue into adolescence and adulthood.[24] Although numerous definitions of stigma are available, it is typically defined as the use of negative labels to identify a person. Individuals vary considerably in the way that they respond to stigmatizing labels, but these can have a substantial and unavoidable impact on self-concept and can become the central factor in a person's identity to the exclusion of other attributes.[25]

One reason for these negative perceptions of the overweight and obese person is the widespread belief in certain societies (such as the UK and the USA) that weight gain and loss are under personal control. The weight gain of obesity is therefore associated with negative stereotypes about personal traits of laziness, lack of self-discipline, and passivity, among others.[26] However, the relationship of obesity-related stigma is complex: obese children and adults have negative attitudes to other obese individuals, and healthcare professionals specialising in obesity also show evidence of this bias.[27] As well as interpersonal discrimination, obese persons also face difficulties in education and employment opportunities; these discriminatory behaviours are particularly evident for obese women in the workplace where at all stages of employment discrimination is evident.[28]

In western societies, women who are overweight often suffer from low self-esteem[29] so that many feel reluctant to participate in normal social life and activities.[30] The changes in body shape that normally occur during pregnancy are often perceived as negative, with leaner women reporting more positive attitudes.[31-33] From their investigations in 183 women, Walker et al[34] confirmed the relationship between postpartum depression and poor body image. Dipietro et al[20] also found that even pregnant women who gained weight within the recommended ranges had negative attitudes about their weight gain, including worry about getting fat at the end of the pregnancy (37%), or feeling unattractive because of the weight gain (14%). Women who gained more weight during their pregnancy were significantly more likely to report negative attitudes about their body image, even when controlling for prepregnancy BMI ($P < 0.01$). Interestingly, women who felt that body changes were a positive consequence of pregnancy had lower levels of psychological distress ($P < 0.05$).

Overweight women reportedly feel more positive about their body image at over 30 weeks' gestation than when they were not pregnant.[35] Other studies also find that, during pregnancy, average-weight women express greater dislike of their body size and shape than do larger women.[36] According to Wiles,[37] the consequence of this is that obese women may feel more relaxed about their diet than they did before they were pregnant and be in a position to gain even more weight during pregnancy.

Why do women continue to eat excessively during pregnancy?

Physiologic changes, plus whether being pregnant was a desired event and the amount of social support that the woman obtains during the pregnancy, are all factors that can affect a woman's diet during pregnancy.[38,39] However, it is unclear which factors may lead women to overeat during pregnancy, and the literature on this question is inconclusive. For example, obese women reportedly are more likely to diet than overeat. Micali et al[40] carried out a longitudinal study in the UK to examine the impact of pregnancy on eating disorders (EDs). In this cohort study, the authors compared women with (1) a recent ED ($n = 57$), (2) a past ED ($n = 395$), and (3) obesity (BMI > 30 before pregnancy) ($n = 681$), as well as non-obese controls (11 184). The obese cohort of women were more likely to diet during pregnancy (as were the recent ED and past ED group) compared with the non-obese controls; the recent ED and the obese women had the highest rates of dieting. Compared with the non-obese controls, obese women reported 'feeling they had put on too much weight' ($P < 0.01$) and a strong desire to lose weight ($P < 0.001$) (as did those with both the recent ED and past ED). At 18 weeks' pregnancy, concerns about weight and body shape declined ($P < 0.001$). As hypothesized by the authors, one explanation for this change at this point may be that concerns over the well-being of the baby become of central importance rather than the initial shape and weight concerns present at the start of pregnancy.

Physiological explanations also have been proposed. For example, animal studies using a pseudo-pregnant rat model have shown that the hormonal changes associated with pregnancy lead to changes in the maternal hypothalamus, thus stimulating food intake and enabling the increased food intake to be maintained.[41] Other explanations for excessive eating during pregnancy may be that pregnancy appears to legitimize increased food intake. For example, Clark and Ogden[42] investigated how pregnancy affects eating behaviours and women's concerns about their weight and looked at the ways in which dietary restraint may influence these changes in pregnant women. In a comparison of 50 pregnant women and 50 nulliparous non-pregnant women living in the UK, the pregnant women reported eating more and showed lower levels of body shape dissatisfaction and dietary restraint, and higher eating self-efficacy, than their non-pregnant counterparts. During pregnancy, compared with the months when they were not pregnant, pregnant women also reported that they were eating more and were less restrained in their eating behaviour.

While there is evidence than some pregnant and obese pregnant women feel legitimized to eat more, this phenomenon also appears to depend upon certain cognitions such as issues of control and beliefs surrounding weight gain. For example, Wiles[30] carried out in-depth interviews of 37 women (mean BMI = 32). It was important to most women not to weigh more after the pregnancy than before. However, beliefs about weight were important in determining the eating practices engaged in by the women. For example, some overweight women were aware of the consequences of giving into temptation and eating what they wanted. However, if they believed they had little control over the amount of weight gained during pregnancy, they tended not to restrict their food intake, believing that the large amount of weight that they were likely to gain was irrespective of their diet, because it was their natural propensity to gain weight.

It is logical to ask what patterns of eating behaviour might contribute to excessive weight gain during pregnancy. In this regard, picking or nibbling at food and binge eating appear important,[43] whereas dietary cravings are less likely to be associated with overeating. Fairburn et al[44] prospectively studied 100 pregnant women in a standardized interview. Although dietary cravings and aversions were common early in pregnancy, they rarely resulted in overeating episodes. Moreover, while the features associated with eating disorders decreased early in pregnancy, they increased later on during the pregnancy.

Does obesity affect the desire for pregnancy?

The question of whether obesity affects the desire for pregnancy is difficult to answer due to the limited research. Most studies on this subject have focused upon sexual desire rather than desire for a pregnancy or family planning. The data on sexual desire in obese women are also complex and replete with conflicting results. Esposito et al[45] investigated the relationship between sexual function, body weight, and distribution of body fat in 52 women who were otherwise healthy but had obtained abnormal scores ($\leq$ 23) for female sexual dysfunction as measured on the Female Sexual Function Index (FSFI), compared with a control group of 66 women (FSFI > 23) matched for menopausal status and age. Desire and pain did not correlate with BMI. However, four additional parameters of sexual function, including arousal, lubrication, orgasm, and satisfaction, did correlate with BMI ($P < 0.001$). However, in 60 obese women preparing for bariatric surgery, significant impairment of sexual function, including sexual desire, arousal, lubrication, orgasm, and satisfaction, were found compared with 50 healthy controls who were matched for age, marital status, and education.[46] Similar findings were reported by Kolotkin et al,[47] who found that higher BMI was associated with lack of enjoyment of sexual activity and desire. Difficulties with sexual performance and avoidance of sexual encounters were also reported, particularly in patients with class III obesity. In a qualitative study of 82 morbidly obese women undergoing gastric banding, reasons for sexual problems were due to lack of self-esteem, poor relationships, and the negative consequences of the stigmatization felt by many obese individuals.[48]

What are the implications of weight-loss programmes?

Although pregnant women may not have specific problems with sexual desire, it appears that, overall, intimate problems may exist in obese women. One of the key problems in targeting maternal obesity is that obese, pregnant women often are unaware of the problems that the excess weight places on their pregnancy.[7] Education and interventions to improve knowledge and cognitions about appropriate weight gain in pregnancy are therefore clearly needed.[37] However, where the intervention should be targeted is not clear. One school of thought is that women who are overweight prior to pregnancy appear to be at greatest risk of gaining excessive weight.[49] Therefore, targeting interventions prior to pregnancy would be most beneficial. In this respect, prior to pregnancy, family planning and more public health campaigns about weight loss and nutrition education would be needed. Indeed, one study has suggested that, although costly, prepregnancy counselling should be provided to all overweight and obese women prior to pregnancy.[50]

However, others have found that interventions are most beneficial during pregnancy. For example, Rossner[51] reported that sustained weight retention 1 year post partum was strongly predicted by the amount of weight gained during pregnancy; in contrast, the weight of women before pregnancy did not predict outcome. This author also suggested that body weight after pregnancy is strongly predicted by changes in lifestyle that occur during the pregnancy, rather than the prepregnancy lifestyle.[51,52]

It has been argued that little is known about the psychosocial influences on behaviour during pregnancy.[10] Of the limited research available, Harris et al[53] investigated whether long-term weight gain was influenced by the behavioural and psychosocial changes that occurred during and after pregnancy in 74 mothers. These investigators found that pregnancy-related weight gain is not simply a question of the amount of retained pregnancy weight but is also associated with the amount gained in the postnatal period and access to food. For example, mothers who said that they ate more had a significantly greater long-term weight gain than those who had not felt that they had increased their food intake ($P = 0.016$), or had greater access to food ($P = 0.032$). Particular lifestyle changes included feeling as though they did less exercise ($P = 0.028$) and low social support ($P = 0.033$). Interestingly, neither maternal depression nor the stress of parenting was significantly associated with long-term weight gain.

During pregnancy, numerous possible interventions have been identified. From the perspective of service users, Thornton et al[54] carried out a qualitative study which found the need for enhanced social support through community-based, family-oriented interventions to promote and sustain healthy lifestyles during pregnancy and the postpartum period. Written information about the appropriate level of weight gain during pregnancy may also be beneficial.[37] In the current and future management of maternal obesity in the UK, the results from one qualitative study revealed that changes to the standard NHS patient information booklet would be beneficial; although it addresses issues related to healthy eating, it fails to address issues about weight gain and BMI-specific dietary requirements.[7] The clinical maternity staff interviewed as part of the study also believed that improving links for the pregnant woman with a dietetic service and weight-management groups would be beneficial. Whether such circumstances exist in other countries is not easy to determine, but it is likely that healthy eating plans are more commonly dispensed by healthcare providers than detailed consequences of poor or inadequate nutrition or factors leading to obesity.

Despite the numerous options available, interventions with obese patients are often difficult and problematic. For example, obesity in women has had a clear impact on access to healthcare,[55] and weight-loss interventions are seldom successful in the long term. As pointed out by Wells,[12] one answer to the problems associated with targeted intervention may be a more sustained approach to educating and supporting women throughout their lifespan, although whether the resources would ever be available to provide such a service is doubtful. In this regard, the rapid acceptance of bariatric surgery underscores the difficulty in follow-through that accompanies traditional programmes that rely on dietary or dietary-exercise interventions alone (see Chapters 12 and 13).

Is obesity considered to be an addiction?

A major and hitherto unsolved problem related to the therapy of obesity is that traditional weight-loss interventions as described above are predominately, if not exclusively, based upon the assumption that, given the right advice and motivation, people can successfully lower their food intake over the long term and therefore lose weight.[56] The sad truth is that this assumption is not grounded in fact. It is equally likely that obesity, at least in many cases, represents a form of addictive behaviour that was not previously recognized, much like the fact that prior generations thought that cigarette smoking was a social nicety, often glamorized in movies and advertisements, rather than the addiction that we now know that it is. The same may be said for the use of caffeine.

The answer to the question posed in the heading of this section is either yes or no. Responsible and well-read authorities could argue either side of the question. Perhaps the more important question is to ask why it should *be considered an addiction*. Recently, it has been argued that eating is an automatic behaviour and that individuals have less control over their eating than the environment in which they live.[56] In such a construct, factors such as the ease with which food can be obtained, the cost of food as a portion of total available disposable income, food visibility and availability, and the constantly increasing portion size of recent years (e.g., the double Big Mac and the 48-oz 'big gulp' portions) strongly influence the amount of food that is eaten in total opposition to the traditional view that humans can self-regulate what they eat.[56]

Discourses such as 'food addiction' and 'food cravings' are often used to support a biological view that humans have little control over their eating behaviour and that physiological mechanisms control appetite and food choices; chocolate and other sweet snacks, such as biscuits and cakes, and other various savoury and salty snacks appear high on the list of craved foods.[57] However, while there may be a biological basis for food cravings, it has been argued that this forms only a small portion of our understanding of eating behaviour, and that a biopsychosocial model is more appropriate for our understanding of the determinants of human eating behaviour and the experiences that accompany eating.[57]

In relation to eating as an automatic behaviour, the degree to which individuals are impulsive has been shown to influence food intake. For example, one study found that healthy women who had a high-impulsive personality ($n = 41$) had a higher food intake and more 'eating disordered' behaviours and thoughts than their low-impulsive personality counterparts ($n = 45$) during a bogus taste test, in which the ingested food was monotonous or varied in taste, texture, colour, and form. No interaction was found between variety and impulsivity or variety.[58] In a later study, the same research team examined whether the effect of the obesogenic environment and impulsivity influenced the amount of food eaten in a group of 78 primary schoolchildren aged 8–10 years.[59] Impulsivity was measured by reward sensitivity and deficient response inhibition (in general, individuals who are impulsive are more reward sensitive and less successful at inhibiting prepotent responses). During a bogus taste test, the study team also manipulated one part of the obesogenic environment; one-half of the children ate food that varied (variety group), and the remaining children tasted food that was monotonous (monotony group). No significant difference was present in food intake between the more and less reward-sensitive children. However, the reward-sensitive children did eat significantly more calories than the less reward-sensitive children, thus leading the investigators to conclude that within the obesogenic environment reward sensitivity may be a causal mechanism of overeating.

Conclusions

Maternal obesity is a widespread problem receiving international attention. Factors such as feeling more relaxed about one's body shape, the belief that pregnancy is a legitimate time in which to put on weight and 'eat for two', and cognitive influences, such as beliefs about the needs of the unborn baby or one's natural propensity to put on weight, have all been identified as possible explanations of maternal obesity. However, in view of the findings of studies on non-pregnant women, more research is needed on the biological mechanisms underpinning appetite, weight control, and the influence of the food environment in order to determine the role that these play in both antenatal and postnatal eating behaviours and obesity.

More research is also needed on the interrelationship of obesity, pregnancy, and psychological well-being. While prepregnancy BMI is an important factor, other possibly confounding factors affecting psychological well-being, such as ethnicity and social support, need to be explored in more detail. Psychological interventions to improve self-esteem, body image, and negative cognitions about obesity in conjunction with more tailored support from dietetic services and maternity staff (particularly on nutrition education, the consequences for both mother and baby of maternal obesity, eating behaviours, and BMI-specific dietary requirements during pregnancy) would be beneficial.

References

1. Siega-Riz AM, Evenson KR, Dole N. Pregnancy-related weight gain – a link to obesity? *Nutr Rev* 2004; **62**:S105–11.
2. Drife JO. Weight gain in pregnancy: eating for two or just getting fat? *BMJ* 1986;**11**:903–4.
3. Visscher TL, Rissanen A, Seidell JC, et al. Obesity and unhealthy life-years in adult Finns: an empirical approach. *Arch Intern Med* 2004;**164**:1413–20.
4. Norman RJ, Clark AM. Obesity and reproductive disorders: a review. *Reprod Fertil Dev* 1998;**10**:55–63.
5. Garbaciak JA Jr, Richter M, Miller S, Barton JJ. Maternal weight and pregnancy complications. *Am J Obstet Gynecol* 1985;**152**:238–45.
6. Gross TL. Operative considerations in the obese pregnant patient. *Clin Perinatol* 1983;**10**:411–21.

7. Heslehurst N, Lang R, Rankin J, et al. Obesity in pregnancy: a study of the impact of maternal obesity on NHS maternity services. *Br J Obstet Gynaecol* 2007;**114**:334–42.

8. Kolotkin RL, Crosby RD, Kosloski KD, Williams GR. Development of a brief measure to assess quality of life in obesity. *Obes Res* 2001;**9**:102–11.

9. Subcommittee on Nutritional Status and Weight Gain During Pregnancy, Institute of Medicine, National Academy of Sciences. *Nutrition During Pregnancy*. Washington, DC: National Academies Press, 1990.

10. Kendall A, Olson CM, Frongillo EA Jr. Evaluation of psychosocial measures for understanding weight-related behaviors in pregnant women. *Ann Behav Med* 2001;**23**:50–8.

11. Rossner S, Ohlin A. Pregnancy as a risk factor for obesity: lessons from the Stockholm pregnancy and weight development study. *Obes Res* 1995;**3** (Suppl 2): 267s–75s.

12. Wells CS, Schwalberg R, Noonan G, Gabor V. Factors influencing inadequate and excessive weight gain in pregnancy: Colorado, 2000–2002. *Matern Child Health J* 2006;**10**:55–62.

13. Caulfield LE, Witter FR, Stoltzfus RJ. Determinants of gestational weight gain outside the recommended ranges among black and white women. *Obstet Gynecol* 1996;**87**:760–6.

14. Lederman SA, Alfasi G, Deckelbaum RJ. Pregnancy-associated obesity in black women in New York City. *Matern Child Health J* 2002;**6**:37–42.

15. Glazener CMA, MacArthur C, Garcia J. Postnatal care: time for change. *Contemp Rev Obstet* 1993;**5**:130–6.

16. O'Hara MW, Zekoski EM, Philips LH, Wright EJ. Controlled prospective study of post-partum mood disorders: comparison of childbearing and non-childbearing women. *J Abnorm Psychol* 1990;**99**:3–15.

17. Amador N, Juárez JM, Guízar JM, Linares B. Quality of life in obese pregnant women: a longitudinal study. *Am J Obstet Gynecol* 2008;**198**:203.e1–5.

18. Carter AS, Baker CW, Brownell KD. Body mass index, eating attitudes, and symptoms of depression and anxiety in pregnancy and the postpartum period. *Psychosom Med* 2000;**62**:264–70.

19. Lacoursiere DY, Baksh L, Bloebaum L, Varner MW. Maternal body mass index and self-reported postpartum depressive symptoms. *Matern Child Health J* 2006;**10**:385–90.

20. Dipietro JA, Millet S, Costigan KA, et al. Psychosocial influences on weight gain attitudes and behaviors during pregnancy. *J Am Diet Assoc* 2003;**103**:1314–19.

21. Cameron RP, Grabill CM, Hobfoll SE, et al. Weight, self-esteem, ethnicity, and depressive symptomatology during pregnancy among inner-city women. *Health Psychol* 1996;**15**:293–7.

22. White MA, O'Neil PM, Kolotkin RL, Karl Byrne T. Gender, race and obesity-related quality of life at extreme levels of obesity. *Obes Res* 2004;**12**:949–55.

23. Venes AM, Krupka LR, Gerad RJ. Overweight/obese patients: an overview. *Practitioner* 1982;**226**:1102–9.

24. Cramer P, Steinwert T. Thin is good, fat is bad: how early does it begin? *J Appl Dev Psychol* 1998;**19**:429–51.

25. Goffman E. *Stigma: Notes on the Management of Spoiled Identity*. Harmondsworth: Pelican Books, 1968.

26. Brown I, Thompson J, Todd A, Jones GL. Obesity, stigma and quality of life: a qualitative study. *Int J Interdiscip Soc Sci* 2006;**1**:169–78.

27. Fabricatore AN, Wadden TA. Psychological aspects of obesity. *Clin Dermatol* 2004;**22**:332–7.

28. Roehling MV. Weight-based discrimination in employment: psychological and legal aspects. *Pers Psychol* 1999;**52**:969–1017.

29. Greaves M. *Big and Beautiful: Challenging the Myths and Celebrating Our Size*. London: Grafton, 1990.

30. Wiles R. The impact of pregnancy on fat women's body image and eating practices. Unpublished PhD thesis, University of Southampton, 1994.

31. Copper RL, DuBard MB, Goldenberg RL, Oweis AI. The relationship of maternal attitude toward weight gain to weight gain during pregnancy and low birth weight. *Obstet Gynecol* 1995;**85**:590–5.

32. Stevens-Simon C, Nakashima I, Andrews D. Weight gain attitudes among pregnant adolescents. *J Adolesc Health* 1993;**14**:369–72.

33. Armstrong JE, Weijohn TT. Dietary quality and concerns about body weight of low-income pregnant women. *J Am Diet Assoc* 1991;**91**:1280–2.

34. Walker L, Timmerman GM, Kim M, Sterling B. Relationships between body image and depressive symptoms during postpartum in ethnically diverse, low income women. *Women Health* 2002;**36**:101–21.

35. Fox P, Yamaguchi C. Body image change in pregnancy: a comparison of normal weight and overweight primigravidas. *Birth* 1997;**24**:35–40.

36. Woollett A, Marshall H. Discourses of pregnancy and childbirth. In: Yardley L, ed. *Material Discourses of Health and Illness*. London: Routledge, 1997.

37. Wiles R. The views of women of above average weight about appropriate weight gain in pregnancy. *Midwifery* 1998;**14**:254–60.

38. Murcott A. On the altered appetites of pregnancy: conceptions of food, body and person. *Sociol Rev* 1988;**36**:733–64.

39. Oakley A. *Social Support and Motherhood*. Oxford: Blackwell, 1992.

40. Micali N, Treasure J, Simonoff E. Eating disorders symptoms in pregnancy: a longitudinal study of women with recent and past eating disorders and obesity. *J Psychosom Res* 2007;**63**:297–303.

41. Augustine RA, Ladyman SR, Grattan DR. From feeding one to feeding many: hormone-induced changes in bodyweight homeostasis during pregnancy. *J Physiol* 2008;**586**:387–97.

42. Clark M, Ogden J. The impact of pregnancy on eating behaviour and aspects of weight concern. *Int J Obes Relat Metab Disord* 1999;**23**:18–24.

43. Abraham S, King W, Llewellyn-Jones D. Attitudes to body weight, weight gain and eating behavior in pregnancy. *J Psychosom Obstet Gynaecol* 1994;**15**:189–95.

44. Fairburn CG, Stein A, Jones R. Eating habits and eating disorders during pregnancy. *Psychosom Med* 1992;**54**:665–72.

45. Esposito K, Ciotola M, Giugliano F, et al. Association of body weight with sexual function in women. *Int J Impot Res* 2007;**19**:353–7.
46. Assimakopoulos K, Panayiotopoulos S, Iconomou G, et al. Assessing sexual function in obese women preparing for bariatric surgery. *Obes Surg* 2006;**16**:1087–91.
47. Kolotkin RL, Binks M, Crosby RD, et al. Obesity and sexual quality of life. *Obesity* 2006;**14**:472–9.
48. Kinzl JF, Trefalt E, Fiala M, et al. Partnership, sexuality, and sexual disorders in morbidly obese women: consequences of weight loss after gastric banding. *Obes Surg* 2001;**11**:455–8.
49. Olafsdottir AS, Skuladottir GV, Thorsdottir I, et al. Maternal diet in early and late pregnancy in relation to weight gain. *Int J Obes* 2006;**30**:492–9.
50. Nankervis AJ, Conn JJ, Knight RL. Obesity and reproductive health. *Med J Aust* 2006;**184**:51.
51. Rössner S. Weight gain in pregnancy. *Hum Reprod* 1997;**12**(Suppl 1): 110–15.
52. Rössner S, Ohlin A. Pregnancy as a risk factor for obesity: lessons from the Stockholm Pregnancy and Weight Development Study. *Obes Res* 1995;**3** (Suppl 2): 267s–75s.
53. Harris HE, Ellison GT, Clement S. Do the psychosocial and behavioral changes that accompany motherhood influence the impact of pregnancy on long-term weight gain? *J Psychosom Obstet Gynaecol* 1999;**20**:65–79.
54. Thornton PL, Kieffer EC, Salabarría-Peña Y, et al. Weight, diet, and physical activity-related beliefs and practices among pregnant and postpartum Latino women: the role of social support. *Matern Child Health J* 2006;**10**:95–104.
55. Drury CA, Louis M. Exploring the association between bodyweight, stigma of obesity and health care avoidance. *J Am Acad Nurse Pract* 2002;**14**:554–61.
56. Cohen D, Farley TA. Eating as an automatic behavior. *Prev Chronic Dis* 2008; **5**:A23.
57. Rogers PJ, Smit HJ. Food craving and food 'addiction': a critical review of the evidence from a biopsychosocial perspective. *Pharmacol Biochem Behav* 2000;**66**:3–14.
58. Guerrieri R, Nederkoorn C, Jansen A. How impulsiveness and variety influence food intake in a sample of healthy women. *Appetite* 2007;**48**: 119–22.
59. Guerrieri R, Nederkoorn C, Jansen A. The interaction between impulsivity and a varied food environment: its influence on food intake and overweight. *Int J Obes* 2008;**32**:708–14.

4 The molecular biology of obesity

David CW Lau

Introduction

Obesity is the most common nutritional problem worldwide, and its prevalence continues to increase.[1] Overweight and obesity are the consequence of a chronic positive energy balance between food intake and energy expenditure. The emerging global obesity epidemic is due mainly to an overabundance of food and decreased physical activity levels. A third of adults in the USA, for example, are obese and one in five children is overweight.[2] Obesity is characterized by excessive body fat to the extent of causing health problems. It is often associated with infertility and can adversely affect reproductive health, especially in females.

Our knowledge of the pathogenesis of obesity has advanced rapidly over the past several decades, and has transformed a rather simplistic view of energy intake exceeding energy expenditure to an infinitely more complex system with an array of sensing and effector controls. The aetiology of obesity is complex, and unravelling the cellular and molecular basis of obesity requires an understanding of energy homeostasis and body fat regulation.[3] Energy homeostasis is meticulously regulated by a sophisticated and complex system involving an integration of humoral and neural signals between the central nervous system and peripheral organs, with redundant circuitry that has evolved as an adaptive defence against extreme fluctuations in body weight. Defects in any of the homeostatic pathways can lead to expansion or contraction of fat mass and changes in body weight and composition.

This chapter reviews the pathophysiology of obesity, focusing mainly on how appetite and body fat mass are regulated, and the diverse functions of adipose tissue in health and obese states.

Diverse functions of adipose tissue

Adipose tissue is distributed throughout the body and comprises white and brown fat. A major function of white adipose tissue is energy storage in the form of triglycerides. Brown fat generates heat and is found mainly in newborns. It gradually disappears within the first few years of life and is present in only a small quantity in adults. Most of the body fat (~85%) is subcutaneous; it can expand inordinately and specializes as a long-term fuel repository. Women have more subcutaneous fat than men, presumably for easy and steady access to energy during pregnancy. Subcutaneous fat also serves as an insulator to prevent heat loss, thereby preserving core body temperature. Another function of fat is cushioning of the joints and extremities, as well as internal organs. Adipose tissue releases high concentrations of fatty acids that are toxic to pathogenic infectious organisms, ranging from viruses to bacteria and fungi, and functions as a barrier to infection. Fat also plays a role in immunity by releasing complement components and inflammatory cytokines as well as chemokines for further protection against infection. Intra-abdominal fat, which accounts for about 15% of total body fat, guards against internal injury by its ability to release pressor, angiogenic, and haemostatic factors. Abdominal fat, notably that in the omental and mesenteric depots, appears to be metabolically more active and releases more of these and other inflammatory factors. Another important function of intra-abdominal, or visceral fat, is to provide short-term storage and rapid energy access to the liver for metabolic processing.

The excess fat in obese persons is usually stored in adipose tissue; where it is distributed in the body is highly variable, however. When body fat can no longer expand to accommodate the surfeit energy, the latter is channelled to other insulin-sensitive organs for storage, resulting in fat deposition in the liver, muscles, and pancreas. The ectopic fat in the affected organs can lead to a myriad of metabolic abnormalities, ranging from hepatic steatosis, insulin resistance, metabolic syndrome, and ultimately type 2 diabetes, to increased cardiovascular disease risk.

People with the same body mass index (BMI) differ markedly with respect to the absolute amount of their body fat, as well as the proportion of subcutaneous and abdominal fat, and its distribution in different subcutaneous depots. The amount of intra-abdominal fat in a given individual is influenced by a combination of total adiposity, gender, age, ethnicity, and physical activity. The clinical relevance of abdominal obesity to insulin resistance, metabolic syndrome, type 2 diabetes, and cardiovascular disease, first reported by the French physician Jean Vague more than 50 years ago, has stimulated intense interest in understanding what controls fat development and growth, as well as its distribution in the body.[4-7]

Research progress over the past several decades clearly indicates that adipose tissue is not merely a passive repository for energy.[5,8] The discovery of leptin as a fat-derived hormone heralded the understanding of the key role that adipose tissue plays in energy homeostasis and body weight regulation. This discovery also helped in the concept that adipose tissue is a highly active metabolic and secretory organ. Adipose tissue expresses and secretes a variety of bioactive peptides that act via endocrine, paracrine, and autocrine mechanisms to store and release energy, as well as coordinating a variety of biological processes, including appetite control, glucose and lipid metabolism, and immune and neuroendocrine functions. As discussed below, a large number of genes are expressed and over 200 proteins are produced during adipogenesis.[9]

Leptin, the fat-derived satiety hormone

Adipose tissue is the main source of leptin, a 16-kDa protein hormone with structural homology to cytokines.[10,11] Mature fat cells express and secrete leptin in direct proportion to adipose tissue mass and nutritional status. How leptin expression and secretion are controlled in fat cells is not well understood, but evidence is accumulating that both endocrine and paracrine pathways operate. In the fed state, circulating leptin levels parallel adipose tissue mass and nutritional status. Leptin acts as a satiety hormone, mediating its inhibitory effects on appetite and energy expenditure centrally via hypothalamic pathways. Weight loss is associated with a decrease in serum leptin levels, and triggers feedback changes to conserve body fat. Hence, leptin, together with insulin, which also plays a role in the central regulation of appetite, functions as a long-term signal for maintenance of body fat and energy balance.

Leptin exerts its effects by binding to its receptors, of which only the long isoform is functional in transmitting the leptin signals in cells.[11,12] Leptin receptors are found predominantly in the hypothalamus but are also present in peripheral tissues and organs, including adipose tissue, ovary, placenta, testis, and prostate.[8]

Central control of energy homeostasis and body weight by leptin and neuropeptides

Leptin acts centrally to reduce food intake and increase energy expenditure by inhibiting the orexigenic and stimulating the anorexigenic pathways, both of which are located in the hypothalamus.[11] Leptin activates the melanocortin pathway, which involves neurons within the arcuate nucleus that express pro-opiomelanocortin (POMC) and cocaine- and amphetamine-regulated transcript (CART), to promote energy expenditure and weight loss (Figure 4.1). In contrast, the orexigenic pathway involving neuropeptide-Y and agouti-related protein (NPY/AgRP) is inhibited by leptin (Figure 4.1). Leptin also influences other orexigenic mediators, such as orexin A, and the endogenous endocannabinoids, such as anandamide.

Leptin also exerts a hypothalamic neurotrophic action during a critical neonatal developmental period. Data obtained from the central administration of ciliary neurotrophic factor suggest that regulated hypothalamic–neurogenesis regulation in adult mice plays a previously unappreciated role in physiology and disease.[13] Furthermore, recent data suggest that leptin actions go beyond known hypothalamic targets with the modulation of mesolimbic dopamine neurons important for the regulation of reward signals and motivated behaviours that influence appetite, locomotor activity, and body weight.[14]

Circulating leptin levels are higher in women than in men and, with the exception of rare cases of congenital leptin deficiency (discussed below), are generally elevated rather than suppressed in most obese people, indicating that obesity is associated with leptin resistance.[11] This finding largely explains why recombinant leptin failed as an effective antiobesity agent in clinical trials.[11,15]

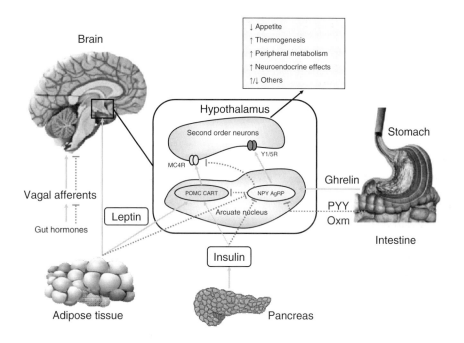

FIGURE 4.1 Complex integration of central and peripheral pathways controlling energy homeostasis, appetite, and body weight. Leptin is an adipose tissue-derived hormone that acts centrally to reduce food intake and increase energy expenditure by inhibiting the orexigenic and stimulating the anorexigenic pathways, both of which are located in the hypothalamus. Leptin activates the pro-opiomelanocortin (POMC) and cocaine- and amphetamine-regulated transcript (CART) neurons located in the arcuate nucleus. POMC neurons project to second-order neurons, where melanocyte-stimulating hormone activates the melanocortin pathway via melanocortin-4 receptors (MC4R) to promote energy expenditure and weight loss. In contrast, leptin inhibits the orexigenic pathway involving neuropeptide-Y and agouti-related protein (NPY/AgRP). The second-order neurons (mainly paraventricular nucleus and lateral hypothalamus) in turn mediate the downstream effects of leptin, which include decreased appetite, and increased thermogenesis and peripheral metabolism, together with neuroendocrine and other effects. Insulin is the other peripheral hormone involved in the long-term regulation of food intake and appetite by inhibiting mainly NPY/AgRP. Ghrelin is a growth hormone-like hormone, secreted mainly by the stomach, that initiates a meal and stimulates the NPY/AgRP pathway, whereas peptide YY (PYY) and oxyntomodulin (Oxm) are satiety hormones that act by inhibiting food intake. These and other gut hormones also mediate their effects via the vagal afferents that relay the peripheral signals centrally to the brain stem and the hypothalamus. Y1/5R denotes the subtypes of NPY receptors. Solid arrows denote stimulatory and dashed arrows inhibitory signals

Human syndromes of deficient leptin signalling

Deficiency of leptin or its receptors results in hyperphagia and early onset severe obesity, as observed in rodents and humans.[10,12] In addition to its effects on energy homeostasis, leptin regulates neuroendocrine, immune, reproductive, and other functions. Congenital leptin deficiency and leptin receptor deficiency are rare missense or nonsense mutations associated with early onset severe obesity, hyperphagia, altered immune function, and delayed puberty due to hypogonadotrophic hypogonadism.[16,17] Low-dose recombinant leptin administration to leptin-deficient patients leads to weight loss, accelerates puberty, and restores normal reproductive and immune function.[17] Animal and human studies strongly suggest that leptin is related to reproductive health and is an important hormonal trigger for the onset of puberty in females.[11]

All known forms of monogenic human obesity involve mutations in the leptin–melanocortin signalling pathway.[18,19] Monogenic forms of obesity at present account for about 7% of children with severe, early onset obesity, that is, less than 0.01% of the population.[18] Mutations involving the *POMC* gene result in a deficiency of some or all of the peptides derived from *POMC*, including α-, β-, and γ-melanocyte-stimulating hormone (MSH), and adrenocorticotrophin (ACTH); most of these deficiencies are manifested as childhood-onset obesity and adrenal insufficiency.[20] Similarly, deficiency of prohormone convertase-1, which cleaves POMC into α-MSH and ACTH, results in the same phenotype.[21]

Melanocortin-4 receptor (MC4R) mutations are the most common form of monogenic obesity, accounting for about 4–6% of massive obesity. Individuals with MC4R deficiency are hyperphagic with severe early onset obesity, as well as increased lean body mass, linear growth, and hyperinsulinaemia.[22]

Disruptions of the transcription factor, single-minded homologue-1 (SIM1), which is required for the development of the paraventricular nucleus (PVN) of the hypothalamus, a principal site of MC4R expression, leads to early onset obesity, hyperinsulinaemia, insulin resistance, and developmental delay.[23]

The gut–brain axis in appetite control

How we decide to eat and how much to eat are affected not only by the circulating levels of leptin and insulin, but also by integrated short-term humoral signals transmitted by the gut hormones, and neural signals from the vagal afferent neurons innervating the gastrointestinal tract to the hypothalamus and the brain stem (see Figure 4.1). The sensation of hunger felt before a meal and satiety in the postprandial state are controlled in part by neural signals transmitted by the mechanoreceptors and chemoreceptors in the gut via the vagal nerve. Ghrelin and peptide YY (PYY) are the respective gut hormone humoral signals affecting hunger and satiety.

Ghrelin is a stomach-derived, 28-amino acid 'hunger hormone' that stimulates food intake by activating the orexigenic NPY/AgRP pathway in the arcuate nucleus of the hypothalamus.[24] It is released from the stomach prior to a meal and is thought to initiate appetite. Circulating ghrelin levels rise before meals and in response to fast or starvation, but are decreased in obese states.[24] Mice deficient in ghrelin have normal body weight but improved insulin sensitivity, suggesting that blocking ghrelin signalling is not a viable target for obesity therapy.

PYY is a 36-amino acid 'satiety' hormone related to NPY, and secreted in the postprandial phase, in proportional to the calories ingested, by the L cells lining the distal small bowel and colon.[24,25] Acute administration of the truncated form, PYY_{3-36}, reduces food intake in both rodents and humans. However, circulating PYY levels are normal and not increased in obese people, pointing to a limited role of this gut peptide as an antiobesity drug target.[24]

Other gut peptides, such as cholecystokinin, pancreatic polypeptide, glucagon-like peptides-1 and -2, amylin, and oxyntomodulin, appear to exert only modest influence on hunger and satiety, but may have other effects, such as the processes of gastric emptying and glucose metabolism, which indirectly contribute to energy and body-weight homeostasis.[24]

Adipose tissue development and growth

During fetal life, adipocytes begin to develop at around 15 weeks of gestation. There is an increase in both adipocyte number and size, both of which accelerate during the third trimester causing body fat to increase from about 5% to 15%. The first year of life, when the size of fat cells nearly doubles without a measurable increase in cell number, may be an important determinant of obesity later in childhood and adolescence. During the early infancy years, the increase in body fat mass is due mainly to an increase in adipocyte size rather than number.

The preschool and early schoolage years are characterized by a period of adiposity rebound, when body fat starts to increase after a period of gradual decline after the first few years of life. The 'rebound' phenomenon occurs at around 5–6 years of age. Lean infants who developed rebound at an earlier age have a greater risk of becoming overweight.

Adolescence represents another critical period of adipose tissue growth. Puberty is associated with an increase in both fat mass and fat-free mass in girls, whereas fat-free mass tends to increase and fat mass decreases with advancing puberty in boys. Childhood obesity is typically associated with increase not only in the size but also the number of adipocytes, leading to the concept of hyperplastic obesity.

The physiology of the critical periods of adipose tissue growth remains poorly understood. Genetic, environmental, and behavioural factors may contribute to accelerated growth during the rebound and critical periods of adipose tissue growth.

Recent data suggest that maternal imprinting may contribute to the development of obesity. Epidemiological studies have shown that infants exposed to increased maternal nutrition before birth are at increased risk of becoming obese in later life. Animal studies suggest that the neural circuitry involved in appetite control may be adversely affected by increased maternal nutrient intake.[26] Failure to upregulate the anoreixgenic regulatory pathway in the brain may be a potential mechanism whereby exposure to maternal overnutrition leads to subsequent increase in childhood and adult obesity.[26] Breastfeeding, on the other hand, appears to offer a protective mechanism against the development of obesity in childhood and adolescence.

Adipose tissue-derived signals involved in energy balance and insulin sensitivity

The recognition that adipose tissue is an active metabolic and endocrine organ has led to the identification of a large number of factors with diverse functions. These factors include free fatty acids (FFAs), with well-described physiological and pathophysiological effects on glucose homeostasis, and proteins termed 'adipokines', which act in an autocrine, paracrine, or endocrine fashion to control various metabolic functions. Some adipokines have been implicated in energy homeostasis and body-weight regulation, as well as in the development of inflammation and insulin resistance, metabolic syndrome, and ultimately diabetes. These compounds may act locally or distally to alter inflammation and insulin sensitivity in insulin-targeted organs, such as muscle and liver, or through neuroendocrine, autonomic, or immune pathways. The relevant and emerging adipokines are discussed here (Table 4.1).

TABLE 4.1 Endocrine and secretory function of adipose tissue

	Proteins	Function	Cell source
Adipokines	Leptin	↓ Appetite, ↑ thermogenesis	A, P
	TNF-α	↓ Adipogenesis, IR	A, P, E, I
	IL-6	Proinflammatory	P, E, SV, I
	CRP	Proinflammatory	A, P, I
Complement and related proteins	Adiponectin	↓ Appetite, ↓ IR	A, P
	Adipsin (complement D)	↑ Angiogenesis	A, E
	Acylation-stimulating protein (C3 desArg)	↑ Triglyceride synthesis	A, P
Lipids and proteins for lipid metabolism	Lipoprotein lipase	↑ Lipogenesis, triglycerides	A, P
	Glycerol-3-phosphate dehydrogenase	↑ Lipogenesis	A, P
	Hormone-sensitive lipase	↑ Lipolysis	A, P
	Cholesterol ester transfer protein	HDL-cholesterol metabolism	A, P
Enzymes involved in steroidogenesis	11β- and 17β-hydroxysteroid dehydrogenase	↑ Cortisol, appetite, IR, ↑ adiposity	A, P

TABLE 4.1 (continued)

	Proteins	Function	Cell source
Proteins involved in glucose metabolism	Resistin	↑ IR	A, P, I
	RBP4	↑ IR, lipid metabolism	A, P
	Visfatin	↓ IR	A, P
	Omentin	↓ IR	A, P
	Vaspin	↓ IR	A, P
Angiogenic proteins involved in vascular function	VEGF	↑ Angiogenesis	E
	FGF-2	↑ Proliferation, ↑ angiogenesis	A, P
	Angiogenin, angiopoietin-2	↑ Proliferation, ↑ angiogenesis	A, P
	PAI-1	Prothrombotic, ↑ IR	A, P, E, I
	Angiotensinogen	↑ BP	A, P, E
Inflammation and chemokines	Macrophage inhibitory factor-1	Proinflammatory	I
	Monocyte chemoattractant protein-1	Proinflammatory	I, E, I
	TIMP-1 and -2	Extracellular matrix metabolism	E, I
Receptors	Leptin	↓ Appetite	A, P
	Insulin	↑ Glucose uptake	A, P
	Growth hormone	Glucose/protein metabolism	A, P
	Glucagon-like peptide-1	↓ Appetite, ↑ glucose uptake	A, P
	Angiotensin II	↑ BP	A, P
	Thyroid and glucocorticoid	Thyroid and steroid hormone	A, P
	Adrenergic β_1-, β_2-, β_3-	↑ Lipolysis	A, P

Adipose tissue is a highly metabolically active and secretory organ producing a large number of bioactive molecules involved in diverse biological processes. Examples of secretory products listed above are derived from different cells found in adipose tissue (A, adipocytes; P, preadipocytes; E, endothelial cells; I, inflammatory cells including macrophages, granulocytes, and mast cells). Abbreviations: IL, interleukin; BP, blood pressure; IR, insulin resistance; TNF-α tumour necrosis factor-α; VEGF, vascular endothelial growth factor; FGF, fibroblast growth factor; PAI-1, plasminogen activator inhibitor-1; TIMP, tissue inhibitor of metalloproteinase.

Adiponectin

The most abundant adipokine produced by fat cells is adiponectin. Adiponectin is a 247-amino acid protein of about 30 kDa that bears structural resemblance to complement C1q; its gene is located on chromosome 3q27 in a region mapped as a susceptibility locus for type 2 diabetes and metabolic syndrome.[27] It exists as a homotrimer, which dimerizes to form the biologically active, high-molecular-weight complex of the hexamer. Adiponectin mediates its effect via two receptors, AdipoR1, which has a higher affinity for the high-molecular-weight forms, and AdipoR2, which has equal affinity for the full-length and high-molecular-weight forms. AdipoR1 is primarily expressed in muscle and, in contrast to adipoR2, which is found mainly in the liver, is also expressed in endothelial cells.[27] Both receptors are present in the hypothalamus, suggesting that adiponectin exerts its effects not only in peripheral tissues but also centrally in the brain.

Adiponectin gene transcription and secretion are regulated by multiple factors. Insulin stimulates adiponectin secretion in rodents. It is conceivable that adiponectin levels are low in obesity because of insulin resistance in the adipocyte. Adiponectin gene transcription and secretion are decreased by tumour necrosis factor α (TNF-α) and interleukin (IL)-6. Its expression is also regulated by peroxisome proliferator-activated receptor-δ-dependent pathways, suggesting that, at least in part, the beneficial effects of thiazolidinedione on insulin sensitivity may be mediated by adiponectin.[27]

Adiponectin modulates insulin sensitivity by stimulating glucose utilization and fatty acid oxidation, and by a decrease in triglyceride content in muscle and liver via the activation and phosphorylation of AMP activated protein kinase (AMPK).[27,28] Adiponectin acts mainly on peripheral targets, although it may have a central action, particularly in the paraventricular nucleus. Administration of adiponectin results in weight loss and increased energy expenditure, as well as improved insulin sensitivity. It also exerts antiatherogenic and anti-inflammatory effects on the vasculature and confers cardioprotective properties.[28]

Circulating plasma levels of adiponectin are 3–30 μg/ml and account for 0.01% of the total plasma protein. These levels are about 1000-fold greater than those of other polypeptide hormones and greater than leptin, which has a plasma level of 2–8 μg/l. Plasma levels of adiponecctin are decreased in obesity, insulin-resistant states with increased cardiometabolic risk, and type 2 diabetes; they increase upon weight loss. Low adiponectin levels are also associated with insulin resistance, dyslipidaemia, and atherosclerosis.

Adiponectin may link adipose tissue to reproductive function by ensuring energy supply and regulating energy needs for normal reproduction and pregnancy. Women with pre-eclampsia have higher plasma concentrations of adiponectin, resistin, and leptin than healthy controls, despite the similar mRNA levels of adiponectin, resistin, and leptin found in abdominal subcutaneous adipose tissue in the two groups. Moreover, leptin mRNA levels are higher in placentas from women with pre-eclampsia than in controls. In another study, adiponectin mRNA levels in abdominal subcutaneous adipose tissue were lower in women with gestational diabetes than in healthy lean pregnant women.[29]

Similarly, plasma adiponectin concentrations in women with gestational diabetes mellitus were 50% lower than those of lean, pregnant controls.[29] Interestingly, cord-blood adiponectin levels are much higher than the serum levels in children and adults, and are positively correlated with fetal birth weights.[29] The relevance of adiponectin and adipokines in general to reproductive function and fetal outcomes clearly deserves further elucidation.

Apelin

Another recently discovered adipose tissue-derived adipokine that confers insulin sensitivity and regulates adiposity is apelin, which was first isolated from the stomach as an endogenous ligand of the seven-transmembrane G-protein-coupled receptor, APJ.[30] Apelin is also found in brain, heart, muscle, and vasculature and, when administered to mice, it increases energy expenditure by upregulating uncoupling protein levels in brown adipose and skeletal tissue. Apelin treatment also increases circulating adiponectin and insulin and, at the same time, decreases leptin levels, thereby improving insulin sensitivity.[30] The physiological function of apelin and whether it plays a role in human obesity remain unknown.

Other adipokines involved in energy balance and insulin resistance

TNF-α is one of the best studied adipokines that decreases adiposity by inhibiting adipocyte differentiation. It also augments insulin resistance by inducing serine phosphorylation of insulin receptor substrate-1 and, thereby, reducing the activity of tyrosine kinase and downstream insulin receptor signalling.[31]

Retinoid-binding protein-4

Retinoid-binding protein-4 (RBP4) was found to be the circulating factor responsible for inducing insulin resistance in muscle and liver in mice lacking adipose tissue-specific glucose transporter-4 (GLUT-4).[32] Mice lacking fat-specific GLUT-4 have a 2.5-fold increase in circulating plasma levels of RBP4, and increased hepatic gluconeogenesis, a hallmark of hepatic insulin resistance. Studies in mice either overexpressing or lacking RBP4 demonstrate that RBP4 attenuates insulin-induced phosphorylation of insulin receptor substrate-1 and the downstream enzyme phosphoinositide 3-kinase (PI3-kinase).[32,33] RBP4 is a 21-kDa protein involved in vitamin A transport, and is thought to be released mainly in the liver. Adipose tissue-derived RBP4 accounts for about a fifth of that of the liver store, and it can be released into the circulation as a diabetogenic signal. RBP4 mRNA expression in adipose tissue is upregulated in mouse models of obesity and type 2 diabetes, whereas decreased RBP4 levels ameliorate insulin resistance in diet-induced obesity. Circulating levels of RBP4 are elevated in people with obesity, impaired glucose tolerance, metabolic syndrome, and type 2 diabetes.[33,34] More recent data suggest that RBP4 is more highly expressed in visceral than in subcutaneous fat tissue by a factor of 5, and that expression is more than 10-fold greater in obese than lean individuals.[35] Moreover, circulating RBP4 levels correlate positively with adipose RBP4 mRNA and intra-abdominal fat, suggesting its potential as a marker of intra-abdominal fat mass.[35]

Resistin

Resistin is a 114-amino acid, 12-kDa hormone, first identified as a transcript induced during adipogenesis and downregulated by thiazolidinedione treatment.[36] Its expression is upregulated in diet-induced obesity as well as in genetic models of obesity and insulin resistance, and it impairs insulin action and glucose tolerance in mice.[36] Resistin is expressed at low levels in human subcutaneous and visceral fat. However, other human studies fail to provide a clear role for resistin in obesity-related inflammatory and insulin-resistant states. Its role in modulation of insulin resistance in human obesity remains to be elucidated.

Adipokines associated with inflammation

One of the key developments in obesity research over the past decade is the recognition that it is characterized by chronic, mild inflammation. The circulating level of several proinflammatory markers is elevated in the obese, including TNF-α, IL-6, C-reactive protein (CRP), macrophage inhibitory factor, haptoglobin, serum amyloid A, and plasminogen activator inhibitor-1 (PAI-1). In some instances, as with CRP and IL-6, a fall in the circulating level occurs on weight reduction. Given the observation that adipose tissue expresses and secretes a number of inflammation-related proteins, it is probable that it is a major source of inflammatory markers in obesity. Adipose-tissue-derived CRP appears to be augmented in obesity and also in omental compared with subcutaneous fat.[7] Fat-derived CRP by its secretion may directly contribute to circulating CRP levels and indirectly upregulate adipokine production, most notably IL-6, the key regulator of hepatic CRP production.[7]

Some inflammatory adipokines are secreted in greater abundance by visceral adipocytes than those from subcutaneous depots, lending support to the epidemiological association of metabolic comorbidities with abdominal obesity. As fat mass expands, inflammation in white adipose tissue is also augmented by the infiltration of macrophages.[37]

Visfatin, omentin, vaspin, and plasminogen activator inhibitor-1

Visfatin is an adipokine more highly expressed in visceral fat than in subcutaneous fat, and is identical to pre-B-cell colony-enhancing factor.[38] Visfatin displays insulin-mimetic effects in vitro and in vivo. Furthermore, adenovirus-mediated high expression of visfatin reduces the plasma levels of glucose and insulin in mice, whereas heterozygous, knockout mice have higher plasma glucose levels and impaired glucose tolerance. Visfatin induces tyrosine phosphorylation of insulin signalling-related molecules, and its effect is additive to that of insulin.[38] It appears that visfatin binds to the insulin receptor and activates insulin signalling separately from insulin. Visfatin may act as an immune modulator with potent proinflammatory properties.[38]

Omentin (also known as intelectin-1) is a protein expressed and secreted by visceral, but not subcutaneous, adipose tissue. It increases insulin sensitivity in humans.[39] Circulating omentin levels inversely correlate with BMI, waist circumference, and insulin resistance. Accordingly, decreased omentin concentrations are present in obesity and insulin resistance.[39] Omentin has also been implicated in inflammation.[39]

Another visceral adipose tissue-derived adipokine is a serine protease inhibitor termed 'vaspin', a 45- to 50-kDa protein belonging to the serpin superfamily.[40] Vaspin is expressed in greater quantity in adipose tissue derived from obese people, and might play a role as a regulator of local inflammation and promoter of insulin sensitivity.[40]

Plasminogen activator inhibitor-1, another member of the serpin superfamily, is also produced in adipose tissue. By inhibiting fibrinolysis and plasminogen activation, PAI-1 may contribute to the procoagulant inflammatory state in obesity, and may also play a role in insulin resistance, angiogenesis, and atherogenesis. Its expression and secretion are increased in visceral fat, and circulating plasma PAI-1 levels are increased in abdominal obesity and metabolic syndrome.[6] PAI-1-deficient, transgenic mice display increased energy expenditure and enhanced insulin sensitivity, and are resistant to diet-induced obesity.[41]

Chemokines

Adipose tissue also releases the chemokine monocyte chemoattractant protein-1 (MCP-1), which has been implicated in the infiltration of macrophages into fat depots in obesity. Its circulating levels are increased in obesity.[37] Adipose-specific overexpression of MCP-1 in transgenic mice leads to macrophage accumulation, whereas loss of function leads to improvement in the metabolic milieu.[42]

Chemerin is a recently reported chemoattractant protein, which is highly expressed in mouse and human adipocytes; circulating concentrations are increased in human obesity. It may be involved in both adaptive and innate immunity, obesity-associated inflammation, and possibly adipogenesis as well.[43]

Future research will undoubtedly identify an increasing number of novel cytokines and chemokines that may contribute to the inflammatory and insulin-resistant states in obesity, and thus be potential new targets for pharmacological intervention.

Adipogenesis and regulation of body fat body distribution

The development of obesity involves extensive adipose tissue remodelling at the cellular level, a process that is dependent on a complex interplay among the various cells present within each fat depot. In response to states of energy surfeits, adipose tissue has to expand to sequester cytotoxic fatty acids as less toxic triglycerides, the storage form of fat. Expansion of the adipose tissue mass can be accomplished by an increase in the cell size, cell number, or both. Mild obesity (WHO classes 1 and 2) is typically associated with increased adipocyte size (hypertrophic obesity), whereas more severe forms of obesity (class 3 obesity) are accompanied by an increase in both fat cell size and number (hyperplastic obesity). Childhood obesity often involves adipocyte hyperplasia and appears to be more refractory to treatment. Weight loss is associated with a decrease in fat cell size through mobilization of triacylglycerols or lipolysis, and liberating free fatty acids and glycerol. It is unclear whether a reduction in the cell number is also observed with weight loss, or whether or not mature fat cells revert to the immature phenotypes (de-differentiation).

An increase in the number of adipocytes is accomplished by formation of new fat cells, or adipogenesis, from their precursors. Adipogenesis occurs throughout the lifetime of an organism, in response both to normal cell turnover, which occurs about every 3 months, and to the stimulus and demand for additional stores to accommodate the surfeit in energy balance.[44] Pleuripotent progenitor cells, collectively known as preadipocytes, are present in all adipose tissue depots and can proliferate and differentiate into the characteristic signet-ring phenotype of mature adipocytes that is easily visible under light microscopy. Depending on the fat depot, preadipocytes may account for 15–50% of cells in adipose tissue.[45]

The differentiation of preadipocytes to mature adipocytes is an orderly but complex and meticulously regulated sequence that is subject to nutritional and hormonal influences.[46] Much of what is known about specific cellular mechanisms associated with preadipocyte proliferation and differentiation comes from studies using established fatty fibroblast or preadipocyte cell lines, or from freshly isolated primary preadipocytes in vitro.[4,46,47] Adipogenesis, or differentiation of preadipocytes, is regulated by an elaborate network of cell-cycle regulators and transcription factors, in concert with specific transcriptional coactivators and corepressors, which coordinate expression of hundreds of proteins as they acquire the mature adipocyte phenotype (Figure 4.2).[47] Adipogenesis in cultured preadipocytes can be induced by the addition of a hormonal cocktail of insulin, glucocorticoids, and appropriate substrates. Before preadipocytes undergo commitment to terminal differentiation, they are usually preceded by two or more cycles of proliferation to expand clonally the cell population.[47] The key regulators of adipogenesis are two principal transcription factors. The first, peroxisome proliferator-activated receptor-δ (PPAR-δ), is a member of the nuclear hormone receptor superfamily that heterodimerizes with retinoid X receptor, another nuclear hormone receptor. The second transcription factor belongs to the basic-leucine zipper family of CCAAT-enhancer-binding proteins (C/EBPs), for which there are six isoforms. C/EBPβ and C/EBPδ are expressed early and may function as early transcription activators, augmenting C/EBPα and PPAR-δ expression in the sequence of events leading to adipocyte differentiation (Figure 4.2). Targeted genetic disruption of C/EBPα and PPAR-δ expression can result in dramatic reduction in the lipid content and mass of adipose tissue. A Proll4Gln mutation in PPAR-δ accelerates adipocyte differentiation and has been reported in a small number of patients with obesity and insulin resistance, whereas Pro12Ala polymorphism decreases receptor activity and is linked to a lower BMI. The cooperative and possibly synergistic interactions between C/EBPα and PPAR-δ

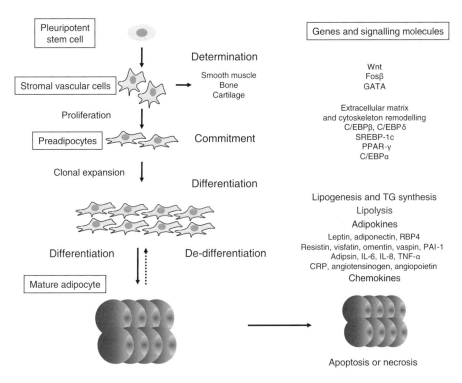

FIGURE 4.2 Model of adipogenesis and apoptosis. Adipogenesis is regulated by an elaborate network of cell-cycle regulators and transcription factors. Pleuripotent stem cells present in all fat depots can differentiate to mesenchymal cells, such as smooth muscle, bone, and cartilage. The first step of determination transforms the stem cells to adipocyte precursor cells or 'adipoblasts', which proliferate exponentially and are found in the stromal vascular cells of adipose tissue. Following commitment, these cells become preadipocytes, expressing early markers of differentiation. After undergoing clonal expansion, preadipocytes change from proliferation to differentiation to become mature adipocytes. CCAAT-enhancer binding proteins (C/EBP-α, -β, and -δ), peroxisome proliferator-activated receptor (PPAR-δ), and SREBP-1c (sterol regulatory element binding protein-1c) are three transcription factors essential for adipogenesis to occur and be maintained. This phase is accompanied by upregulation of many gene products as well as downregulation of antiadipogenic transcription factors and proteins such as GATA, Wnt, and Fosβ. During adipogenesis, preadipocytes gradually accumulate increasing amounts of cellular lipids, and start to round up and lose their fibroblastoid appearance. These morphological changes are accompanied by remodelling of the extracellular matrix and cytoskeleton to enable the differentiating cells to expand more freely in size and shape. Differentiating cells eventually become unilocular and acquire the characteristic phenotype of mature adipocytes. Developing and mature fat cells produce a large number of enzymes involved in lipogenesis, triglyceride synthesis, and lipolysis, as well as mitogenic, differentiation-promoting, angiogenic, and proinflammatory mediators. Mature fat cells turn over slowly via apoptosis, necrosis, and, to a limited extent, de-differentiation.

CRP, C-reative protein; IL, interleukin; PAI-1, plasminogen activator inhibitor-1; RBP4, retinoid-binding protein-4; TG, triglyceride; TNF, tumour necrosis factor.

have been described by in vitro and in vivo studies, suggesting a relevant physiological role for these transcription factors during adipocyte differentiation. A third transcription factor, adipocyte determination and differentiation factor-1 (ADD1), also known as steroid-binding protein-1c (SREBP-1c), is a member of the basic helix–loop–helix family of transcription factors. ADD1/SREBP-1c appears to promote adipogenesis by augmenting the transcriptional activity of PPAR-δ, as well as inducing differentiation-dependent lipogenic enzymes, such as fatty acid synthase and lipoprotein lipase.[47]

PPAR-δ and C/EBP initiate gene expression by binding to response elements in target genes where they recruit appropriate coactivators after dissociation from corepressors. One PPAR-δ coactivator, PGC-1, also stimulates brown fat adipogenesis and may play a potential role in the transformation of white into brown fat.[48] In contrast, signalling pathways have recently been described that inhibit adipogenesis. The Wnt pathway, for example, favours the differentiation of progenitors into other mesenchymal cells, such as bone and muscle cells, as opposed to adipocytes.[49] Transgenic mice overexpressing *Wnt10b* in adipocytes have less adipose tissue when maintained on a normal chow diet and are resistant to diet-induced obesity.[49] Other recently reported inhibitors of adipogenesis are GATA-2 and GATA-3, two members of the GATA family of transcription factors, which are zinc-finger DNA-binding proteins involved in developmental processes. GATA-2 and GATA-3 interfere with PPAR-δ and C/EBP activity and thereby suppress differentiation.[50] Both are expressed in preadipocytes and are normally downregulated during adipogenesis.

Regional control of body fat body distribution

The propensity of preadipocytes to proliferate and differentiate, and undergo apoptosis, is influenced by extrinsic factors such as circulating hormones and nutrients. Insulin, glucocorticoids, growth hormone, thyroid hormones, insulin-like growth factor-1, and oestrogens are known activators of preadipocyte differentiation.[46] Preadipocyte replication and/or differentiation is also influenced by an extensive cross-talk among the cells within each fat depot via paracrine signalling pathways, extracellular components, and direct cell–cell interactions (Figure 4.3). Mature adipocytes account for 90% of the volume but less than 85% of the total cell number in adipose tissue. Preadipocytes and endothelial cells lining the capillaries are present in all fat depots and may contribute as much as 10–30% of the total cell number. The remainder of the cells in adipose tissue are made up of fibroblasts and inflammatory–immune cells such as macrophages, granulocytes, lymphocytes, mast cells, and nerve cells. During embryogenesis, adipocytes arise from mesenchymal stems cells clustered around vascular structures, suggesting that adipogenesis and angiogenesis are temporally and spatially coupled events. Early evidence for paracrine regulation of angiogenesis came from cell culture studies, in which we observed that capillary endothelial cells from different fat depots differ in their proliferative capacity, suggesting that fat cells play a role in modulating angiogenesis.[51] Furthermore, not only do fat-

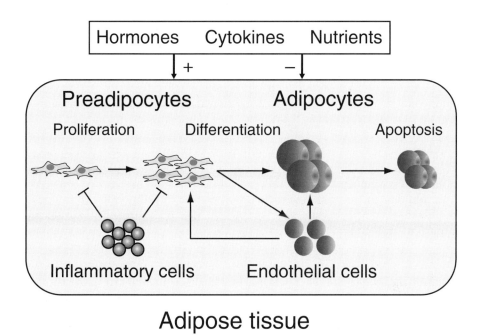

FIGURE 4.3 Regional control of body fat mass. Adipose tissue growth is achieved by an increase in the size and number of mature adipocytes and is influenced by circulating levels of hormones, cytokines, and nutrients. Growth within each adipose tissue depot is also modulated by extensive cross-talk, via paracrine and autocrine mediators, among mature adipocytes, preadipocytes, and capillary endothelial and inflammatory cells

derived capillary endothelial cells stimulate preadipocyte proliferation in culture,[4,51] but their secreted extracellular matrix components also induce preadipocyte differentiation.[52] However, the fact that medium conditioning by mature fat or preadipocytes has little influence on preadipocyte replication suggests a synergistic paracrine interaction between capillary endothelial cells and preadipocytes via angiogenic factors elaborated locally within the fat depot.[53] Inhibition of angiogenesis in vivo by vascular endothelial growth factor receptor-2-blocking antibody not only reduced neovascularization and fat tissue growth but also inhibited adipogenesis.[54] Recent studies provide further support that angiogenic factors such as leptin, adipsin, and fibroblast growth factor-2 also modulate fat tissue growth via paracrine signalling pathways.[55] Preadipocytes from different fat depots differ in replicative potential in culture and retain these differences in successive passages, thus suggesting inherent differences among fat depots in both rodents and humans that may include epigenetic mechanisms.[4] Rat cells from the retroperitoneal depot proliferate more excessively than cells from the epididymal depots.[51,56] The latter phenomenon is reflected by a greater increase in retroperitoneal than epididymal fat cell numbers during depot growth in vivo.[57] Preadipocytes from human abdominal subcutaneous depots are capable of more extensive replication than from the mesenteric or omental depots.[58] Interestingly, preadipocytes from massively obese people have a greater propensity to proliferate than cells from lean individuals, and these cells also release mitogens that stimulate proliferation of preadipocytes via paracrine mechanisms.[56,59] In addition, media conditioned by mature fat cells also induce preadipocyte differentiation, lending further support to the hypothesis that fat cell growth is modulated by paracrine factors elaborated locally.[60] These adipocyte differentiation induction factors, including a 53-kDa protein, show that fat begets more fat in a given depot and may at least partly explain the regional variation in fat tissue development and growth.[61]

In addition to the region-specific differences in preadipocyte cell dynamics (proliferation, adipogenesis, and apoptosis), the pool size of preadipocytes appears to differ among various fat depots in rodents and humans. Hence, adipose tissue mass can expand not only by altering the proliferative and adipogenic properties of preadipocytes, but also by the turnover of the preadipocyte pool. Evidence for this is adduced from studies in lean, and diet-induced and genetically obese rodents.[62,63] Diets high in fats, especially saturated fats, greatly induce adipocyte proliferation and differentiation, with a disproportionate increase in intra-abdominal fat depots.[62,63]

A recent discovery has provided new insight into the plasticity of adipose tissue growth. For the past three decades, it has been known that preadipocytes are found throughout the life of an organism, and that these cells arise from unipotent adipoblasts derived from pleuripotent mesenchymal stem cells. Current data indicate that bone marrow-derived progenitor cells originating outside adipose tissue can contribute to an increase in adipocyte number.[64] Thiazolidinedione treatment of mice fed a high-fat diet promoted the trafficking of circulating bone marrow-derived stem cells into adipose tissue, where they differentiate into multilocular fat cells expressing many genes that are known markers of the mature adipocyte phenotype.[64]

It is evident that the inhibition of adipogenesis and formation of new fat cells are a potential target for controlling regional as well as total body fat mass, thus opening a new avenue for treating obesity. Parallel effort has been undertaken in search of novel genes responsible for the regional differences in adipogenesis. One notable finding is the fat mass- and obesity-associated gene *FTO*, which was discovered as part of a genome-wide search for a type 2 diabetes susceptibility gene. A common variant of the *FTO* gene is associated with high BMI and predisposes to the development of childhood and adult obesity.[65] The *FTO* gene is of unknown function and is expressed in fetal and adult tissues. Future research will yield new understanding of the mechanisms and pathways whereby the *FTO* variant gene increases the risk of obesity.[65]

Conclusion

Obesity is a common phenotypical expression of excess body fat arising from multifactorial aetiologies. The exciting and rapid advances in the molecular biology of obesity over the past decades have revealed the complex and dynamic interplay of the forces of nature and nurture in energy homeostasis, control of appetite, and deposition of both regional and total body fat. Human obesity is rarely caused by single-gene defects, but is the result of complex interactions among adipose tissue, the gut, and the brain. Leptin and insulin clearly are the major humoral signals to the brain for long-term energy homeostasis. Appetite is controlled by a complex interplay of humoral and neural signals between the periphery tissues (fat and the gut) and the brain. Adipose tissue development and growth are influenced by regional differences in adipose tissue composition, preadipocyte proliferation, adipogenesis, angiogenesis, and release of adipokines and paracrine factors. Bone marrow-derived stem cells can populate in adipose tissue and alter the size of preadipocyte pool and adipogenesis. Finally, the search for genes responsible for the various pathways controlling energy homeostasis, and regional and total body fat mass, will pave the way for novel and effective strategies to treat and prevent obesity. While awaiting exciting research breakthroughs, lifestyle intervention aiming at a modest 5–10% body-weight loss remains the mainstay treatment for obesity and related complications.

References

1. Lau DCW. Synopsis of the 2006 Canadian clinical practice guidelines on the management and prevention of obesity in adults and children. *Can Med Assoc J* 2007;**176**:1103–6.
2. Ogden CL, Carroll MD, Curtin LR, et al. Prevalence of overweight and obesity in the United States, 1999–2004. *JAMA* 2006;**205**:1549–55.
3. Lau DCW, Douketis JD, Morrison K, et al. Obesity Canada Clinical Practice Guidelines Expert Panel. 2006 Canadian clinical practice guidelines on the management and prevention of obesity in adults and children [summary]. *Can Med Assoc J* 2007;**176**(Suppl 8):S1–14.
4. Lau DC, Schillabeer G, Li ZH, et al. Paracrine interactions in adipose tissue development and growth. *Int J Obes Relat Metab Disord* 1996;**20**(Suppl 3): S16–25.
5. Lau DCW. Adipose tissue growth and differentiation: view from the chair. *Int J Obes Relat Metab Disord* 2000;**24**(Suppl 4):S20–2.
6. Lau DCW, Dhillon B, Yan H, et al. Adipokines: molecular links between obesity and atherosclerosis. *Am J Physiol Heart Circ Physiol* 2005;**288**: H2031–41.
7. Lau DCW, Yan H, Dhillon B. Metabolic syndrome: a marker of patients at high cardiovascular risk. *Can J Cardiol* 2006;**22**(Suppl B):85B–90B.
8. Kershaw EE, Flier JS. Adipose tissue as an endocrine organ. *J Clin Endocrinol Metab* 2004;**89**:2548–56.

9. Gomez-Ambrosi J, Catalan V, Diez-Caballero A, et al. Gene expression profile of omental adipose tissue in human obesity. *FASEB J* 2004;**18**:215–17.

10. Friedman JM, Halaas JL. Leptin and the regulation of body weight in mammals. *Nature* 1998;**395**:763–70.

11. Ahima RS, Flier JS. Leptin. *Annu Rev Physiol* 2000;**62**:413–37.

12. Vydelingum S, Shillabeer G, Hatch G, et al. Overexpression of the obese gene in the genetically obese JCR:LA-corpulent rat. *Biochem Biophys Res Commun* 1995;**216**:148–53.

13. Kokoeva MV, Yin H, Flier JS. Neurogenesis in the hypothalamus of adult mice: potential role in energy balance. *Science* 2005;**310**:679–83.

14. Fulton S, Pissios P, Manchon RP, et al. Leptin regulation of the mesoaccumbens dopamine pathway. *Neuron* 2006;**51**:811–22.

15. Heymsfield SB, Greenberg AS, Fujioka K, et al. Recombinant leptin for weight loss in obese and lean adults. A randomized, controlled, dose-escalation trial. *JAMA* 1999;**282**:1568–75.

16. Farooqi IS, Wangensteen T, Collins S, et al. Clinical and molecular genetic spectrum of congenital deficiency of the leptin receptor. *N Engl J Med* 2007;**356**:237–47.

17. Montague CT, Farooqi IS, Whitehead JP, O'Rahilly S. Congenital leptin deficiency is associated with severe early-onset obesity in humans. *Nature* 1997;**387**:903–8.

18. Farooqi IS, O'Rahilly S. Monogenic obesity in humans. *Annu Rev Med* 2005;**56**:443–58.

19. Rankinen T, Zuberi A, Chagnon YC, et al. The human obesity gene map: the 2005 update. *Obesity* 2006;**14**:529–644.

20. Krude H, Biebermann H, Luck W, et al. Severe early-onset obesity, adrenal insufficiency and red hair pigmentation caused by POMC mutations in humans. *Nat Genet* 1998;**19**:155–7.

21. Jackson RS, Creemers JWM, Ohagi S, et al. Obesity and impaired prohormone processing associated with mutations in the human prohormone convertase 1 gene. *Nat Genet* 1997;**16**:303–6.

22. Farooqi IS, Keogh JM, Yeo GSH, et al. Clinical spectrum of obesity and mutations in the melanocortin 4 receptor gene. *N Engl J Med* 2003;**348**:1085–95.

23. Holder JL Jr, Butte NF, Zinn AR. Profound obesity associated with a balanced translocation that disrupts the SIM1 gene. *Hum Mol Genet* 2000;**9**:101–8.

24. Murphy KG, Bloom SR. Gut hormones and the regulation of energy homeostasis. *Nature* 2006;**444**:854–9.

25. Korner J, Leibel RL. To eat or not to eat – how the gut talks to the brain. *N Engl J Med* 2003;**349**:926–8.

26. Muhlhausler BS, Adam CL, Findlay PA, et al. Increased maternal nutrition alters development of the appetite-regulating network in the brain. *FASEB J* 2006;**20**:1257–9.

27. Yamauchi T, Kamon J, Waki H, et al. The fat-derived hormone adiponectin reverses insulin resistance associated with both lipoatrophy and obesity. *Nat Med* 2001;**7**:941–6.

28. Szmitko PE, Teoh H, Stewart DJ, Verma S. Adiponectin and cardiovascular disease: state of the art? *Am J Physiol Heart Circ Physiol* 2007;**292**:H1655–63.
29. Haugen F, Drevon CA. The interplay between nutrients and the adipose tissue. *Proc Nutr Soc* 2007;**66**:171–82.
30. Higuchi K, Masaki T, Gotoh K, et al. Apelin, an APJ receptor ligand, regulates body adiposity and favors the messenger ribonucleic acid expression of uncoupling proteins in mice. *Endocrinology* 2007;**148**:2690–7.
31. Hotamisligil GS, Peraldi P, Budavari A, et al. IRS-1-mediated inhibition of insulin receptor tyrosine kinase activity in TNF-alpha- and obesity-induced insulin resistance. *Science* 1996;**271**:665–8.
32. Yang Q, Graham TE, Mody N, et al. Serum retinol binding protein 4 contributes to insulin resistance in obesity and type 2 diabetes. *Nature* 2005;**436**:356–62.
33. Wolf G. Serum retinol-binding protein: a link between obesity, insulin resistance, and type 2 diabetes. *Nutr Rev* 2007;**65**:251–6.
34. Graham TE, Yang Q, Bluher M, et al. Retinol-binding protein 4 and insulin resistance in lean, obese, and diabetic subjects. *N Engl J Med* 2006;**354**:2552–63.
35. Klöting N, Graham TE, Berndt J, et al. Serum retinol-binding protein is more highly expressed in visceral than in subcutaneous adipose tissue and is a marker of intra-abdominal fat mass. *Cell Metab* 2007;**6**:79–87.
36. Steppan CM, Bailey ST, Bhat S, et al. The hormone resistin links obesity to diabetes. *Nature* 2001;**409**:307–12.
37. Weisberg SP, McCann D, Desai M, et al. Obesity is associated with macrophage accumulation in adipose tissue. *J Clin Invest* 2003;**112**:1796–1808.
38. Fukuhara AM, Nishizawa M, Segawa K, et al. Visfatin: a protein secreted by visceral fat that mimics the effects of insulin. *Science* 2005;**307**:426–43.
39. de Souza Batista CM, Yang RZ, Lee MJ, et al. Omentin plasma levels and gene expression are decreased in obesity. *Diabetes* 2007;**56**:1655–61.
40. Hida K, Wada J, Eguchi J, et al. Visceral adipose tissue-derived serine protease inhibitor: a unique insulin-sensitizing adipocytokine in obesity. *Proc Natl Acad Sci USA* 2005;**102**:10610–15.
41. Ma LJ, Mao SL, Taylor KL, et al. Prevention of obesity and insulin resistance in mice lacking plasminogen activator inhibitor 1. *Diabetes* 2004;**53**:336–46.
42. Kanda H, Tateya S, Tamori Y, et al. MCP-1 contributes to macrophage infiltration into adipose tissue, insulin resistance, and hepatic steatosis in obesity. *J Clin Invest* 2006;**116**:1494–1505.
43. Bozaoglu K, Bolton K, McMillan J, et al. Chemerin is a novel adipokine associated with obesity and metabolic syndrome. *Endocrinology* 2007;**148**:4687–94.
44. Strawford A, Antelo F, Christiansen M, Hellerstein MK. Adipose tissue triglyceride turnover, de novo lipogenesis, and cell proliferation in humans measured with ^2H_2O. *Am J Physiol* 2004;**286**:E577–88.
45. Kirkland JL, Hollenberg CH, Kindler S, Gillon WS. Effects of age and anatomic site on preadipocyte number in rat fat depots. *J Gerontol* 1994;**49**:B31–5.

46. Lau DC. Nature and nurture in adipocyte development and growth. *Int J Obes* 1990;**14**(Suppl 3):153–7.
47. Farmer SR. Transcriptional control of adipocyte formation. *Cell Metab* 2006;**4**:263–73.
48. Rosen ED, Spiegelman BM. Adipocytes as regulators of energy balance and glucose homeostasis. *Nature* 2006;**444**:847–53.
49. Ross SE, Hemati N, Longo KA, et al. Inhibition of adipogenesis by Wnt signaling. *Science* 2000;**289**:950–3.
50. Tong Q, Dalgin G, Xu H, et al. Function of GATA transcription factors in preadipocyte–adipocyte transition. *Science* 2000;**290**:134–8.
51. Lau DC, Wong KL, Tough SC. Regional differences in the replication rate of cultured rat microvascular endothelium from retroperitoneal and epididymal fat pads. *Metabolism* 1987;**36**:631–6.
52. Varzaneh FE, Shillabeer G, Wong KL, Lau DC. Extracellular matrix components secreted by microvascular endothelial cells stimulate preadipocyte differentiation in vitro. *Metabolism* 1994;**43**:906–12.
53. Lau DC, Shillabeer G, Wong KL, et al. Influence of paracrine factors on preadipocyte replication and differentiation. *Int J Obes* 1990;**14**(Suppl 3): 193–201.
54. Fukumura D, Ushiyama A, Duda DG, et al. Paracrine regulation of angiogenesis and adipocyte differentiation during in vivo adipogenesis. *Circ Res* 2003;**93**:e88–97.
55. Cao Y. Angiogenesis modulates adipogenesis and obesity. *J Clin Invest* 2007;**117**:2362–8.
56. Lau DC, Roncari DA, Hollenberg CH. Release of mitogenic factors by cultured preadipocytes from massively obese human subjects. *J Clin Invest* 1987;**79**:632–6.
57. Wang H, Kirkland JL, Hollenberg CH. Varying capacities for replication of rat adipocyte precursor clones and adipose tissue growth. *J Clin Invest* 1989;**83**:1741–6.
58. Tchkonia T, Tchoukalova YD, Giorgadze N, et al. Abundance of two human preadipocyte subtypes with distinct capacities for replication, adipogenesis, and apoptosis varies among fat depots. *Am J Physiol* 2005;**288**:E267–77.
59. Roncari DAK, Lau DCW, Kindler S. Exaggerated replication in culture of adipocyte precursors from massively obese persons. *Metabolism* 1981;**30**:425–7.
60. Shillabeer G, Forden JM, Lau DC. Induction of preadipocyte differentiation by mature fat cells in the rat. *J Clin Invest* 1989;**84**:381–7.
61. Li ZH, Carraro R, Gregerman RI, Lau DC. Adipocyte differentiation factor (ADF): a protein secreted by mature fat cells that induces preadipocyte differentiation in culture. *Cell Biol Int* 1998;**22**:253–70.
62. Shillabeer G, Forden JM, Russell JC, Lau DC. Paradoxically slow preadipocyte replication and differentiation in corpulent rats. *Am J Physiol* 1990;**258**(2 Pt 1):E368–76.
63. Shillabeer G, Lau DC. Regulation of new fat cell formation in rats: the role of dietary fats. *J Lipid Res* 1994;**35**:592–600.

64. Crossno JT Jr, Majka SM, Grazia T, et al. Rosiglitazone promotes development of a novel adipocyte population from bone marrow-derived circulating progenitor cells. *J Clin Invest* 2006;**116**:3220–8.
65. Frayling TM, Timpson NJ, Weedon MN, et al. A common variant in the FTO gene is associated with body mass index and predisposes to childhood and adult obesity. *Science* 2007;**316**:889–94.

Section 2

Obesity and Reproduction

5 Obesity and conception

Erica E Marsh and Randall B Barnes

Introduction

Obesity is defined as a body mass index (BMI) of over 30 kg/m². According to the World Health Organization (WHO) estimates, almost 30 million people worldwide were categorized as obese in 2003.[1] In the USA, 32% of the overall population are obese and another 34.1% are overweight.[2] When race and gender are overlaid on these findings, striking disparities are seen, with 30% of non-Hispanic white women, 42.3% of Mexican–American women, and 53.9% of non-Hispanic black women categorized as obese in the USA.[2] In Europe, 150 000 000 adults and 15 000 000 children carry the diagnosis of obesity.[3] Given the well-known impact of obesity on poor health outcomes, these findings make obesity one of the focus areas of the US Department of Health and Human Services[1] Healthy People 2010 agenda.[4] In addition to its negative impact on cardiac, pulmonary, endocrine, and vascular disease, obesity has a similar impact on fertility, fecundity, and fecundability.[5,6]

Fertility is broadly defined as the ability to conceive, whereas infertility is more specifically defined as the inability to conceive after having regular, unprotected intercourse for 12 months. The infertility rate in the USA is 10%, and more than 15% of reproductive-aged women in the USA have at one time received infertility services.[7] It is of great importance that infertility rates in obese women are higher than those of normal-weight women,[8,9] and those who are not intrinsically infertile take longer to achieve pregnancy.[10] These findings recur in several large epidemiologic studies. The British Birth Study found that obese women at age 23 years were less likely to conceive within 12 months of unprotected intercourse.[11] The Nurses Health Study II found 25% of ovulatory infertility in the USA to be attributable to women being overweight.[8] Obesity is thought to affect fertility through various physiologic mechanisms. In this chapter, we begin by reviewing the pathophysiology of obesity as it relates to conception, including hyperandrogenism and hyperinsulinemia in the physiology of conception. We then discuss the clinical ramifications of the physiologic dysfunctions caused by obesity, including anovulation, amenorrhea, and polycystic ovarian syndrome (PCOS). Next we describe the psychosocial factors of obesity and infertility, and finally we conclude with a discussion of available treatment regimens (and their associated success rates) for obese women desiring conception.

Pathophysiology of obesity and infertility

The association of obesity, hyperinsulinemia, hyperandrogenism, and other endocrine disruptions is well established. Obesity is known to cause hyperinsulinemia and insulin resistance. Increased circulating insulin causes several physiologic changes that lead to hyperandrogenism, which, in turn, subsequently leads to follicular atresia and anovulatory cycles. Specifically, insulin decreases sex hormone-binding globulin (SHBG) and insulin-like growth factor-binding protein 1 (IGFBP-1) levels, leading to increased circulating androgens, estrogens, and growth factors. Insulin also directly stimulates theca cells, leading to increased production of androstenedione and testosterone. Hyperandrogenism leads to follicular atresia, and the circulating estrogens (from the decreased SHBG levels and aromatized from increased androstenedione levels) lead to decreased follicle-stimulating hormone (FSH) levels and increased lutenizing hormone (LH) levels. Finally, the increased LH levels stimulate the theca cells, which in turn increase androgen production, leading to more follicular atresia and subsequent infertility.

Clinical sequelae – anovulation and PCOS

PCOS is the most common endocrinopathy in reproductive-aged women. The polycystic ovary as a marker of disease was first described in 1935 by Stein and Leventhal and was associated with obesity, amenorrhea, hirsutism, and infertility.[12] Because of the wide ranges of presentation, both the European Society for Human Reproduction and Embryology (ESHRE) and the American Society for Reproductive Medicine (ASRM) had a consensus meeting in 2003, whereby the following criteria for diagnosis were proposed[13]:

1. Anovulation or oligomenorrhea
2. Clinical or biochemical hyperandrogenism
3. Polycystic ovaries on ultrasound examination.

When any two of these three criteria are present, and other causes of anovulation and hyperandrogenism have been ruled out, the diagnosis of PCOS can be made.

Although PCOS has an overall prevalence of 4–8%, its prevalence in obese women is much higher, with one study in a population of Spanish women reporting a prevalence of 28%.[14–16] Interestingly, an American study looking at prevalence of PCOS by BMI over time found that the risk of PCOS was only minimally increased in obese women and that, although the percentage of women with obesity and PCOS has increased, the increase is similar to the increase in obesity in the general population.[17] As one might expect, the percentage of PCOS patients who are obese is much higher than the percentage of obese patients with PCOS. In the US population, 60% of women with PCOS are obese.[14]

Clearly, although the 'what comes first?' question about obesity and PCOS may not yet have an answer, what is presently apparent is that obesity results in worse PCOS sequelae. For example, menstrual abnormalities are more common in obese women with PCOS than in normal-weight women with PCOS. Moreover, obese women with PCOS are also more likely than lean women with PCOS to develop the metabolic sequelae associated with the disease such as hypertension, type 2 diabetes mellitus (DM), and lipid abnormalities, i.e., the metabolic syndrome. In addition, obese women with PCOS have been consistently shown to have lower SHBG levels and higher circulating androgen levels than their normal-weight counterparts. Taken together, these findings certainly suggest that, although obesity may not cause PCOS, it certainly pushes women to a more severe presentation of the syndrome.

Psychosocial factors of obesity and infertility

A host of psychosocial and sociobiological factors affect women's ability to achieve pregnancy. These include sex drive, sexual function, and frequency of intercourse. Many of these factors are affected negatively in overweight women.

Sexual dysfunction

Obese people have higher rates of sexual dysfunction. In one study from Greece, 60 obese women and 50 nonobese women were administered the Female Sexual Function Index (FSFI) and completed the Hospital Anxiety and Depression Scale (HADS). The obese women had significantly worse scores on most of the domains of sexual function – arousal, orgasm, sexual desire, lubrication, and satisfaction – than normal-weight controls.[18]

Frequency of intercourse

Several studies have found that obese women have less sexual intercourse than normal weight women. As fecundity is driven by both normal reproductive physiology and frequency of intercourse, decreased sexual activity can negatively affect conception rates. Another study examining the frequency of sexual intercourse and masturbation as they relate to slimness in young adults found that slimmer hip size was associated with a greater frequency of sexual intercourse.[19]

Treatments

Weight loss

Weight loss remains the first-line treatment for infertility in overweight patients, especially, but not exclusively, in women who have anovulatory amenorrhea. In 1989, a study of 20 obese, hyperandrogenic, amenorheic women who ate a hypocaloric diet for an average of 8 months found that they had significant decreases in their plasma testosterone and LH levels, and 33% became ovulatory. Hirsutism and acanthosis nigracans also improved significantly in the women, and four pregnancies occurred.[20] A 1992 study by Kiddy et al found that even a modest weight loss of ≥5% was associated with improvements in fertility and decreases in hirsutism.[21] In a small 1995 study by Clark et al, 13 obese women with anovulatory infertility participated in a 6-month weight-loss-treatment program.[22] After the program, 12 of the 13 women resumed ovulation and 11 achieved pregnancy. Five of the pregnancies were spontaneous. In a larger follow-up study by the same group, 67 infertile obese women participated in a similar 6-month weight-loss-treatment program.[23] This study population had infertility from multiple causes, unlike the first study, in which all the women had anovulatory infertility. Sixty of the 67 women resumed spontaneous ovulation, 52 achieved pregnancy, and 18 had spontaneous pregnancies. In their review of reproductive performance, obesity, and weight management, Norman et al nicely summarize the effects of obesity and overweight on reproductive functions.[24] These authors recommend weight management as the first-line therapy offered to all overweight and obese women, and that the weight-loss strategy include dietary intervention, increased physical activity, lifestyle modifications, and regular support from a dietitian. Nelson and Fleming recommend not only caloric and activity interventions, but also pharmacologic and surgical interventions if indicated.[25] In summary, weight loss should be the first-line treatment in obese patients, as there is a clear benefit with even a modest reduction in weight.

These and other study findings have led to inclusion of BMI and/or weight modification as guidelines in countries where infertility treatment costs are covered by national health insurance. For example, the National Institute for Health and Clinical Excellence in the UK commissioned the National Collaborating Centre for Women's and Children's Health to develop guidelines for fertility assessment and treatment.[26] These include initial recommendations that women with a BMI over 29 who are not ovulating be counseled that weight loss is likely to increase their chance of conception. Women with a BMI over 29 are also advised that they will take longer to conceive. The British Fertility Society recommends that fertility treatments be deferred until a BMI of under 35 kg/m^2 is achieved.[27] In those with more time, if FSH levels are within normal limits and the patient is under 37 years old, the society recommends targeting a BMI under 30 kg/m^2. More formal guidelines are in place in New Zealand. Here, patients are ranked for publicly funded elective procedures by the clinical priority access criteria (CPAC), which include age, duration of infertility, smoking status, basal FSH levels, and the sterilization status of the couple.[28] Under this system, only women with BMIs of 18–32 kg/m^2 are eligible to receive a prioritization score outright. Women outside this range are required to undergo weight normalization programs and to have achieved weight modification.[29]

Clomiphene citrate

Clomiphene citrate is a selective estrogen receptor modulator (SERM) that is used to treat anovulation and infertility by increasing FSH levels by blocking estradiol negative feedback at the level of the hypothalamus and pituitary gland. It has been used since the early 1960s.[30,31] Clomiphene citrate is successful in inducing ovulation in obese women; however, its effects are attenuated by increasing BMI and increased doses are required.[31,32] A prospective cohort study published in 1998 by Imani et al found that increasing BMI, among other factors, significantly decreased response to clomiphene citrate.[33] However, in comparison to metformin, clomiphene citrate is superior in achieving live birth rates in women with PCOS. In a randomized controlled trial, 626 women with PCOS and average BMIs of 34–36 were randomized to receive clomiphene citrate alone, metformin alone, or both.[34] The live birth rate was 22.5% in the clomiphene citrate group, 7.2% in the metformin group, and 26.8% in the combination-therapy group. Among pregnancies, the rate of multiple pregnancy was 6.0% in the clomiphene citrate group, 0% in the metformin group, and 3.1% in the combination-therapy group. The rates of first-trimester pregnancy loss did not differ significantly among the groups. However, the conception rate among women who ovulated was significantly lower in the metformin group (21.7%) than in either the clomiphene citrate group (39.5%) or the combination-therapy group (46.0%). Thus, clomiphene citrate is superior to metformin in achieving live birth in infertile women with PCOS, although multiple births are a complication.

Metformin

As the pathophysiology of PCOS began to be elucidated in the 1990s, and the central role of hyperinsulinemia made clear, investigators began to look at insulin-sensitizing medications as a possible treatment for PCOS. Metformin is an oral biguanide that lowers insulin levels by both increasing peripheral sensitivity to insulin and decreasing liver production of glucose. The first study of metformin in obese PCOS patients was performed in 1994 by Velasquez et al; it demonstrated that metformin can significantly decrease insulin, LH, and testosterone levels in this population. In addition, most of the women had some degree of menstrual cycle improvement.[35] In 1996, Nestler et al published a placebo-controlled trial that demonstrated that meformin treats hyperandrogenism at least in part by reducing ovarian cytochrome P450c17α.[36] A follow-up study looked at the effect of metformin on the ovulatory response to clomiphene citrate.[37] Sixty-one obese women with PCOS were given either clomiphene citrate and a placebo or clomiphene citrate plus metformin. Ninety percent of the women who received clomiphene citrate plus metformin ovulated versus 8% of the patients who received the placebo and clomiphene citrate, thus demonstrating that metformin can potentiate the effects of clomiphene citrate. In addition, the women who received clomiphene citrate plus metformin had a significantly lower insulin area under the effect (AUE) curve after their treatment, while the placebo group had no significant difference in their insulin AUE values.

Despite the early success of the metformin studies, several large randomized controlled trials, including the Legro study discussed above, have shown that clomiphene citrate is superior to metformin in inducing ovulation in women with PCOS.[34] A randomized trial of 225 Dutch women with PCOS who were given either clomiphene citrate plus placebo or clomiphene citrate plus metformin showed that there were no significant differences in pregnancy or ovulation rates between the two groups.[38] In 2008, the ESHRE and the ASRM published a consensus statement on guidelines for the treatment of PCOS. Their recommendations regarding metformin were that it should be restricted to patients with glucose intolerance, that it is less effective than clomiphene citrate, and that there is no advantage to adding metformin to clomiphene citrate in women with PCOS.[39]

Laparoscopic ovarian drilling

After the original case series describing the association of polycystic ovaries, hirsutism, obesity, and infertility in the 1930s, the recommended treatment was ovarian wedge resection, after which ovulation was restored in a number of instances.[40] Wedge resection has been largely replaced by the less invasive laparoscopic approach of ovarian tissue destruction with monopolar electrosurgery or laser. The mechanism of the benefit is presumed to be the destruction of androgen-producing tissue in the ovary, as androgen levels decrease in women after the procedure. The procedure appears to be of particular benefit in women with PCOS who do not respond to clomiphene citrate. In women with clomiphene citrate-resistant PCOS, outcomes after laparoscopic ovarian drilling (LOD) are similar to those after gonadotropin treatment, without the associated risks of multiple gestations and ovarian hyperstimulation syndrome (OHSS). In 2002, a randomized controlled trial with a 6 month follow-up after LOD versus three cycles of gonadotropin therapy found no significant difference in pregnancy or miscarriage rates in these women between the two groups.[41] A Cochrane Review arrived at similar conclusions.[41] In addition, LOD has been shown to be an economically superior option to gonadotropin.[43,44] The 2008 ESHRE/ASRM PCOS Treatment Guidelines conclude that LOD can achieve monofollicular ovulation without the associated risks of OHSS; additionally, the intensive monitoring required with gonadotropin treatment is not necessary. The guidelines further support LOD as an alternative to gonadotropin therapy for PCOS patients who are resistant to clomiphene citrate.[39]

Controlled ovarian hyperstimulation and intrauterine insemination

Very few studies in the literature address this treatment modality, as it specifically pertains to obesity. A retrospective study by Dodson et al reviewed the charts of 333 ovulatory women who underwent ovulation with gonadotropins followed by intrauterine insemination (IUI) and grouped the subjects by BMI.[45] This study found that there was no difference in the number of follicles matured, days of stimulation, or cycle fecundity among obese, overweight, and normal-weight subjects. There was a significant difference in the total dose of gonadotropin used between the obese and normal-weight subjects (1814 vs 1353 IU). There was also a statistical difference in estradiol levels between the groups, obese women having lower levels (742 pg/ml) than overweight (1004 pg/ml) and normal-weight (980 pg/ml) subjects. Another study by Balen et al reviewed 335 women with anovulatory infertility who failed to ovulate or conceive on clomiphene citrate and their response to gonadotropins. Similarly, this study found that increasing BMI was associated with increasing gonadotropin requirement, but not with ovulation or pregnancy rates.[46]

A retrospective cohort study examined 2040 patients undergoing 5089 initiated cycles or 4509 completed cycles (cancellation rate, 11.4%) of IUI treated between 1990 and 2000 at a tertiary infertility center at the University of Adelaide, Australia. Patients were stratified into five BMI (kg/m^2) groups: underweight (BMI < 20), normal weight (20–24.9), overweight (25–29.9), obese (30–34.9), and very obese (≥ 35). Fecundity was defined as the probability of achieving at least one pregnancy throughout the course of IUI treatment, which usually consisted of 2–4 insemination cycles.[47] Overall, 28.4% of women achieved at least one pregnancy after treatment. Across the five BMI groups, fecundity increased significantly ($P < 0.001$) from the underweight group to the obese group and remained high even in very obese women (not significant).

Assisted reproductive technologies

Although obesity is known to have negative effects on fertility, the effect of obesity on assisted reproductive technologies (ARTs) is less clear. Although some studies have shown that obesity is associated with a lower pregnancy rate, others have not.[48–50] A review of 5019 in vitro fertilization (IVF) or intracytoplasmic sperm injection (ICSI) treatments in 2660 couples found a cumulative live birth rate within three treatment cycles of 41.4% in obese women with BMI of at least 30 kg/m^2 and 50.3% in normal-weight women with BMI of 18.5–24.9 kg/m^2. Obesity was associated with an increased risk of early pregnancy loss before 6 weeks' gestation. A positive correlation between BMI and gonadotropin requirement during stimulation and a negative correlation between BMI and number of collected oocytes were observed.[49]

However, Dechaud et al found that, while obese patients require a higher recombinant FSH dose to achieve follicular maturation than normal-weight patients, obesity does not negatively affect the results of IVF.[50] In this study, 573 patients underwent 789 IVF cycles or ICSI. The patients were classified into four BMI groups: < 20 kg/m^2 (264 cycles), 20–25 kg/m^2 (394 cycles), > 25–30 kg/m^2 (83 cycles), and ≥ 30 kg/m^2 (48 cycles). All parameters of ovarian response were comparable except the total required recombinant FSH dose. This dose was statistically higher in the group with BMI of ≥ 30 than in the other groups ($P = 0.0003$). All parameters of IVF outcome were comparable, including the cancellation rate, the implantation rate, and pregnancy rates. However, Lashen et al found no difference between obese and control women in gonadotropin dosage during ovarian stimulation, and a similar number follicles was retrieved.[51] However, this study did report significantly lower estradiol levels in the obese women than in normal-weight controls.

A systematic review assessed the effects of obesity on the outcome of ARTs.[52] Interpretation of the results was compromised by variations in the methods used to define overweight and obese populations, and inconsistencies in the choice and definition of outcome measures. Compared with women with BMI under 25 kg/m², women with BMI of at least 25 kg/m² have a lower chance of pregnancy following IVF (odds ratio [OR] 0.71, 95% CI: 0.62, 0.81), require a higher dose of gonadotropin (weighed mean difference 210.08, 95% CI 149.12, 271.05), and have an increased miscarriage rate (OR 1.33, 95% CI 1.06, 1.68). The authors concluded that there is insufficient evidence of the effect of BMI on live birth, cycle cancellation, oocyte recovery, and OHSS, and that further well-designed studies are needed.

Conclusion

Obesity negatively affects many aspects of human physiology, and reproduction is no exception. Whether as part of the constellation of PCOS or as an independent condition, obesity has a wide range of negative effects on a woman's fertility. Although its impact is complex and many questions remain to be answered, what is clear is that weight loss is a first-line therapy for obesity that has benefits that go far beyond any medications or procedural interventions. Lifestyle modifications should ideally be made prior to making the decision to achieve pregnancy, thereby improving the patient's health status and decreasing the overall risk to the patient.

References

1. World Health Organization. Information sheets on obesity and overweight. Available at: www.who.int/mediacentre/factsheets/fs311/en/index.html.
2. Ogden CL, Carroll MD, Curtin LR, et al. Prevalence of overweight and obesity in the United States, 1999–2004. *JAMA* 2006;**295**:1549–55.
3. Deitel M. The European Charter on counteracting obesity. *Obes Surg* 2007;**17**:143–4.
4. US Department of Health and Human Services. *Healthy People 2010*, 2nd edn. *Understanding and Improving Health and Objectives for Improving Health*, 2 vols. Washington, DC: US Government Printing Office, 2000.
5. Gesink Law DC, Maclehose RF, Longnecker MP. Obesity and time to pregnancy. *Hum Reprod* 2007;**22**:414–20.
6. Bolúmar F, Olsen J, Rebagliato M, et al. Body mass index and delayed conception: a European Multicenter Study on Infertility and Subfecundity. *Am J Epidemiol* 2000;**151**:1072–9.
7. Abma J, Chandra A, Mosher W, et al. Fertility, family planning, and women's health: new data from the 1995 National Survey of Family Growth. National Center for Health Statistics. *Vital Health Stat 23* 1997;**19**:1–114.
8. Rich-Edwards JW, Spiegelman D, Garland M, et al. Physical activity, body mass index, and ovulatory disorder infertility. *Epidemiology* 2002;**13**:184–90.
9. Jensen TK, Scheike T, Keiding N, et al. Fecundability in relation to body mass and menstrual cycle patterns. *Epidemiology* 1999;**10**:422–8.
10. Ramlau-Hansen CH, Thulstrup AM, Nohr EA, et al. Subfecundity in overweight and obese couples. *Hum Reprod* 2007;**22**:1634–7.

11. Lake JK, Power C, Cole TJ. Women's reproductive health: the role of body mass index in early and adult life. *Int J Obes Relat Metab Disord* 1997;**21**:432–8.

12. Stein IF, Leventhal NL. Amenorrhea associated with bilateral polycystic ovaries. *Am J Obstet Gynecol* 1935;**29**:181–91.

13. Rotterdam ESHRE/ASRM-Sponsored PCOS Consensus Workshop Group. Revised 2003 consensus on diagnostic criteria and long-term health risks related to polycystic ovary syndrome. *Fertil Steril* 2004;**81**:19–25.

14. Azziz R, Woods KS, Reyna R, et al. The prevalence and features of the polycystic ovary syndrome in an unselected population. *J Clin Endocrinol Metab* 2004;**89**:2745–9.

15. Asunción M, Calvo RM, San Millán JL, et al. A prospective study of the prevalence of the polycystic ovary syndrome in unselected Caucasian women from Spain. *J Clin Endocrinol Metab* 2000;**85**:2434–8.

16. Alvarez-Blasco F, Botella-Carretero JI, San Millán JL, Escobar-Morreale HF. Prevalence and characteristics of the polycystic ovary syndrome in overweight and obese women. *Arch Intern Med* 2006;**166**:2081–6.

17. Yildiz BO, Knochenhauer ES, Azziz R. Impact of obesity on the risk for polycystic ovary syndrome. *J Clin Endocrinol Metab* 2008;**93**:162–8.

18. Assimakopoulos K, Panayiotopoulos S, Iconomou G, et al. Assessing sexual function in obese women preparing for bariatric surgery. *Obes Surg* 2006;**16**:1087–91.

19. Brody S. Slimness is associated with greater intercourse and lesser masturbation frequency. *J Sex Marital Ther* 2004;**30**:251–61.

20. Pasquali R, Antenucci D, Casimirri F, et al. Clinical and hormonal characteristics of obese amenorrheic hyperandrogenic women before and after weight loss. *J Clin Endocrinol Metab* 1989;**68**:173–9.

21. Kiddy DS, Hamilton-Fairley D, Bush A, et al. Improvement in endocrine and ovarian function during dietary treatment of obese women with polycystic ovary syndrome. *Clin Endocrinol (Oxf)* 1992;**36**:105–11.

22. Clark AM, Ledger W, Galletly C, et al. Weight loss results in significant improvement in pregnancy and ovulation rates in anovulatory obese women. *Hum Reprod* 1995;**10**:2705–12.

23. Clark AM, Thornley B, Tomlinson L, et al. Weight loss in obese infertile women results in improvement in reproductive outcome for all forms of fertility treatment. *Hum Reprod* 1998;**13**:1502–5.

24. Norman RJ, Noakes M, Wu R, et al. Improving reproductive performance in overweight/obese women with effective weight management. *Hum Reprod Update* 2004;**10**:267–80.

25. Nelson SM, Fleming R. Obesity and reproduction: impact and interventions. *Curr Opin Obstet Gynecol* 2007;**19**:384–9.

26. National Institute for Health and Clinical Excellence. *Clinical Guideline 11. Fertility: Assessment and treatment for people with fertility problems.* London: NICE, 2004.

27. Balen AH, Anderson RA, and Policy and Practice Committee of the BFS. Impact of obesity on female reproductive health: British Fertility Society, Policy and Practice Guidelines. *Hum Fertil (Camb)* 2007;**10**:195–206.

28. Gillett WR, Putt T, Farquhar CM. Prioritising for fertility treatments – the effect of excluding women with a high body mass index. *Br J Obstet Gynaecol* 2006;**113**:1218–21.

29. Farquhar CM, Gillett WR. Prioritising for fertility treatments – should a high BMI exclude treatment? *Br J Obstet Gynaecol* 2006;**113**:1107–9.

30. Greenblatt RB, Barfield WE, Jungck EC, Ray AW. Induction of ovulation with MRL/41. Preliminary report. *JAMA* 1961;**178**:101–4.

31. Kousta E, White DM, Franks S. Modern use of clomiphene citrate in induction of ovulation. *Hum Reprod Update* 1997;**3**:359–65.

32. Lobo RA, Gysler M, March CM, et al. Clinical and laboratory predictors of clomiphene response. *Fertil Steril* 1982;**37**:168–74.

33. Imani B, Eijkemans MJ, te Velde ER, et al. Predictors of patients remaining anovulatory during clomiphene citrate induction of ovulation in normogonadotropic oligoamenorrheic infertility. *J Clin Endocrinol Metab* 1998;**83**:2361–5.

34. Legro RS, Barnhart HX, Schlaff WD, et al and Cooperative Multicenter Reproductive Medicine Network. Clomiphene, metformin, or both for infertility in the polycystic ovary syndrome. *N Engl J Med* 2007;**356**:551–66.

35. Velazquez EM, Mendoza S, Hamer T, et al. Metformin therapy in polycystic ovary syndrome reduces hyperinsulinemia, insulin resistance, hyperandrogenemia, and systolic blood pressure, while facilitating normal menses and pregnancy. *Metabolism* 1994;**43**:647–54.

36. Nestler JE, Jakubowicz DJ. Decreases in ovarian cytochrome P450c17α activity and serum free testosterone after reduction in insulin secretion in polycystic ovary syndrome. *N Engl J Med* 1996;**335**:617–23.

37. Nestler JE, Jakubowicz DJ, Evans WS, Pasquali R. Effects of metformin on spontaneous and clomiphene-induced ovulation in the polycystic ovary syndrome. *N Engl J Med* 1998;**338**:1876–80.

38. Moll E, Bossuyt PM, Korevaar JC, et al. Effect of clomifene citrate plus metformin and clomifene citrate plus placebo on induction of ovulation in women with newly diagnosed polycystic ovary syndrome: randomised double blind clinical trial. *BMJ* 2006;**332**:1485.

39. The Thessaloniki ESHRE/ASRM-Sponsored PCOS Consensus Workshop Group. Consensus on infertility treatment related to polycystic ovary syndrome. *Hum Reprod* 2008;**23**:462–77.

40. Stein IF, Cohen MR. Surgical treatment of bilateral polycystic ovaries. *Am J Obstet Gynecol* 1939;**38**:465–73.

41. Farquhar CM, Williamson K, Gudex G, et al. A randomized controlled trial of laparoscopic ovarian diathermy versus gonadotropin therapy for women with clomiphene citrate-resistant polycystic ovary syndrome. *Fertil Steril* 2002;**78**:404–11.

42. Farquhar C, Lilford RJ, Marjoribanks J, Vandekerckhove P. Laparoscopic 'drilling' by diathermy or laser for ovulation induction in anovulatory polycystic ovary syndrome. *Cochrane Database Syst Rev* 2007;**3**:CD001122.

43. Farquhar CM, Williamson K, Brown PM, Garland J. An economic evaluation of laparoscopic ovarian diathermy versus gonadotrophin therapy for women with clomiphene citrate resistant polycystic ovary syndrome. *Hum Reprod* 2004;**19**:1110–15.

44. van Wely M, Bayram N, van der Veen F, Bossuyt PM. An economic comparison of a laparoscopic electrocautery strategy and ovulation induction with recombinant FSH in women with clomiphene citrate-resistant polycystic ovary syndrome. *Hum Reprod* 2004;**19**:1741–5.

45. Dodson WC, Kunselman AR, Legro RS. Association of obesity with treatment outcomes in ovulatory infertile women undergoing superovulation and intrauterine insemination. *Fertil Steril* 2006;**86**:642–6.

46. Balen AH, Platteau P, Andersen AN, et al. The influence of body weight on response to ovulation induction with gonadotrophins in 335 women with World Health Organization group II anovulatory infertility. *Br J Obstet Gynaecol* 2006;**113**:1195–202.

47. Wang JX, Warnes GW, Davies MJ, Norman RJ. Overweight infertile patients have a higher fecundity than normal-weight women undergoing controlled ovarian hyperstimulation with intrauterine insemination. *Fertil Steril* 2004;**81**:1710–12.

48. van Swieten EC, van der Leeuw-Harmsen L, Badings EA, van der Linden PJ. Obesity and clomiphene challenge test as predictors of outcome of in vitro fertilization and intracytoplasmic sperm injection. *Gynecol Obstet Invest* 2005;**59**:220–4.

49. Fedorcsák P, Dale PO, Storeng R, et al. Impact of overweight and underweight on assisted reproduction treatment. *Hum Reprod* 2004;**19**:2523–8.

50. Dechaud H, Anahory T, Reyftmann L, et al. Obesity does not adversely affect results in patients who are undergoing in vitro fertilization and embryo transfer. *Eur J Obstet Gynecol Reprod Biol* 2006;**127**:88–93.

51. Lashen H, Ledger W, Bernal AL, Barlow D. Extremes of body mass do not adversely affect the outcome of superovulation and in-vitro fertilization. *Hum Reprod* 1999;**14**:712–15.

52. Maheshwari A, Stofberg L, Bhattacharya S. Effect of overweight and obesity on assisted reproductive technology – a systematic review. *Hum Reprod Update* 2007;**13**:433–44.

6 Maternal risks: hypertension, thromboembolism, and gestational diabetes

Daghni Rajasingam and Hannah Rickard

Thou seest I have more flesh than another man, and therefore more frailty.
Henry IV, Part I, Act III, scene iii

Introduction

Obesity in the non-pregnant population is associated with numerous health problems, including increased risk of hypertension, cardiovascular disease, and diabetes. On an annual basis, obesity in non-pregnant populations is responsible for more than 30 000 deaths in the UK[1] (6% of all deaths) and 280 000 in the USA[2] after having reduced a person's life expectancy by 9 years.[1] The relative risk of hypertension in obese women is 4.2, of type 2 diabetes 12.7, and of having a stroke 1.3.

Globally, the prevalence of obesity, especially in the young, is increasing rapidly. In the UK in 2003, 16% of females aged 16–34 were obese and 24% were overweight (total 2.4 million). It is predicted that, by 2010, this will have risen to 22% obese and 22% overweight.[3] Maternal body mass index (BMI) at pregnancy onset is increasing. One Scottish cohort showed that BMI at the first antenatal visit increased by 1.37 kg/m² over a 12-year period. Even more striking was the proportion of women classified as obese (BMI > 30 kg/m²), which had more than doubled from 9.4% to 18.9% in the same time period.[4] In the USA, 61.6% of women aged over 20 are overweight or obese, and these figures are continuing to rise.[5] The mean weight at the first antenatal visit has also increased by 20% in the past 20 years in the USA.[6] Racial differences in the incidence of obesity in women are extensive, the highest levels consistently being seen in non-white female populations, notably African-Caribbean populations.[5,7]

In pregnancy, the risks associated with obesity are compounded by physiological and metabolic changes related to pregnancy. Not only is the risk of developing pregnancy-related medical complications increased, but also the overall risk of morbidity and mortality to the mother and fetus. In the UK Confidential Enquiry into Maternal and Child Health (CEMACH) 2003–5, more than half of all women who died from direct or indirect causes for whom information was available were either overweight or obese. Of these, 15% were morbidly obese (BMI > 40).[8]

BMI is the most commonly used measure for defining an individual's weight relative to height. It is calculated as the weight in kilograms divided by the height in metres squared (kg/m^2). According to the WHO, a BMI of 25–30 kg/m^2 is classified as being overweight and one over 30 is taken as obese. This is then subclassified into class I (BMI 30–34.9), class II (BMI 35–39.9), and class III (morbid obesity: BMI $\geq$ 40).

This chapter explores the maternal risks of obesity, including pathogenesis, disease monitoring, treatment, and prevention.

Hypertension

In early pregnancy, blood pressure falls as a result of vasodilatation. It continues to decrease in the second trimester until about 22–24 weeks' gestation, after which it rises steadily to prepregnant values at term. Postpartum, the blood pressure declines immediately and then increases until about 4 days.

Hypertension is the most common medical problem in pregnancy, occurring in 10–15% of all pregnancies, and is a leading cause of maternal morbidity and mortality worldwide. In South Africa, for example, complications of hypertension in pregnancy are the most common direct cause of death and the second most common cause of all maternal deaths (19.1%) after HIV.[9] In the UK, the CEMACH 2003–5 report listed 14 deaths over the 3-year period related to hypertensive complications.[8]

Blood pressure monitoring represents an additional problem in obese women, with a risk of overestimating blood pressure if a small sphygmomanometer cuff is used. Even when a correct cuff size is selected, the phase V (Korotkoff sound) should be taken as the diastolic reading, as this is reproducible and better related to outcome.[10]

Pre-existing hypertension

Pre-existing hypertension in the general adult population is a major risk factor for cardiovascular and cerebrovascular disease. It affects 1–5% of pregnancies[11] and increases the risk of pre-eclampsia, abruption, and neonatal compromise. The incidence of hypertension increases with age and is multifactorial in aetiology. Genetic influences, race, diet, and obesity are common risk factors. In obese pregnancies, the incidence of pre-existing hypertension increases to 4.3%.[12] Pre-existing hypertension is defined as a systolic blood pressure of 140 mmHg or greater, and/or a diastolic blood pressure of 90 mmHg or more, either prepregnancy or at an early visit (around 12–16 weeks' gestation).[13] In any young woman with hypertension, a secondary cause must be excluded prior to treatment.

Assessment should include thorough history, clinical examination, and appropriate laboratory investigations. Clinical examination must include the cardiovascular system, examination for radiofemoral delay (coarctation of the aorta), and auscultation for renal bruits (renal artery stenosis). Investigations should be performed selectively to exclude renal disease, a common cause of secondary hypertension, cardiac disease, and endocrine causes (Conn's syndrome, Cushing's syndrome, adrenal hyperplasia, and phaeochromocytoma).

Appropriate examinations include renal and liver profile, serum electrolytes, fasting state lipids, and blood glucose as well as electrocardiogram and, if required, echocardiogram. If serum urea or creatinine levels are elevated, more specific renal investigations include creatinine clearance and renal ultrasound. If phaeochromocytoma is suspected, urinary catecholamines should be measured. An elevated glucose level always requires further investigation for diabetes (gestational or pre-existing).

Management

If all causes are excluded and non-pharmacological methods of blood pressure control, such as reducing dietary salt intake and weight loss, fail, medical treatment should be considered. When the patient is trying to conceive or is pregnant, appropriate medication recognized to be safe in pregnancy should be used. Prepregnancy counselling in women with pre-existing hypertension should include switching medication to a recommended drug regimen during the pregnancy (Table 6.1).

TABLE 6.1 Suggested drug treatments for hypertension in pregnancy and the puerperium[34]

Drug	Indication	Starting dose	Maximum dose	Contra-indications	Safe in breast-feeding?
Methyldopa	First-line therapy	250 mg twice daily	1 g three times daily	Depression	Yes
Nifedipine SR	Second-line therapy	10 mg twice daily	40 mg twice daily		Yes
Hydralazine	Second-line therapy	25 mg three times daily	75 mg four times daily		Yes
Labetalol	Third-line therapy	100 mg twice daily	600 mg four times daily	Asthma	Yes
αBlockers, e.g., doxazocin	Third-line therapy	1 mg once daily	8 mg twice daily		No*
ACE inhibitors, e.g., enalapril	Postpartum only	2.5 mg once daily	40 mg once daily		Yes

*Accumulates in breast milk; manufacturer advises avoidance.

ACE, angiotensin-converting enzyme

Pregnancy-induced hypertension

Pregnancy-induced hypertension (PIH) is defined as hypertension developing after 20 weeks' gestation and resolving within 6 weeks of delivery. It complicates 5–10% of pregnancies, but, with increasing maternal weight and obesity, this risk increases greatly.[12,14-17]

Management

Routine antenatal care should include a record of blood pressure at the initial and every subsequent prenatal visit. It is important to monitor patients for emerging pre-eclampsia with urinalysis and blood tests. Antihypertensive medication is not usually indicated, but moderate and severe hypertension do require treatment and persistent monitoring. Treatment is recommended if the systolic pressure exceeds 160 mmHg or the diastolic exceeds 110 mmHg (Table 6.1). Methyldopa is the first-line antihypertensive in pregnancy. Labetalol, nifedipine SR, and hydralazine are also used. Angiotensin-converting enzyme (ACE) inhibitors and angiotensin-receptor antagonists should be avoided, as they have been associated with congenital abnormalities and fetal death.[18]

Pre-eclampsia

Pre-eclampsia is a multisystemic disorder, most commonly making its appearance in the second half of pregnancy.[10] Its manifestations are widespread and involve the renal, hepatic, neurological, and haematological systems. Classically, it includes the triad of high blood pressure, proteinuria, and oedema. High blood pressure is diagnosed as blood pressure above 140/90 mmHg on two separate occasions 4 h apart, or a single diastolic pressure ≥ 110 mmHg. The appearance of hypertension is usually but not always in association with new-onset proteinuria of ≥ 2 on a dipstick or quantified proteinuria 0.3 g/24 h.

The risk factors for pre-eclampsia are numerous, including a history in first-degree relatives, multiple pregnancy, pre-existing hypertension, increased maternal age, primiparity, and coexisting medical conditions. Obesity is a well-recognized risk factor, and data from Europe, America, and the Middle East show a clear association between maternal obesity and increasing incidence of hypertensive disorders in pregnancy (Figure 6.1).[7,15-17,19,20-22] The incidence and adjusted relative risk of developing pre-eclampsia increase concomitantly with increasing BMI in all these studies. In a review of 13 studies, totalling over 1.3 million women,[23] the risk of pre-eclampsia doubled with each 5 to 7-unit increase in BMI. A similar picture is seen with increasing early pregnancy waist circumference.[21,24] This latter phenomenon acts as a sensitive marker for identifying women at risk of pre-eclampsia. Racial differences come into play as well, Bodnar et al[17] having found that obese white women have a higher risk of pre-eclampsia and hypertension than obese African–Caribbean women, whereas, in normal-weight women, this trend is reversed and white women have a lower risk of hypertensive disorder.

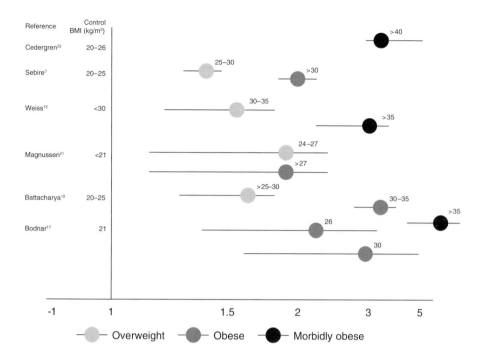

FIGURE 6.1   Risk of pre-eclampsia in pregnancy, classified by prepregnant BMI. Comparison of cited papers. Control BMI is reference group for that study.

Pathogenesis

The exact pathogenesis of pre-eclampsia is unknown, but it is thought to involve a failure of adequate placentation and an abnormal inflammatory response[25] by the mother to the pregnancy and the fetus. Increased levels of many cytokines, including tumour necrosis factor α (TNF-α), interleukin 1 (IL-1), and IL-6, characterize pre-eclampsia. The inflammatory response causes widespread endothelial dysfunction,[25,26] resulting in hypertension due to vasoconstriction, proteinuria due to renal glomerular dysfunction, and generalized peripheral and facial oedema due to increased vascular permeability. The pulmonary circulation is particularly vulnerable, and these women are at high risk of developing pulmonary oedema.

In obese women, high body fat levels correlate with increased levels of inflammatory mediators, making such individuals more susceptible to the condition (Figure 6.2). Adipose tissue produces proinflammatory cytokines, including leptin and C-reative protein (CRP),[27] and triglycerides. Elevated levels of these in early pregnancy correlate with and are thought to contribute to increased risk of developing pre-eclampsia later in pregnancy.[27,28]

Sattar et al[29] speculate that patients with central abdominal obesity have increased insulin resistance and dyslipidaemia (Figure 6.2). The associated

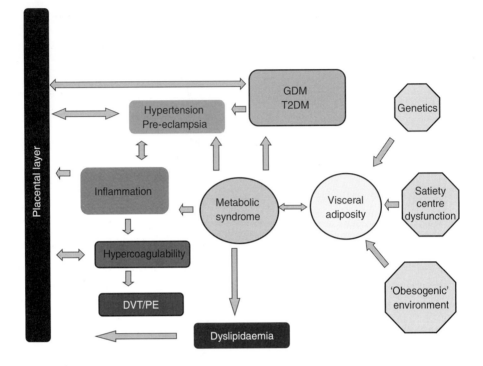

FIGURE 6.2 The interacting factors that contribute to poor maternal outcomes in obese pregnant women. DVT: deep vein thrombosis; GDM: gestational diabetes mellitus; PE: pulmonary embolism; T2DM: type 2 diabetes mellitus.

hyperinsulinaemia leads to increased lipid breakdown in visceral fat, increased concentration of fatty acids in the portal circulation, and thus abnormal synthesis of triglycerides in the liver and the accumulation of free triglyceride in hepatocytes, leading to liver dysfunction and 'fatty liver'. The increased synthesis of very-low-density lipoprotein (VLDL) and low-density lipoprotein (LDL) by the liver contributes to pre-eclampsia, as these particles promote endothelial cell activation and expression of adhesion molecules and decreased levels of high-density lipoprotein (HDL)-cholesterol, and stimulate antioxidant prostacyclin (PGI$_2$). Bodnar et al[28] have shown that inflammation and increased triglyceride levels account for only about 30% of the effect that prepregnancy BMI has on pre-eclampsia risk. It is still unclear exactly which other factors play the most significant part in the development and progression of pre-eclampsia.

Women who have pre-existing cardiovascular risk factors, such as hypertension or high triglycerides or cholesterol, are at increased risk of developing pre-eclampsia at their first antenatal visit.[21] Furthermore, women who suffer from pre-eclampsia are also at increased lifetime risk of hypertension and vascular disease.[30] These facts add weight to suggestions that pre-eclampsia and vascular diseases are linked by a common mechanism of chronic inflammation and endothelial dysfunction.

Severe pre-eclampsia may develop rapidly into eclampsia, characterized by severe hypertension and seizures. Other life-threatening consequences include renal and hepatic failure, DIC (disseminated intravascular coagulation), and HELLP (haemolysis elevated liver enzymes and low platelets) syndrome. The fetus may be growth restricted as a result of poor placental function. Eclampsia occurs in about 1–2% of women with pre-eclampsia in the developed world, equating to 0.05% of all pregnancies. It remains an important cause of maternal mortality globally.

Management

It is important to identify risk factors, such as obesity, family history, or multiple pregnancy, early and closely follow these women. Antiplatelet agents, such as low-dose aspirin (75 mg once daily), have small-to-moderate benefits when used early for prevention of pre-eclampsia and its complications in women at risk. While there are no data for its effect in obese women, the rationale for considering its use exists.[31] Given the role of nutrient deficiency, oxidative stress, and inflammation in pre-eclampsia, a role for antioxidants, especially vitamin C and vitamin E, in its prevention has been suggested. An initial pilot study showed a reduction in pre-eclampsia in normal-weight women taking multivitamins.[32] However, in a large, randomized controlled trial, Vitamins in Pregnancy (VIP), no reduction in pre-eclampsia was found in women taking vitamin C and E supplementation.[33] The trial also included a small cohort of obese women in whom vitamin supplementation also was not associated with a decrease in pre-eclampsia.

Early recognition and management of women with symptoms and signs of pre-eclampsia, such as headache, visual disturbances, oedema, and epigastric pain, are crucial. Quantification of proteinuria is done by collecting urine over a 24-h period. If protein excretion is of new onset and is over 0.3 g in the absence of a renal disorder, it is diagnostic of pre-eclampsia. Patients with underlying renal disease should have their baseline 24-h protein excretion level checked at the first antenatal visit. Monthly monitoring of full blood count, liver function, renal function, electrolytes, and serum urate is appropriate. If thrombocytopenia is present, clotting studies should be performed. Urinary tract infections should be excluded by microscopy and culture. Fetal well-being should be monitored by repeated ultrasound scanning (see Chapter 8). Uterine artery Doppler ultrasonography performed in the second trimester can predict a high risk of developing pre-eclampsia and is indicative of fetal health.

Antihypertensive therapy is the same as recommended for PIH (Table 6.1). The only definitive, curative treatment of pre-eclampsia is delivery of the baby and placenta.

Gestational diabetes mellitus

Diabetes mellitus is a disease in which glucose homeostasis is abnormal. Pre-existing diabetes mellitus is classified into types 1 and 2. Type 2 diabetes often occurs in older, overweight or obese patients. Although all racial groups are affected in the UK, diabetes is more common in Asian, African–Caribbean, and Middle Eastern immigrants. In the USA, the Latin American and African–American populations are also at high risk (see Chapter 14). South Asians have two- to fourfold higher rates of type 2 diabetes, develop it, on average, 10 years earlier, and have more cardiovascular disease than their European counterparts. Although African–Caribbeans in the UK also share this higher prevalence of type 2 diabetes, they tend to have more favourable lipid profiles and thus a lower prevalence of cardiovascular disease. Kumari et al found that in obese patients the risk of pre-existing diabetes mellitus was 10.8 times higher than in normal-weight controls.[12] It is axiomatic that the problem of undiagnosed type 2 diabetes is intimately correlated with the global obesity epidemic. It is equally true that obesity is more common in women from socioeconomically deprived areas, thereby compounding the problem of undiagnosed type 2 diabetes and obesity.

During pregnancy, glucose handling is significantly altered. The fasting glucose levels are decreased and postprandial levels are higher. Glucose tolerance decreases with increasing gestation, and most women are in an insulin-resistant state in the last trimester. The placenta contributes to these changes by secreting anti-insulin hormones, particularly glucagons, cortisol, human placental lactogen, and placental growth hormone (Figure 6.2). In addition, the renal tubular threshold for glucose declines. As the pregnancy advances, many women experience episodes of glycosuria, but glycosuria in the first half of pregnancy is likely to indicate glucose intolerance.

Gestational diabetes mellitus (GDM) is defined as 'carbohydrate intolerance of variable severity with onset or first recognition during the present pregnancy' (National Diabetes Data Group 1985). Its prevalence in developed countries has risen from 2.9% to 8.8% over the past two decades, albeit variably, depending on the level of glucose intolerance used to define the condition and the ethnicity and demographics of the population.[35] In the UK, for example, the prevalence of GDM is increased threefold in the African–Caribbean population, sixfold in the Arab/Mediterranean population, eightfold in the south-east Asian population, and eleven-fold in women from the Indian subcontinent. Because a small proportion (0.1%) of women diagnosed with GDM may actually have had pre-existing undiagnosed type 2 diabetes, it is important that all women have postnatal glucose tolerance tests and screening for fetal abnormalities in subsequent pregnancies.

As of this writing, no international consensus is available on when and how to screen, and whom to screen, for GDM. Many units screen on clinical risk factors, such as previous GDM, family history, obesity, previous macrosomic baby, glycosuria, polyhydramnios, maternal age, and previous stillbirth. Some units advocate universal screening depending on the prevalence in the local population. The timing of screening also lacks agreement. Higher detection rates will occur later in pregnancy, but later screening clearly misses the opportunity to treat hyperglycaemia early and thereby improve outcomes.

Pre-existing diabetes mellitus is higher in women with obesity, and the incidence of GDM increases proportionally to the BMI. A meta-analysis of studies of obesity found that the unadjusted odds ratios (ORs) of developing GDM were 2.14 (95% CI 1.82–2.53), 3.56 (3.05–4.21), and 8.56 (5.07–16.04) among overweight, obese, and severely obese compared with normal-weight pregnant women, respectively.[36] In certain morbidly obese women, the incidence of GDM is as high as 24.5% (OR 22.6).[12] GDM, like pre-existing diabetes mellitus, is associated with increased perinatal morbidity and mortality, including infant macrosomia, hyperinsulinaemia, polycythaemia, neonatal intensive care unit (NICN) admissions, and maternal pre-eclampsia. Women who develop GDM are at increased risk of type 2 diabetes in the long term, and 40–60% develop it within 10–15 years.

Management

Obese mothers should be referred early and seen by a team of dedicated obstetricians, nurses, midwives, and dietitians. They should have random blood glucose levels checked in early pregnancy, and again at midtrimester. If levels are elevated, they should be referred for a glucose tolerance test and HbA1c and be taught to monitor their blood glucose levels at home. Exact cut-off levels for diagnosis vary regionally, but, in the USA, the levels used are usually over 95 mg/dl fasting, and over 155 mg/dl at 2 h.[37]

The exact management of gestational diabetic mothers has been much debated. The ACHOIS trial randomized women with GDM to routine antenatal care or intensive monitoring and blood glucose optimization, and found the group managed with intensive interventions had improved perinatal outcomes.[38] On the basis of this large trial, it would seem appropriate to screen and treat intensively all women with GDM.

Treatment involves trying to maintain normoglycaemia. Women should be advised to increase daily exercise, lose weight, and adopt a low-calorie, low-fat diet. They should eliminate sugary drinks, decrease salt intake, and increase fibre and complex carbohydrate consumption. If blood glucose levels remain elevated despite dietary changes, patients should be started on antiglycaemics. The first-line treatment is usually insulin, and the exact regimen depends on local guidelines.

Traditionally, oral hypoglycaemic agents are not recommended for use in pregnancy as they cross the placenta and cause fetal hypoglycaemia. However, data from retrospective trials of women treated with metformin for polycystic ovarian syndrome (PCOS) who continued taking it during part or all of their pregnancy show that it is relatively safe in pregnancy without increased risk of neonatal hypoglycaemia, fetal anomalies, or malformations.[39,40] Initial data from the MiG study comparing insulin with metformin have also shown that metformin is potentially safe, and may reduce insulin resistance.[41] Sulphonylureas are prescribed, especially in the USA, and are potentially as safe and effective as insulin in GDM.[42] However, in obese women with optimal gylcaemic control on diet, adverse pregnancy outcomes such as metabolic complications, macrosomic infants, or NICU admissions are two- to threefold higher than in obese patients treated with insulin.[43]

Postnatally, women with GDM can stop their medication immediately. A repeat glucose tolerance test (GTT) should be performed at 6 weeks, to establish whether underlying type 2 diabetes is present. All patients with GDM should be counselled about their increased risk of diabetes in future pregnancies, and advised to seek preconception counselling to ensure adequate glycaemic control. They should also be given dietary and exercise advice with the aim of reducing their risk of type 2 diabetes later in life.

Venous thromboembolism

The overall risk of developing venous thromboembolism (VTE) either during or after pregnancy is about 0.1%. This is approximately three times the risk in the non-pregnant population aged under 40. A study from Scotland estimated 0.7 deep vein thrombosis (DVT) and 0.21 pulmonary embolism (PE) per 1000 deliveries.[44] In obese, pregnant women, however, the incidence of developing DVT is higher than in the non-obese population, although relatively few studies have looked specifically at this, possibly because the numbers of both conditions are so small. In a large study of pregnant women in the UK, the prevalence of PE in overweight women was 0.07% and in obese women 0.08% compared with 0.04% in normal-weight women. Although clinically important, this difference was not significant from a statistical point of view.[7] In a Danish study of 126 783 women, obesity in early pregnancy was found to increase significantly the risk of VTE (OR 5.3, CI 2.1, 13.5).[45] The UK Obstetric Surveillance System Report 2007 found that BMI over 30 is a major risk factor for PE (OR 2.8, CI 1.12, 7.02).[46] One suggested reason for this increase is that obese women have more sedentary lifestyles and are overall less likely to participate in any form of exercise.

Thromboembolic disease is a leading cause of direct maternal death across the world, and is the most common cause in the UK. In the UK CEMACH report of 2003–5, 33 deaths were recorded from PE and 8 from cerebral vein thrombosis (1.56 per 100 000).[8] In Australia, there were 2 direct deaths from VTE in the 750 000 births from 2000–2.[47] PE has a mortality rate of about 2.5%, so, for each fatal PE, there are 40 non-fatal PEs (UKOSS).

Of the 33 who died from PEs in the UK in 2003–5, only 25 had weight recorded in their notes, and only 21 a calculated BMI. Of those, four were overweight (BMI 25–29.5), four were obese (BMI 30–34.5), and eight were morbidly obese (BMI > 35).[8] The correlation between obesity and risk of PE is evident, and must be taken into consideration when caring for women, especially when evaluating for thromboprophylaxis. In the non-pregnant population, obesity, diabetes, and dyslipidaemia have been associated with increased incidence of DVT.[48] Patients who have suffered DVT also have elevated haemorrheological parameters such as plasma viscosity, fibrinogen, triglycerides, and erythrocyte aggregation.[49]

Pathogenesis

In pregnancy, the maternal coagulation and fibrinolytic systems change dramatically as a physiological adaptation in preparation for the need for haemostasis following delivery of the baby and placenta. Synthesis of procoagulant factors, such as factors VIII, IX, and X, increases fibrinogen levels by 50%, along with a suppression of fibrinolysis and reduction in antithrombin and protein S levels. The result is a shift in the balance of the clotting system in favour of a 'hypercoagulable' state, and for this reason, pregnant and recently delivered women are at increased risk of venous thrombosis.

For a thrombus to arise, the classic Virchow's triad of venous stasis, hypercoagulability, and injury to the intima of veins must be present. Venous flow normally decreases by 50% in all pregnancies, and stasis is exacerbated by prolonged periods of bed rest, immobility after caesarean section, or long-haul travel. Pregnancy itself represents a hypercoagulable state, which is further increased in many disorders, such as inherited and acquired thrombophilia, chronic medical conditions, and underlying malignancy. In pregnancy, 70% of DVT lesions are located in the iliofemoral region, compared with 9% in non-pregnant women, with the majority of these on the left side due to the compression of the left iliac vein by the overlying right iliac and ovarian arteries.

Obese women have increased venous stasis, as they are relatively less active. Injury to the vascular endothelium, especially of the pelvic veins, may also occur during the delivery or at the time of caesarean section. Relatively little is known about the physiological reasons for the increased risk of VTE in obese mothers. The theories include increased activation of endothelial cells, increased inflammatory mediators, and reduction in antithrombotic agents, such as PGI_2, which is produced by vessel endothelial cells and acts as an inhibitor of platelet aggregation (Figure 6.2). Studies have shown that PGI_2 levels are reduced in obese patients and in pre-eclamptic pregnancies, and there is speculation that this may contribute to the risk.

Clinical features of DVT include calf pain and tenderness, leg swelling and oedema, overlying skin warmth, and superficial venous dilatation. Venous thromboses sometimes begin in the leg veins, which then extend proximally where they attach to the vein wall, limiting venous return, or they may remain loose in the vessel lumen. These latter thrombi are particularly dangerous, as they potentially do not cause venous obstruction or present with any clinical features. As such, they are difficult to detect clinically until they embolize to the pulmonary circulation. Two-thirds of patients with PEs do not have any symptoms of DVT.

A PE presents clinically with breathlessness, pleuritic chest pain, cough, and haemoptysis. Clinical examination may reveal tachycardia, tachypnoea, and hypoxia, especially on exertion. In cases of severe PE, the patient may present shocked or collapsed, and there may be signs of right heart strain, increased jugular venous pressure (JVP), and right ventricular heave. Atypical presentations are common, and a high index of suspicion in pregnancy is required.

Management

If DVT is suspected, imaging is necessary, and the diagnosis must be confirmed, as there are major implications for this pregnancy and future pregnancies. Investigations should include the following:

- *Venous Doppler ultrasonography*: this is normally the first-line investigation. It is sensitive for detection of most above-knee DVT, but its use is limited in very obese patients due to their large body habitus and subcutaneous fat layer.
- *Venography:* if available, this study is preferable in obese patients, but it is an invasive investigation, and involves significant radiation exposure.
- *D-dimers:* this is not a useful investigation, as they are invariably elevated in all pregnancies.

The diagnosis of PE should involve a full range of tests to exclude other causes of chest pain and breathlessness, as in the following:

- *Chest radiography* may be normal, but signs to look for include pleural effusion, lobar collapse, or areas of translucency due to hypoperfusion.
- *Arterial blood gas analysis* may reveal hypoxaemia and hypocapnia (due to hyperventilation).
- *Electrocardiography* may be normal except for sinus tachycardia. Some patients may have signs of right heart strain, including right-axis deviation, right bundle-branch block, and peaked P-waves.
- *Full blood count (FBC)*: the white cell and neutrophil counts are often raised in patients with PEs. It should not be taken as false reassurance that breathlessness is due to infection.
- *Computed tomography pulmonary angiogram (CT/PA)*: this investigation is safe in pregnancy, as the radiation dose to the fetus is minimal, whereas maternal breast tissue is exposed to moderate radiation.
- *Lung perfusion (Q) or ventilation–perfusion (V/Q) scans:* inhalation of radioactive xenon-133 combined with intravenous technetiu-99 identifies areas of mismatch and potential hypoperfusion.
- *Pulmonary angiography* involves the highest radiation exposure. Doses of exposure are shown in Table 6.2.

Thromboprophylaxis

Thromboprophylaxis against VTE in the antenatal period should be offered on the basis of the individual woman's risk profile. If a woman has had a previous VTE, and is known to have underlying thrombophilia or three or more persisting risk factors for VTE, aspirin or low-molecular-weight heparin (LMWH) can be offered, depending on the risk profile. Aspirin reduces the incidence of VTE by 36% in orthopaedic patients postoperatively, but this use has not been studied in pregnancy. LMWH is more commonly used. The

TABLE 6.2 Estimated radiation dose to the fetus with investigations for thromboembolism.[34] Maximum exposure recommended in pregnancy is 50 000 μGy

Investigation	Radiation (μGy)
Chest radiography	<10
Limited venography	<500
Unilateral venography without abdominal shield	3140
Perfusion lung scan	60–120
Ventilation lung scan	
Xenon-133	40–190
Technetiu-99m	10–350
CT/PA	60–1000
Pulmonary angiography	
Brachial route	<500
Femoral route	2210–3740

CT/PA: computed tomography pulmonary angiogram.

prophylactic dose for normal-weight women is 40 mg enoxaparin once daily/500 U dalteparin once daily/4500 U tinzaparin once daily. If patients weigh over 90 kg, it is recommended that this dose be given twice daily (e.g., enoxaparin 40 mg once daily)[50] (Table 6.3).

Post partum, women who have had caesarean section should be given LMWH prophylaxis for the duration of their inpatient stay, irrespective of their weight. In obese women (BMI > 30) or women aged over 35 who have had vaginal deliveries and have other current risk factors for VTE, such as immobility, pre-eclampsia, prolonged labour, excessive blood loss, or instrumental delivery, LMWH prophylaxis should be given for 3–5 days post partum. The postnatal prophylactic dose regimens are the same as those used antenatally. Thromboprophylaxis should be given as soon as possible after delivery, provided that there is no postpartum haemorrhage, and it must be at least 4 h after the insertion or removal of spinal or epidural anaesthesia. If an obese woman is discharged home prior to completing her course of LMWH, she should be given the remaining doses to self-administer at home.[50]

Good clinical practice should encourage all women to keep well hydrated and to mobilize early. Women who are inpatients should also be advised to wear class I graduated compression stockings while in hospital. It is important to educate women that LMWH is safe in breastfeeding, as it does not pass into breast milk. At each antenatal visit, obese pregnant women should be reassessed for risk of thrombosis; if admitted, they should be given thromboprophylaxis.

TABLE 6.3 Suggested prophylactic and treatment doses of LMWH in the antenatal and postnatal periods.[34,50,51] Weight based on pre/early pregnancy weight

	Enoxaparin	**Dalteparin**	**Tinzaparin**
Prophylaxis – normal weight	40 mg once daily	5000 units once daily	4500 units once daily
Prophylaxis – obese	40 mg twice daily	5000 units twice daily	4500 units twice daily
Treatment – antenatal	1 mg/kg twice daily	100 units/kg twice daily	90 units/kg twice daily *or* 175 units/kg once daily
Treatment – postnatal	1.5 mg/kg once daily	10 000–18 000 units once daily depending on weight	175 units/kg once daily

LMWH: low-molecular-weight heparin.

Treatment of VTE

The treatment of confirmed VTE is usually LMWH (Table 6.3). The dosage depends on the patient's body weight and whether treatment is antenatal or post partum. In pregnancy, the pharmacokinetic properties of some LMWHs are altered, so a twice-daily dosage regimen is recommended (enoxaparin 1 mg/kg twice daily, dalteparin 100 U/kg twice daily). Treatment should begin before any investigations if there is a high clinical index of suspicion. These medications are safe for the fetus and do not cross into breast milk. Unstable or collapsed patients should be treated by a multidisciplinary team, including senior obstetricians and the on-call medical team. Intravenous unfractionated heparin is the treatment of choice, but, in extreme circumstances, immediate thrombolysis, embolectomy, or thoracotomy may be considered. An inferior venal filter can be considered in patients presenting with recurrent PEs.

When VTE is confirmed, screening for acquired and inherited thrombophilia is required, including protein C, protein S, factor V Leiden, antithrombin deficiency, antiphospholipid antibodies, lupus anticoagulant, and anticardiolipin antibodies. The patient must be treated for 3 months, including 6 weeks postnatally. Either LMWH or warfarin can be offered as a long-term thromboprophylaxis postnatally, as both are safe in breastfeeding. Warfarin is usually started on day 3 post partum due to the risk of bleeding. LMWH must be continued until an adequate international normalized ratio (INR) is achieved.[51]

Prevention of gestational obesity

Prevention of obesity in women of childbearing age should be high on the national public health agenda and should be based on the following:

- prepregnancy education
- prepregnancy weight optimization
- prevention of excessive weight gain during pregnancy
- postnatal avoidance of interpregnancy weight gain.

All health professionals, including nurses, who have contact with obese women should undertake prepregnancy counselling whenever possible. Although more than 77% of non-pregnant women are trying to lose or maintain their weight, only 21% of these actually use the recommended combination of calorie restriction and increased physical activity.[52] The increased maternal and fetal risks for obese women during pregnancy must be effectively disseminated to all groups of women at risk in a way that is culturally and socially acceptable to them.

During pregnancy, it is recommended that underweight women put on 4–10 kg, normal-weight women (BMI 20–24.9) 2–10 kg, overweight women under 9 kg (BMI 25–29.9), and obese women (BMI > 30) under 6 kg.[53] Higher weight gain than recommended can lead to large-for-gestational-age infants and increased risk of GDM and pre-eclampsia. Obese women who put on only a small amount of weight during pregnancy (<8 kg) have a lower risk of pre-eclampsia and caesarean section;[54] however, women who begin pregnancy as overweight are nearly twice as likely as women who are normal or underweight to gain more than the recommended amount. These women are also more likely to retain their gestational weight gain postnatally, African–Caribbean women being the most likely to do so.[55] Advice about healthy diet, exercise, and weight gain during pregnancy is beneficial in reducing excessive weight gain in normal-weight women, but not in overweight women.[56] Several studies with small cohorts of pregnant and non-pregnant women at risk of obesity who receive intensive interventions show benefit in optimization of weight.[57,58] Data show that regular exercise can result in decreased levels of circulating inflammatory mediators,[59] although it is not clear whether exercise alone will lead to a reduction in risk.

Interpregnancy weight changes can have a significant impact on subsequent maternal and neonatal outcomes. In a large study of women in consecutive pregnancies, an increase in BMI by over 3 units between pregnancies was associated with an increase in risk of developing pre-eclampsia (OR 1.78), PIH (OR 1.76), and GDM (OR 2.09).[60] The increase in risk was seen, with an increase in BMI, even if, overall, the women's BMI was still normal. This implies that all women should be discouraged from gaining weight between pregnancies.

There is an urgent need for large randomized trials of interventions that are effective in reducing levels of obesity in women of childbearing age. Research on health-promotion strategies, including social health marketing, is required to negate the impact of obesity on pregnancy and perinatal outcomes.

References

1. National Audit Office. *Tackling Obesity in England*. Report by the Comptroller and Auditor General. London: Stationery Office, 2001.

2. Allison DB, Fontaine KR, Manson JE, et al. Annual deaths attributable to obesity in the United States. *JAMA* 1999;**282**:1530–8.
3. Department of Health. Forecasting obesity to 2010. *Health Survey for England.* London: DH, 2005.
4. Kanagalingam MG, Forouhi NG, Greer IA, Sattar N. Changes in booking body mass index over a decade: retrospective analysis from a Glasgow Maternity Hospital. *Br J Obstet Gynaecol* 2005;**112**:1431–3.
5. Hedley AA, Ogden CL, Johnson CL, et al. Prevalence of overweight and obesity Among US children, adolescents, and adults, 1999–2002. *JAMA* 2004;**291**:2847–50.
6. Lu GC, Rouse DJ, DuBard M, et al. The effect of the increasing prevalence of maternal obesity on perinatal morbidity. *Am J Obstet Gynecol* 2001;**185**:845–9.
7. Sebire NJ, Jolly M, Harris JP, et al. Maternal obesity and pregnancy outcome: a study of 287 213 pregnancies in London. *Int J Obes* 2001;**25**:1175–82.
8. Lewis G, ed. *The Confidential Enquiry into Maternal and Child Health (CEMACH). Saving Mothers' Lives: Reviewing Maternal Deaths to Make Motherhood Safer – 2003–2005.* The Seventh Report on Confidential Enquiries into Maternal Deaths in the United Kingdom. London: CEMACH, 2007.
9. South African Department of Health. *Saving mothers – report on confidential enquiries into maternal deaths in South Africa.* South African Department of Health, 2002–2004. Available at: www.doh.gov.za/docs/reports/2004/savings.pdf.
10. Action on Pre-Eclampsia (APEC). Pre-eclampsia community guideline. Middlesex: Action on Pre-Eclampsia (APEC), 2004.
11. National High Blood Pressure Education Program Working Group. Report on high blood pressure in pregnancy. *Am J Obstet Gynecol* 1990;**163**:1691–1712.
12. Kumari AS. Pregnancy outcome in women with morbid obesity. *Int J Gynecol Obstet* 2001;**73**:101–7.
13. Brown MA, Lindheimer MD, de Swiet M, et al. The classification and diagnosis of the hypertensive disorders of pregnancy: statement from the International Society for the Study of Hypertension in Pregnancy (ISSHP). *Hypertens Pregnancy* 2001;**20**:9–14.
14. Thadhani R, Stampfer MJ, Hunter DJ, et al. High body mass index and hypercholesterolaemia: risk of hypertensive disorders in pregnancy. *Obstet Gynecol* 1999;**94**:543–50.
15. Weiss JL, Malone FD, Emig D, et al. Obesity, obstetric complications and caesarean delivery rate – a population-based screening study. *Am J Obstet Gynecol* 2004;**190**:1091–7.
16. Gaultier-Dereure F, Montpeyroux F, Boulot P, et al. Weight excess before pregnancy: complications and cost. *Int J Obes* 1995;**19**:443–38.
17. Bodnar LM, Catov JM, Klebanoff MA, et al. Pre-pregnancy body mass index and the occurrence of severe hypertensive disorders of pregnancy. *Epidemiology* 2007;**18**:234–9.

18. Friedman JM. ACE inhibitors and congenital anomalies. *N Engl J Med* 2006;**354**:2498–500.

19. Bhattacharya S, Campbell DM, Liston WA, Bhattacharya S. Effect of body mass index on pregnancy outcomes in nulliparous women delivering singleton babies. *BMC Public Health* 2007;**7**:168.

20. Bodnar LM, Ness RB, Markovic N, Roberts JM. The risk of pre-eclampsia rises with increasing pre-pregnancy body mass index. *Ann Epidemiol* 2005;**15**:475–82.

21. Magnussen EB, Vatten LJ, Lund-Nilsen TI, et al. Pre-pregnancy cardiovascular risk factors as predictors of pre-eclampsia: population based cohort study. *BMJ* 2007;**335**:978–81.

22. Cedergren MI. Maternal morbid obesity and the risk of adverse pregnancy outcome. *Obstet Gynecol* 2004;**103**:219–24.

23. O'Brien TE, Ray JG, Chan W-S. Maternal Body mass index and risk of pre-eclampsia: a systematic review. *Epidemiology* 2003;**14**:368–74.

24. Sattar N, Clark P, Holmes A, et al. Antenatal waist circumference and hypertension risk. *Obstet Gynecol* 2001;**97**:268–71.

25. Freeman DJ, McManus F, Brown EA, et al. Short- and long-term changes in plasma inflammatory markers associated with pre-eclampsia. *Hypertension* 2004;**43**:708–14.

26. Roberts JM. Endothelial dysfunction in pre-eclampsia. *Semin Repro Endocrinol* 1998;**16**:5–15.

27. Wolf M, Kettyle E, Sandler L, et al. Obesity and pre-eclampsia: the potential role of inflammation. *Obstet Gynecol* 2001;**98**:757–62.

28. Bodnar LM, Ness RB, Harger GF, Roberts JM. Inflammation and triglycerides partially mediate the effect of prepregnancy body mass index on the risk of pre-eclampsia. *Am J Epidemiol* 2005;**162**:1198–206.

29. Sattar N, Gaw A, Packard CJ, Greer IA. Potential pathogenic roles of aberrant lipoprotein and fatty acid metabolism in pre-eclampsia. *Br J Obstet Gynaecol* 1996;**103**:614–20.

30. Bellamy L, Casas J-P, Hingorani AD, Williams DJ. Pre-eclampsia and risk of cardiovascular disease and cancer in later life: systematic review and meta-analysis. *BMJ* 2007;**335**:974–7.

31. Askie LM, Duley L, Henderson-Smart DJ, Stewart LA and PARIS Collaborative Group. Antiplatelet agents for prevention of pre-eclampsia: a meta-analysis of individual patient data. *Lancet* 2007;**369**:1791–8.

32. Bodnar LM, Tang G, Ness RB, et al. Periconceptional multivitamin use reduces the risk of pre-eclampsia. *Am J Epidemiol* 2005;**164**:470–7.

33. Poston L, Briley AL, Seed PT, et al and VIP Trial Consortium. Vitamin C and vitamin E in pregnant women at risk for pre-eclampsia (VIP trial): randomised placebo-controlled trial. *Lancet* 2006;**367**:1145–54.

34. Nelson-Piercy C. *Handbook of Obstetric Medicine*, 3rd edn. Informa Healthcare, 2006.

35. Confidential Enquiry into Maternal and Child Health (CEMACH). *Pregnancy in women with type 1 and type 2 diabetes 2002–2003: England, Wales and Northern Ireland*. London: CEMACH, 2005.

36. Chu SY, Callaghan WM, Kim SY, et al. Maternal obesity and risk of gestational diabetes mellitus. *Diabetes Care* 2007;**30**:2070–6.

37. National Diabetes Information Clearinghouse (NDIC), National Institute of Diabetes and Kidney Diseases, NIH. Available at: diabetes.niddk.nih.gov/index.htm.

38. Crowther CA, Hiller JE, Moss JR, et al for ACHOIS Collaborative Group. Effect of treatment of mild gestational diabetes mellitus on pregnancy outcomes. The ACHOIS randomized controlled trial. *N Engl J Med* 2005;**352**:2477–86.

39. Homko CJ, Reece EA. Insulins and oral hypoglycemic agents in pregnancy. *J Matern Fetal Neonatal Med* 2006;**19**:679–86.

40. Ho FL, Liew CF, Cunanan EC, Lee KO. Oral hypoglycaemic agents for diabetes in pregnancy – an appraisal of the current evidence for oral anti-diabetic drug use in pregnancy. *Ann Acad Med Singapore* 2007;**36**:672–8.

41. Simmons D, Walters BN, Rowan JA, McIntyre HD. Metformin therapy and diabetes in pregnancy – MiG Study. *Med J Aust* 2004;**180**:462–4.

42. Jacobson GF, Ramos GA, Ching JY, et al. Comparison of glyburide and insulin for the management of gestational diabetes in a large managed care organization. *Am J Obstet Gynecol* 2005;**193**:118–24.

43. Langer O, Yogev Y, Xenakis EMJ, Brustman L. Overweight and obese in gestational diabetes. *Am J Obstet Gynecol* 2005;**192**:1768–76.

44. McColl MD, Ramsey JE, Tait RC et al. Risk factors for pregnancy associated venous thromboembolism. *Thromb Haemost* 1997;**78**:1183–8.

45. Larsen TB, Sorensen HT, Gislum M, Johnsen SP. Maternal smoking, obesity and risk of venous thromboembolism during pregnancy and the puerperium: a population-based nested case-control study. *Thromb Res* 2007;**120**:505–9.

46. Knight M, Kurinczuk JJ, Spark P, Brocklehurst P. *United Kingdom Obstetric Surveillance System (UKOSS) Annual Report 2007*. Oxford: National Perinatal Epidemiology Unit, 2007.

47. Australian Institute of Health and Welfare. *Maternal deaths in Australia 2000–2002*. Available at: www.aihw.gov.au/publications/index.cfm/title/10207.

48. Tsai AW, Cushman M, Rosamond WD, et al. Cardiovascular risk factors and venous thromboembolism incidence: the longitudinal investigation of thromboembolism aetiology. *Arch Intern Med* 2002;**162**:1182–9.

49. Vaya A, Falco C, Simo M, et al. Influence of lipids and obesity on haemorrheological parameters in patients with deep vein thrombosis. *Thromb Haemost* 2007;**98**:621–6.

50. Royal College of Obstetricians and Gynaecologists. *Thromboprophylaxis During Pregnancy, Labour and After Vaginal Delivery*. Green Top Guidelines. London: RCOG, 2004.

51. Royal College of Obstetricians and Gynaecologists. *Thromboembolic Disease in Pregnancy and the Puerperium: Acute Management.* Green Top Guidelines. London: RCOG, 2007.
52. Cogswell ME, Perry GS, Schieve LA, Dietz WH. Obesity in women of childbearing age: risks, prevention and treatment. *Prim Care Update Obstet Gynecol* 2001;**8**:89–105.
53. Cedergren MI. Optimal gestational weight gain for body mass index categories. *Obstet Gynecol* 2007;**110**:759–64.
54. Cedergren M. Effects of gestational weight gain and body mass index on obstetric outcome in Sweden. *Int J Gynaecol Obstet* 2006;**93**:269–74.
55. Parker JD, Abrams B. Difference in post-partum weight retention between black and white mothers. *Obstet Gynecol* 1993;**81**:867–74.
56. Polley BA, Wing RR, Sims CJ. Randomised controlled trail to prevent excessive weight gain in pregnant women. *Int J Obes* 2002;**26**:1494–1502.
57. Eiben G, Lissner L. Health Hunters – an intervention to prevent overweight and obesity in high-risk women. *Int J Obes* 2006;**30**:691–6.
58. Olson CM, Strawderman MS, Reed RG. Efficacy of an intervention to prevent excessive gestational weight gain. *Am J Obstet Gynecol* 2004;**191**:530–6.
59. Petersen AMW, Pedersen BK. The anti-inflammatory effect of exercise. *J Appl Physiol* 2005;**98**:1154–62.
60. Villamor E, Cnattingius S. Interpregnancy weight change and risk of adverse pregnancy outcomes: a population-based study. *Lancet* 2006;**368**:1164–70.

7 Fetal risks: early and late pregnancy, and long-term complications in adult life

Eyal Sheiner and Adi Y Weintraub

Introduction

The increase in obesity rates among pregnant women is a significant public health concern with various implications for prenatal care and supervision of delivery. From a public health perspective, obesity represents an important modifiable risk factor for adverse pregnancy outcome,[1–5] with serious obstetric complications for the mother and the fetus,[6–12] including increased incidence of malformation, fetal macrosomia (birth weight of 4 kg and above), and long-term complications in adult life.[6–17] Figure 7.1 presents the distribution of maternal obesity during pregnancy in 1988–2000, in southern Israel. As our data are population based, this microcosmic picture reflects the global nature of the problem facing the obstetric community. This chapter discusses fetal risks of obese parturients during early and late pregnancy, as well as long-term complications in adult life.

Fetal complications during early pregnancy: abortion and congenital malformation

Abortions

A large population-based study comparing all pregnancies of obese and nonobese patients in the Negev, southern Israel, was conducted in order to investigate the pregnancy outcome of obese patients not suffering from hypertensive disorders or diabetes mellitus.[10] In 1988–2002, there were 126 080 deliveries, of which 1769 (1.4%) occurred in obese patients (body mass index [BMI] >30 kg/m²). Recurrent abortions were significantly more common among the obese than the nonobese population (7.4% vs 4.8%; odds ratio [OR] = 1.5, 95% confidence interval (CI) 1.2–1.9; $P < 0.001$) (Table 7.1). This association was significant for patients undergoing fertility treatments as well as for these who conceived spontaneously.

Lashen et al[18] in the UK performed a nested, case–control study, and compared obese women with an age-matched control group with normal BMI (18.5–24.9). Only primiparous women were included in order to avoid including a given woman more than once, and for correct identification of recurrent miscarriages.

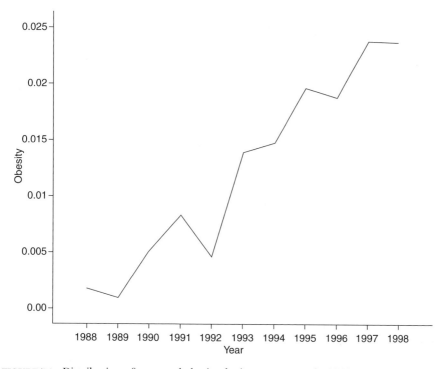

FIGURE 7.1 Distribution of maternal obesity during pregnancy in 1988–2000, in southern Israel.

TABLE 7.1 Short-term fetal outcome of obese and nonobese patients: results from a population-based study from southern Israel

Characteristics	Obese (%) ($n = 1769$)	Nonobese (%) ($n = 124\,311$)	OR	95% CI	P
Recurrent abortion	7.1	4.8	1.5	1.2–1.9	<0.001
Birth weight > 4000 g	6.4	4.5	1.5	1.2–1.8	<0.001
Meconium-stained amniotic fluid	21.5	16.2	1.4	1.2–1.6	<0.001
Malpresentation	9.2	5.9	1.6	1.3–1.9	<0.001
Cesarean delivery	27.8	10.8	3.2	2.9–3.5	<0.001
Apgar 1 min <7	4.4	4.3	1.0	0.8–1.3	0.93
Apgar 5 min <7	0.6	0.6	1.0	0.5–1.8	0.94
Perinatal mortality	1.7	1.3	1.3	0.9–1.8	0.18
Shoulder dystocia	0.3	0.2	1.6	0.7–4.0	0.25
Congenital malformations	4.0	3.9	1.0	0.8–1.3	0.74

Adapted from Sheiner et al.[10]

CI, confidence interval, OR, odds ratio.

A total of 1644 obese and 3288 age-matched, normal-weight controls were included. The risks of early miscarriage (OR 1.2, 95% CI 1.01–1.46; $P = 0.04$) and recurrent abortions (OR 3.5, 95% CI 1.03–12.01; $P = 0.04$) were significantly higher among the obese patients. These authors concluded that obesity was associated with increased risk of first-trimester and recurrent miscarriage.[18] Similar results were noted in a former cohort of 383 patients conceiving after in vitro fertilization (IVF) or intracytoplasmic sperm injection (ICSI).[19] Obese patients had fewer oocytes collected (median: 8 vs 10; $P = 0.03$), higher abortion rates during the first 6 weeks (22% vs 12%; $P = 0.03$), and lower live birth rates (63% vs 75%; $P = 0.04$). The relative risk of abortion before week 6 was 1.77 (95% CI 1.05–2.97). Multivariate logistic regression analysis revealed that obesity and low oocyte count were independently associated with spontaneous abortion. In the obese group, low oocyte number was associated with a more profound increase in the risk of abortion than was present among lean patients. Interestingly, the effects of age, history of past pregnancies, or infertility diagnosis on the probability of miscarriage were not significant. These authors concluded that obesity is an independent risk factor for early pregnancy loss.[19] Given the findings of these two investigations, weight loss before conception should be strongly recommended in obese patients considering assisted reproductive therapy.[20]

At the same time, when implantation rates, continuing pregnancy rates, or spontaneous miscarriage rates were compared in an obese and normal-weight population of women attempting conception through oocyte donation, no difference was found in implantation rates or pregnancy outcome.[21] Stated another way, BMI has no adverse impact on implantation or reproductive outcome in donor oocyte recipients,[21] a finding that suggests that obesity does not exert a negative effect on endometrial receptivity.[21,22]

No clear explanation exists for these findings. Experience with polycystic ovary syndrome patients showed that insulin resistance is related to early pregnancy loss as well as to infertility.[19] Obesity is known to be a risk factor for infertility, mainly due to anovulation,[10] and even mild weight loss can restore ovulation.[10] Thus, maternal obesity should be addressed directly not only to reduce associated morbidities, but also in order to increase fertility. The preconception counseling of obese patients should include pointing out the increased risk of subfertility as well as the risk of recurrent early abortions. Primary care physicians would do well to point this out as part of their general health counseling.

Congenital malformation

Controversy exists regarding the association between obesity and congenital malformation. Some studies do not find such an association,[10,11] but others suggest that obesity is indeed a risk factor for malformation, primarily neural tube defects (NTDs).[23–25] Other reported anomalies include congenital heart defects,[26] multiple anomalies,[24] other defects of the central nervous system, great vessel defects, ventral wall defects, and intestinal defects.[27]

Most studies, however, show an increased risk of NTDs associated with prepregnancy maternal obesity.[23–25] Few studies have investigated the relationship between maternal prepregnancy obesity and overweight and birth defects, Watkins et al[24] explored the relationship for several birth defects and obesity in a population-based, case–control study, using data from the Atlanta Birth Defects Risk Factor Surveillance Study. Mothers who delivered an infant with and without selected birth defects in a five-county metropolitan Atlanta area between January 1993 and August 1997 were interviewed. The risks for obese women (BMI $\geq$ 30) and overweight women (BMI 25.0–29.9) were compared with those of average-weight women (BMI 18.5–24.9). Obese women were more likely than average-weight women to have an infant with spina bifida (unadjusted OR 3.5, 95% CI 1.2–10.3), omphalocele (OR 3.3, 95% CI 1.0–10.3), heart defects (OR 2.0, 95% CI 1.2–3.4), or multiple anomalies (OR 2.0, 95% CI 1.0–3.8). Overweight women were more likely than average-weight women to have infants with heart defects (OR 2.0, 95% CI 1.2–3.1) or multiple anomalies (OR 1.9, 95% CI 1.1–3.4). These authors concluded that obesity was significantly associated with these congenital malformations.

The reasons for the association between birth defects and maternal obesity are poorly understood, although it is hypothesized that an association exists with undetected pregestational diabetes mellitus, increases in serum insulin, triglycerides, uric acid and insulin resistance, technical problems with the ultrasound detection (resulting in less early terminations), and lower folic acid levels.[22] Most authors recognize that there are other potential explanations yet to be identified.[22]

Pregestational diabetes mellitus is a well-established risk factor for congenital anomalies,[28,29] and the association between this condition and obesity is significant.[10,20,22] Our group investigated the association between obesity and congenital malformations after excluding patients with diabetes mellitus, and did not find such an association[10] (see Table 7.1). The results support that the association between obesity and congenital malformation might be attributed to pregestational diabetes mellitus, and not to the obesity itself.

The increased prevalence of NTDs in the offspring of pregnant obese population was thought to be related to lower circulating levels of folic acid.[22] However, the higher risk of NTDs associated with obesity remained even after universal folic acid flour fortification.[23] By late 1997, it became mandatory in Canada that all refined wheat flour be fortified with folic acid. Because overweight women may consume greater quantities of refined wheat flour, Ray and coauthors questioned whether their risk of NTDs changed after flour fortification.[23] The presence of NTDs was systematically detected, both antenatally and postnatally, among Ontarian women who underwent antenatal maternal screening at 15–20 weeks' gestation. A total of 292 open NTDs were detected among 420 362 women. The adjusted OR for NTD was 1.2 (95% CI 1.1–1.3) per 10-kg incremental rise in maternal weight. The interaction between elevated maternal weight and the presence of folic acid flour fortification was of borderline significance ($P = 0.09$). Before fortification, greater maternal weight was associated with a modestly increased risk of NTD (adjusted OR 1.4, 95% CI 1.0–1.8); after flour fortification, this effect was more pronounced (adjusted OR 2.8, 95% CI 1.2–6.6). These data emphasize the higher risk of NTDs associated with increased maternal weight, even after universal folic acid flour fortification. The problem is not as simple in the USA, where the anticipated reduction in NTDs after the mandatory fortification regulation in the early 1990s was not forthcoming. It is now thought that at least part of this shortfall may be due to the fact that a large portion of the Hispanic population prefer daily consumption of products made from corn flour, which was not included in the 1992 fortification regulation. It is noteworthy that maternal serum α-fetoprotein (AFP) levels at 15–20 weeks of pregnancy are significantly related to maternal weight ($r = 0.24$, $P < 0.0001$[30]) probably due to greater plasma volume in obese patients. It is possible that the results of serum markers for NTDs in obese women are harder to interpret.

Ultrasound in obese women is often suboptimal.[31] Sonograms from 1622 consecutively scanned singleton pregnancies at a mean gestational age of 28.5 weeks were analyzed to determine whether maternal obesity affected visualization of fetal anatomy. Fetal head (cerebral ventricles), heart (four-chamber view), stomach, kidneys, bladder, diaphragm, intestines, spinal column, extremities, and umbilical cord were classified as visualized or suboptimally visualized. Maternal BMI was used as a measure of relative leanness. No significant impairment of ultrasound visualization was noted in the vast majority of patients. With a BMI beyond the 90th percentile, visualization fell by an average of 14.5%. Reduction in visualization was most marked for the fetal heart, umbilical cord, and spine. Among obese women (BMI > 30), BMI was the best predictor of visualization.[32] Likewise, Hendler et al[33] examined the impact of maternal obesity on the rate of suboptimal ultrasound visualization of fetal anatomy and determined the optimal timing of prenatal ultrasound examination for the obese gravidas. More than 11 000 pregnancies were studied, of which 38.6% of the patients were obese. Patients were divided into four groups and categorized by BMI: nonobese (BMI < 30), class I obesity (BMI > 30 but ≤ 35), class II obesity (BMI > 35 but ≤ 40), and extreme obesity (BMI ≤ 40). The rate of suboptimal ultrasound visualization of the fetal structures was higher for obese than for nonobese women. Increased severity of maternal obesity was associated with suboptimal visualization rates for both the cardiac (nonobese 18.7% [1275/6819], class I 29.6% [599/2022], class II 39.0% [472/1123], and extreme obesity 49.3% [580/1055]; $P < 0.0001$) and the craniospinal structures (nonobese 29.5% [2012/6819], class I 36.8% [744/2022], class II 43.3% [486/1123], and extreme obesity 53.4% [563/1055]; $P < 0.0001$). Even after adjustment for gestational age and the type of ultrasound machine, obese women had a greater risk of suboptimal ultrasound visualization of the fetal cardiac and craniospinal structures than nonobese women. The optimal gestational age for visualization of fetal cardiac and craniospinal anatomy in obese patients may be beyond 18–20 weeks' gestation. These authors also suggested that repeated ultrasound examination for suboptimal ultrasound visualization of the fetal heart at a later gestational age dramatically reduces the overall rate of suboptimal ultrasound visualization.[34]

Fetal complications during late pregnancy: macrosomia, and stillbirth

Macrosomia

Obesity is recognized to be associated with fetal macrosomia, leading to potential adverse maternal (induction of labor, cesarean section) and neonatal outcomes (shoulder dystocia, birth injuries).[10-12,20,31] Obesity and diabetes mellitus are independently associated with increased risk of macrosomic and large infants.[31] Macrosomic infants have hyperinsulinemia.[35] Macrosomia is a predictor of hyperinsulinemia and vice versa ($R^2 = 0.26$).[35] Maternal anthropometric factors as well as hyperinsulinemia are correlated with macrosomia, and the macrosomia may be causally related to the high insulin levels. Moreover, obesity is associated with increased maternal insulin resistance and fetal hyperinsulinemia even in the absence of maternal diabetes.[35]

In a previous retrospective analysis by our group, birth weight was significantly higher among obese than nonobese patients and was associated with higher rates of fetal macrosomia (birth weight ≥ 4 kg).[10] This association was noted even after bariatric surgery.[11] Obese patients were also more likely to have meconium-stained amniotic fluid, malpresentations, and cesarean deliveries (CDs) than nonobese patients (Table 7.1). Likewise, Weiss et al aimed to determine whether obesity was associated with obstetric complications and CDs. They studied a large, prospective, multicenter database from which patients were divided into three groups: BMI under 30 (control), 30–34.9 (obese), and 35 or greater (morbidly obese). Their study included 6102 patients: 3752 control, 1473 obese, and 877 morbidly obese patients. Obesity and morbid obesity had a statistically significant association with fetal birth weight greater than 4000 g (OR 1.7 and 1.9, respectively) and greater than 4500 g (OR 2.0 and 2.4, respectively).[36]

Shoulder dystocia complicates 0.13–2.1% of all deliveries and is associated with adverse pregnancy outcome.[37,38] One of the risk factors for this condition is maternal obesity.[39] However, it has been questioned whether this association is related to the correlation of obesity with diabetes mellitus, a known risk factor for shoulder dystocia,[37,39] or acts independently. Indeed, diabetic patients are at increased risk of shoulder dystocia, even after controlling for birth weight.[40] Robinson et al[41] concluded that the strongest predictor for shoulder dystocia is fetal macrosomia, and for obese, nondiabetic parturients no increased risk of shoulder dystocia is present unless the fetus is macrosomic. However, after excluding patients with diabetes mellitus, our group[10] did not find such an association, despite higher rates of fetal macrosomia in our study population.

Fetal distress and perinatal mortality

No agreement was found in the literature regarding these outcomes. Indeed, maternal obesity has been linked to fetal distress, meconium aspiration, and perinatal mortality.[20,42] Kristensen et al evaluated the association between maternal prepregnancy BMI and the risk of stillbirth and neonatal death.[42] Maternal obesity was associated with a more than doubled risk of stillbirth (OR 2.8, 95% CI 1.5–5.3) and neonatal death (OR 2.6, 95% CI 1.2–5.8) compared with women of normal weight. No single cause of death explained the higher risk of perinatal mortality. In contrast, Rode et al[43] found no differences between obese and nonobese women with regard to neonatal morbidity estimated by Apgar score, umbilical cord pH, or admission to a neonatal intensive care unit.[43]

Importantly, after the exclusion of hypertensive disorders and diabetes mellitus, our group did not find maternal obesity associated with an increased rate of adverse perinatal outcome.[10] No significant differences were found regarding low Apgar scores, perinatal mortality, congenital malformation, or preterm delivery (Table 7.1). The increased risk found in other studies[42] may be due to the significant contribution of diabetes mellitus and hypertension to the adverse perinatal outcome, rather than obesity itself.[44] Obviously, women with diabetes and hypertensive disorders should be monitored closely, especially as we know that, in obese women with gestational diabetes mellitus, pregnancy outcome is compromised regardless of the level of obesity or treatment modality.[45] Nevertheless, in obese parturients without comorbidities the cost/potential benefit of more extensive evaluation is speculative.

Long-term complications in adult life

Maternal weight affects neonatal outcomes in several ways. With regard to reports of higher preterm delivery rates in obese women,[8,46,47] most of these are probably elective due to maternal complications (such as hypertensive disorders) rather than being spontaneous preterm births. Regardless of the etiology, such preterm infants have an increased risk of neonatal mortality, and the surviving offspring are likely to have an increased risk of long-term disability due to chronic respiratory problems and neurodevelopmental impairment.[46,47] Obesity is a risk factor for macrosomia,[10,31,48] as are pregestational and gestational diabetes, which are also more common among overweight and obese patients. In the immediate postnatal period, macrosomic babies are at increased risk of birth trauma and metabolic issues, including hypoglycemia and hyperbilirubinemia. Shoulder dystocia is increased in obese patients.[39,48]

Converging lines of evidence from epidemiologic studies and animal models now indicate that the origins of obesity and related metabolic disorders lie not only in the interaction between genes and traditional adult risk factors, such as unbalanced diet and physical inactivity, but also in the interplay between genes and the embryonic, fetal, and early postnatal environment.[49] Convincing evidence supports the contention that, in both human and animal models, the in utero environment affects fetal developmental processes, altering offspring homeostatic regulatory mechanisms (see Chapter 2). 'Gestational programming' may result in altered cell number, organ structure, hormonal set points, or gene expression, with effects being permanent or expressed only at certain offspring ages (e.g., newborn, childhood, adolescence, adulthood).[49]

It has been suggested that intrauterine overnutrition affects lifelong risk of obesity. According to this hypothesis, high maternal plasma concentrations of glucose, free fatty acids, and amino acids result in permanent changes in appetite control, neuroendocrine functioning, or energy metabolism in the developing fetus and thus lead to obesity in later life. Since maternal BMI is positively associated with insulin resistance and glucose intolerance, and therefore higher plasma concentrations of glucose and free fatty acids, fetal overnutrition is more likely among mothers with greater BMI during pregnancy.[50]

Growth in utero is roughly summarized by birth weight, which, if related to fatness later in life, might implicate the fetal environment in the development of obesity.[51] The relationship between birth weight and fatness, measured in childhood or adulthood, is generally positive, albeit variable in magnitude.[52,53] A possible reason for this variability is that the strength of the relationship may depend on the age at which fatness is measured. More importantly, several factors, such as gestational age, parental body size, and socioeconomic status, may confound the relationship between birth weight and later fatness.[51] Parsons et al[51] examined the influence of birth weight on BMI at different stages of later life in order to determine whether this relationship persists after accounting for potential confounding factors. These investigators found that, in adulthood, BMI increased with increasing birth weight mainly at the heaviest birth weights. The relationship between birth weight and BMI was influenced markedly by the mother's weight and BMI but was unaffected by the mother's height, age, or smoking habits, or by the father's weight or social class.[51]

Few studies have been designed to investigate the direct association between maternal and offspring overweight or obesity, but several have found one. Laitinen et al[54] reported that children of overweight or obese mothers had higher mean BMI at each age point tested than children born to underweight or normal-weight mothers. At 31 years, overweight and obesity were more common in progeny whose mothers were overweight or obese before pregnancy (men: 43% overweight and 12% obese; women: 27% overweight and 14% obese) than in progeny whose mothers were underweight or of normal weight (men: 39% overweight and 7% obese; women: 18% overweight and 7% obese; $P < 0.001$). Circumferences of the waist and hip and waist-to-hip ratios of the offspring at 31 years increased as maternal BMI increased.[54] Some of the studies reporting a positive association between maternal and offspring overweight or obesity[50,51,54-57] are presented in Table 7.2.

Large cohort studies on obesity describe a J-shaped curve when an association with birth weight is made (a slightly greater BMI among subjects born small but a much greater prevalence of overweight and obesity in those born large).[58,59] The increased prevalence of adolescent obesity is related to increased later risk of metabolic syndrome. The increased incidence of obesity accounts for the increase in type 2 diabetes, particularly among the young. Most diabetic adolescents (type 2 diabetes) are overweight or obese. Many obese young children (4–10 years) have impaired glucose tolerance.[60] Given these circumstances, the epidemic of obesity and subsequent risk of diabetes and components of metabolic syndrome may begin in utero with fetal overgrowth/adiposity rather than undergrowth. The presence of two different mechanisms has been suggested for development

TABLE 7.2 Studies reporting a positive association between maternal and offspring overweight or obesity

Study				Subjects			Maternal biometry	Offspring biometry	Results
Reference	Primary Author	Year of publication	Study design	Place of birth	Number of subjects	Year of birth			
51	Parsons TJ	2001	Longitudinal study	England, Scotland and Wales	10 683	1958	Maternal height was measured, and weight before pregnancy was reported by the mother, shortly after the birth of the cohort member	Body mass index at ages 7, 11, 16, 23, and 33 years	The relationship between birth weight and adult BMI was largely accounted for by maternal weight or BMI
54	Laitinen J	2001	Longitudinal study	Northern Finland	12 063	1966	The mothers' weight before pregnancy was recorded during her first visit to the antenatal clinic (on average around week 16). Height was measured or self-reported	Body weight and height were measured at birth and at 1 and 31 years, but were self-reported at 14 years	Children of overweight or obese mothers had higher mean BMI at each age point than did children born to underweight or normal-weight mothers

TABLE 7.2 continued...

Study				Subjects			Maternal biometry	Offspring biometry	Results
Reference	Primary Author	Year of publication	Study design	Place of birth	Number of subjects	Year of birth			
55	Eriksson J	2003	Birth cohort study	Helsinki, Finland	4515	1934 –44	Data from birth records that included height and maternal body weight measured on admission in labor	Maximum BMI ascertained from a postal questionnaire	A higher maternal BMI in pregnancy was associated with a more rapid childhood growth and an increased risk of becoming obese in adult life
56	Whitaker RC	2004	Retrospective cohort study	Cincinnati, Ohio	8494 From the Special Supplemental Nutrition Program for Women, Infants, and Children (WIC) in Ohio	1992 –96	Height and weight measurements collected in WIC during the first trimester of pregnancy	Children who were enrolled in the WIC were followed from the first trimester of gestation until 24–59 months of age. Height and weight measurements occurred at enrollment and at 6-month intervals	After controlling for confounders, the relative risk of childhood obesity associated with maternal obesity in the first trimester of pregnancy was 2.0 (95% CI 1.7–2.3) at 2 years of age, 2.3 (95% CI 2.0–2.6) at 3 years of age, and 2.3 (95% CI 2.0–2.6) at 4 years of age.

TABLE 7.2 continued...

| Study | | | | | Subjects | | | Maternal biometry | Offspring biometry | Results |
Reference	Primary Author	Year of publication	Study design		Place of birth	Number of subjects	Year of birth			
57	Li C	2005	Longitudinal survey		United States	2636	1986–2000	Maternal prepregnancy BMI was calculated based on self-reported height and weight just before pregnancy	Children's height and weight were measured	After adjusting for potential confounders, children whose mothers were obese before pregnancy were at a greater risk of becoming overweight than children whose mothers had normal BMI (adjusted OR 4.1; 95% CI, 2.6–4; $P < 0.001$)
50	Lawlor DA	2007	Prospective study		South Brisbane, Australia	3,340	1981–84	Height and weight reported by the mother at her first antenatal clinic visit	Measurements of weight and height taken at the 5- and 14-year follow-up	There was statistical support for a difference in the magnitude of the association between maternal-offspring BMI and paternal-offspring BMI in all confounder-adjusted models tested (all $P < 0.0001$)

of glucose intolerance: one at the higher end of the birth-weight spectrum that may be associated with maternal hyperglycemia, and the other at the lower end, probably caused by different mechanisms.[61]

Maternal pregravid weight and diabetes exert an independent effect not only on birth weight but also on the adolescent risk of obesity. Langer and colleagues[62] reported that, in obese women with gestational diabetes mellitus (GDM) whose glucose was well controlled on diet alone, the odds of fetal macrosomia were significantly increased (OR 2.12) compared with women with normal BMI and well-controlled (diet only) GDM with normal BMI. Similar results were reported in women with GDM who were poorly controlled on diet or insulin. In well-controlled, insulin-requiring GDM, no significant increased risk of macrosomia was associated with increasing pregravid BMI. Additionally, Dabelea et al[63] reported that the mean adolescent BMI was 2.6 kg/m^2 greater in sibling offspring of diabetic pregnancies than in the index siblings born when the mother previously had normal glucose tolerance. Hence, maternal pregravid obesity as well as the presence of maternal diabetes may independently affect the risk of adolescent obesity in the offspring.

The risk of the development of metabolic syndrome in adolescents was addressed by Boney et al[64] in a longitudinal cohort study of appropriate-for-gestational age (AGA) and large-for-gestational age (LGA) infants of women with normal glucose tolerance and GDM. The metabolic syndrome was defined as the presence of two or more of the following components: obesity, hypertension, glucose intolerance, and dyslipidemia. Maternal obesity was defined as a pregravid BMI greater than 27.3. Interestingly, these authors found that exposure of children to maternal obesity was as strong a predictor of risk of MS as LGA status (1.81, 95% CI 1.03–3.19; P <0.04 and 2.19, 95% CI 1.25–3.82; P <0.01, respectively). This suggests that, among obese mothers without clinical GDM, fetal hyperinsulinemia might develop because of mild maternal hyperglycemia that is below the threshold for a diagnosis of GDM or occurs later in the pregnancy, after screening. This possibility is consistent with other studies showing that maternal obesity is a risk factor for LGA birth in the absence of frank GDM.[65]

Conroy et al[66] conducted an integrative review of Canadian, childhood, obesity-prevention programs, finding a significant lack of prenatal or infancy obesity-prevention programs to address early obesogenesis. Such programs would be innovative and are much needed in an effort to stem the alarming increase in obesity in children and adults. Research is warranted to assess prenatal intervention in the prevention of childhood and adult obesity.

Conclusions

Obesity poses a significant risk of early and late fetal adverse outcome, including early abortions, congenital malformation (mainly NTDs), and fetal macrosomia and its consequences. Interpretation of serum markers in obese women is more difficult because of the changes in the volume of distribution of these markers. Likewise, the ability of ultrasound to detect fetal malformations is significantly limited. Delaying evaluation until after 18 weeks' gestation and repeated ultrasound examination for suboptimal ultrasound visualization of the fetal heart at a later gestational age may be of some value, although overall maternal obesity still limits visibility of the fetus. The preconception counseling of obese patients should include pointing out the increased risk of subfertility as well as the risk of recurrent early abortions, malformation, and fetal macrosomia, and long-term risks of metabolic syndrome and childhood obesity. It is recommended that primary-care physicians give this counseling as part of general health advice. Prenatal obesity prevention programs to address early obesogenesis are lacking. Such programs would be innovative and are much needed to stem the alarming increase in obesity in children and adults.

References

1. National Heart, Lung, and Blood Institute. *Clinical guidelines on the identification, evaluation and treatment of obesity in adults: the evidence report.* Washington, DC: US Department of Health and Human Services, 1998.
2. Mokdad AH, Serdula MK, Dietz WH, et al. The spread of the obesity epidemic in the United States, 1991–1998. *JAMA* 1999;**282**:1519–22.
3. Ehrenberg HM, Dierker L, Milluzzi C, Mercer BM. Prevalence of maternal obesity in an urban center. *Am J Obstet Gynecol* 2002;**187**:1189–93.
4. Gross T, Sokol RJ, King KC. Obesity in pregnancy: risks and outcome. *Obstet Gynecol* 1980;**56**:446–50.
5. Allison DB, Fonatine KR, Manson JE, et al. Annual deaths attributable to obesity in the United States. *JAMA* 1999;**282**:1530–8.
6. Isaacs JD, Magnon EF, Martin RW, et al. Obstetric challenges of massive obesity complicating pregnancy. *J Perinatol* 1994;**14**:10–14.
7. Ratner RE, Hamner LH, Isada NB. Effects of gestational weight gain in morbidly obese women: fetal morbidity. *Am J Perinatol* 1990;**7**:295–9.
8. Cnattingius S, Bergstrom R, Lipworth L, Kramer MS. Prepregnancy weight and the risk of adverse pregnancy outcomes. *N Engl J Med* 1998;**338**: 147–52.
9. Kumari AS. Pregnancy outcome in women with morbid obesity. *Int J Gynaecol Obstet* 2001;**73**:101–7.
10. Sheiner E, Levy A, Menes TS, et al. Maternal obesity as an independent risk factor for caesarean delivery. *Paediatr Perinat Epidemiol* 2004;**18**:196–201.
11. Sheiner E, Levy A, Silverberg D, et al. Pregnancy after bariatric surgery is not associated with adverse perinatal outcome. *Am J Obstet Gynecol* 2004;**190**: 1335–40.
12. Sheiner E, Menes TS, Silverberg D, et al. Pregnancy outcome of patients with gestational diabetes mellitus following bariatric surgery. *Am J Obstet Gynecol* 2006;**194**:431–5.
13. Castro LC, Avina RL. Maternal obesity and pregnancy outcome. *Curr Opin Obstet Gynecol* 2002;**14**:601–6.

14. Robinson H, Tkatch S, Mayes DC, et al. Is maternal obesity a predictor of shoulder dystocia? *Obstet Gynecol* 2003;**101**:24–7.

15. Lu GC, Rouse DJ, DuBard M, et al. The effect of the increasing prevalence of maternal obesity on perinatal morbidity. *Am J Obstet Gynecol* 2001;**185**:845–9.

16. Bo S, Menato G, Signorile A, et al. Obesity or diabetes: what is worse for the mother and for the baby? *Diabetes Metab* 2003;**29**:175.

17. Sebire NJ, Jolly M, Harris JP, et al. Maternal obesity and pregnancy outcome: a study of 287,213 pregnancies in London. *Int J Obes Relat Metab Disord* 2001;**25**:1175–82.

18. Lashen H, Fear K, Sturdee DW. Obesity is associated with increased risk of first trimester and recurrent miscarriage: matched case-control study. *Hum Reprod* 2004;**19**:1644–6.

19. Fedorcsak P, Storeng R, Dale PO, et al. Obesity is a risk factor for early pregnancy loss after IVF or ICSI. *Acta Obstet Gynecol Scand* 2000;**79**:43–8.

20. Catalano PM. Management of obesity in pregnancy. *Obstet Gynecol* 2007;**109**:419–33.

21. Styne-Gross A, Elkind-Hirsch K, Scott RT Jr. Obesity does not impact implantation rates or pregnancy outcome in women attempting conception through oocyte donation. *Fertil Steril* 2005;**83**:1629–34.

22. Krishnamoorthy U, Schram CM, Hill SR. Maternal obesity in pregnancy: is it time for meaningful research to inform preventive and management strategies? *Br J Obstet Gynaecol* 2006;**113**:1134–40.

23. Ray JG, Wyatt PR, Vermuelen MJ, et al. Greater maternal weight and the ongoing risk of neural tube defects after folic acid flour fortification. *Obstet Gynecol* 2005;**105**:261–5.

24. Watkins ML, Rasmussen SA, Honein MA, et al. Maternal obesity and risk for birth defects. *Pediatrics* 2003;**111**:1152–8.

25. Watkins ML, Scanlon KS, Mulinare J, Khoury MJ. Is maternal obesity a risk factor for anencephaly and spina bifida? *Epidemiology* 1996;**7**:507–12.

26. Cedergren MI, Kallen BA. Maternal obesity and infant heart defects. *Obes Res* 2003;**11**:1065–71.

27. Waller DK, Mills JL, Simpson JL, et al. Are obese women at higher risk of producing malformed offspring? *Am J Obstet Gynecol* 1995;**172**:245–7.

28. Jenkins KJ, Correa A, Feinstein JA, et al. Noninherited risk factors and congenital cardiovascular defects: current knowledge. A Scientific Statement from the American Heart Association Council on Cardiovascular Disease in the Young. Endorsed by the American Academy of Pediatrics. *Circulation* 2007;**115**:2995–3014.

29. Galindo A, Burguillo AG, Azriel S, Fuente Pde L. Outcome of fetuses in women with pregestational diabetes mellitus. *J Perinat Med* 2006;**34**:323–31.

30. Wald N, Cuckle H, Boreham J, et al. The effect of maternal weight on maternal serum alpha-fetoprotein levels. *Br J Obstet Gynaecol* 1981;**88**:1094–6.

31. Yu CK, Teoh TG, Robinson S. Obesity in pregnancy. *Br J Obstet Gynaecol* 2006;**113**:1117–25.

32. Wolfe HM, Sokol RJ, Martier SM, Zador IE. Maternal obesity: a potential source of error in sonographic prenatal diagnosis. *Obstet Gynecol* 1990;**76**:339–42.

33. Hendler I, Blackwell SC, Bujold E, et al. The impact of maternal obesity on midtrimester sonographic visualization of fetal cardiac and craniospinal structures. *Int J Obes Relat Metab Disord* 2004;**28**:1607–11.

34. Hendler I, Blackwell SC, Bujold E, et al. Suboptimal second-trimester ultrasonographic visualization of the fetal heart in obese women: should we repeat the examination? *J Ultrasound Med* 2005;**24**:1205–9.

35. Hoegsberg B, Gruppuso PA, Coustan DR. Hyperinsulinemia in macrosomic infants of nondiabetic mothers. *Diabetes Care* 1993;**16**:32–6.

36. Weiss JL, Malone FD, Emig D, et al. FASTER Research Consortium. Obesity, obstetric complications and cesarean delivery rate: a population based screening study. *Am J Obstet Gynecol* 2004;**190**:1091–7.

37. Sheiner E, Levy A, Hershkovitz R, et al. Determining factors associated with shoulder dystocia: a population-based study. *Eur J Obstet Gynecol Reprod Biol* 2006;**126**:11–15.

38. Levy A, Sheiner E, Hammel RD, et al. Shoulder dystocia: a comparison of patients with and without diabetes mellitus. *Arch Gynecol Obstet* 2006;**273**:203–6.

39. Christoffersson M, Rydhstroem H. Shoulder dystocia and brachial plexus injury: a population-based study. *Gynecol Obstet Invest* 2002;**53**:42–7.

40. Wagner RK, Nielsen PE, Gonik B. Shoulder dystocia. *Obstet Gynecol Clin North Am* 1999;**26**:371–83.

41. Robinson H, Tkatch S, Mayes DC, et al. Is maternal obesity a predictor of shoulder dystocia? *Obstet Gynecol* 2003;**101**:24–7.

42. Kristensen J, Vestergaard M, Wisborg K, et al. Pre-pregnancy weight and the risk of stillbirth and neonatal death. *Br J Obstet Gynaecol* 2005;**112**:403–8.

43. Rode L, Nilas L, Wojdemann K, Tabor A. Obesity related complications in Danish singleton cephalic term pregnancies. *Obstet Gynecol* 2005;**105**:537–42.

44. Gonzalez-Quintero VH, Istwan NB, Rhea DJ, et al. The impact of glycemic control on neonatal outcome in singleton pregnancies complicated by gestational diabetes. *Diabetes Care* 2007;**30**:467–70.

45. Yogev Y, Langer O. Pregnancy outcome in obese and morbidly obese gestational diabetic women. *Eur J Obstet Gynecol Reprod Biol* 2008;**137**:21–6.

46. Kelly C, Allison, David B Sarwer, Emmanuelle Paré. Issues related to weight management during pregnancy among overweight and obese women. *Expert Rev Obstet Gynecol* 2007;**2**:249–54.

47. Smith GC, Shah I, Pell JP, et al. Maternal obesity in early pregnancy and risk of spontaneous and elective preterm deliveries: a retrospective cohort study. *Am J Public Health* 2007;**97**:157–62.

48. Usha Kiran TS, Hemmadi S, Bethel J, Evans J. Outcome of pregnancy in a woman with an increased body mass index. *Br J Obstet Gynaecol* 2005;**112**:768–72.

49. Taylor PD, Poston L. Developmental programming of obesity in mammals. *Exp Physiol* 2007;**92**:287–98.

50. Lawlor DA, Smith GD, O'Callaghan M, et al. Epidemiologic evidence for the fetal overnutrition hypothesis: findings from the Mater University study of pregnancy and its outcomes. *Am J Epidemiol* 2007;**165**:418–24.

51. Parsons TJ, Power C, Manor O. Fetal and early life growth and body mass index from birth to early adulthood in 1958 British cohort: longitudinal study. *BMJ* 2001;**323**:1331–5.

52. Parsons TJ, Power C, Logan S, Summerbell CD. Childhood predictors of adult obesity: a systematic review. *Int J Obes Relat Metab Disord* 1999;**23**(Suppl 8):S1–107.

53. Whitaker RC, Dietz WH. Role of the prenatal environment in the development of obesity. *J Pediatr* 1998;**132**:768–76.

54. Laitinen J, Power C, Järvelin MR. Family social class, maternal body mass index, childhood body mass index, and age at menarche as predictors of adult obesity. *Am J Clin Nutr* 2001;**74**:287–94.

55. Eriksson J, Forsén T, Osmond C, Barker D. Obesity from cradle to grave. *Int J Obes Relat Metab Disord* 2003;**27**:722–7.

56. Whitaker RC. Predicting preschooler obesity at birth: the role of maternal obesity in early pregnancy. *Pediatrics* 2004;**114**:e29–e36.

57. Li C, Kaur H, Choi WS, et al. Additive interactions of maternal prepregnancy BMI and breast-feeding on childhood overweight. *Obes Res* 2005;**13**:362–71.

58. Curhan GC, Willett WC, Rimm EB, et al. Birth weight and adult hypertension, diabetes mellitus, and obesity in US men. *Circulation* 1996;**94**:3246–50.

59. Curhan GC, Chertow GM, Willett WC, et al. Birth weight and adult hypertension and obesity in women. *Circulation* 1996;**94**:1310–15.

60. Sinha R, Fisch G, Teague B, et al. Prevalence of impaired glucose tolerance among children and adolescents with marked obesity. *N Engl J Med* 2002;**346**:802–10.

61. Oken E, Gillman MW. Fetal origins of obesity. *Obes Res* 2003;**11**:496–506.

62. Langer O, Yogev Y, Xenakis EM, Brustman L. Overweight and obese in gestational diabetes: the impact on pregnancy outcome. *Am J Obstet Gynecol* 2005;**192**:1768–76.

63. Dabelea D, Hanson RL, Lindsay RS, et al. Intrauterine exposure to diabetes conveys risks for type 2 diabetes and obesity: a study of discordant sibships. *Diabetes* 2000;**49**:2208–11.

64. Boney CM, Verma A, Tucker R, Vohr BR. Metabolic syndrome in childhood: association with birth weight, maternal obesity and gestational diabetes mellitus. *Pediatrics* 2005;**115**:e290–6.

65. Schäfer-Graf UM, Dupak J, Vogel M, et al. Hyperinsulinism, neonatal obesity and placental immaturity in infants born to women with one abnormal glucose tolerance test value. *J Perinat Med* 1998;**26**:27–36.

66. Conroy S, Ellis R, Murray C, Chaw-Kant J. An integrative review of Canadian childhood obesity prevention programmes. *Obes Rev* 2007;**8**:61–7.

SECTION 3

Preconceptual, Antenatal, and Postnatal Care

8 Antenatal care and ultrasound monitoring

Rebecca Black

Introduction

Women who are overweight or obese are at increased risk of developing problems in the antenatal period (Tables 8.1 and 8.2). It is therefore appropriate to tailor antenatal care to the needs of such women. Ideally, the type and pattern of antenatal care should be adjusted according to the degree of obesity. The reasons for any additional intervention or surveillance need to be thoroughly explained and understood by the woman and her family.

TABLE 8.1 Antenatal maternal and fetal risks of obesity

Maternal	Fetal
Miscarriage	Congenital abnormality
Pre-eclampsia	Stillbirth
Hypertensive disorders	Macrosomia
Diabetes	Birth injury
Venous thromboembolism	
Urinary tract infection	
Cholelithiasis	
Induction of labour	
Caesarean section	

TABLE 8.2 Examples of studies examining the magnitude of antenatal risks of overweight and obesity

Study type	Participants	Results				
Population based, USA[1]	16 102 singletons	Incidence (%)	BMI < 30	BMI 30–34.9	BMI > 35	
		Gestational HT	4.8	10.2	12.3	
		PET	2.1	3.0	6.3	
		GDM	2.3	6.3	9.5	
		CS (nullips only)	20.7	33.8	47.4	
Retrospective population-based, London, UK[2]	287 213 singleton pregnancies	OR compared with normal-weight women (99% CI)				
			BMI 25–9.9		BMI ≥ 30	
		GDM	1.68 (1.53–1.84)		3.6 (3.25–3.98)	
		PET	1.44 (1.28–1.62)		2.14 (1.85–2.47)	
		IOL	2.14 (1.85–2.47)		1.70 (1.64–1.76)	
		Emergency CS	1.30 (1.25–1.34)		1.83 (1.74–1.93)	
		UTI	1.17 (1.04–1.33)		1.39 (1.18–1.63)	
		IUD	1.10 (0.94–1.28)		1.40 (1.14–1.71)	
Population-based cohort, Aberdeen, UK[3]	24 241 singleton nullips	Incidence (%)	Normal weight	BMI 25–9.9	BMI 30–4.9	BMI ≥ 35
		PET	5	8.1	14.7	28.2
		IOL	27.2	33.4	42.8	49.0
		CS rate	16.4	24.1	30.8	42.7

TABLE 8.2 (continued)

Study type	Participants	Results			
Tertiary referral centre, Brisbane, Australia[4]	18 401 singletons	AOR compared with normal women (95% CI)			
			BMI 25.01–30	BMI 30.01–40	BMI >40
		HT disease	1.74 (1.45– 2.15)	3.00 (2.40– 3.74)	4.87 (3.27– 7.24)
		GDM	1.78 (1.25– 2.52)	2.95 (2.05– 4.25)	7.44 (4.42– 12.54)
		CS	1.50 (1.36– 1.66)	2.02 (1.79– 2.29)	2.54 (1.94– 3.32)

AOR, adjusted odds ratio; BMI, body mass index; CS, caesarean section; GDM, gestational diabetes mellitus; HT, hypertension; IOL, induction of labour; IUD, intrauterine death; nullips: nulliparous; OR, odds ratio; PET, pre-eclampsia; UTI, urinary tract infection.

Prepregnancy weight

More than half of women of childbearing age in the USA are overweight or obese. Obesity in pregnancy includes women who gain excess weight antenatally, or who carry excess weight prior to conception. Obesity in pregnancy affects all racial and ethnic groups, although non-Hispanic black women in the USA have the highest rate of obesity and weight gain, according to the CDC Pediatric and Pregnancy Nutrition Surveillance System.[5] Obesity in pregnancy is more common in lower socioeconomic groups.[2] For example, 43% of women in the WIC (Women, Infants, and Children) programme in the USA, which supports low-income, pregnant women, are overweight or obese prior to pregnancy, an increase of 19% in 20 years.[6]

Overweight and obesity constitute a worldwide public health problem. Pregnancy itself is too late to initiate weight-reduction programmes. The concept of provision of population-wide preconception care is rapidly taking hold, and, in 2005, the US Centers for Disease Control and Prevention (CDC) and the March of Dimes Charity convened a 3-day summit to discuss multiple issues surrounding preconception care programmes, research, and policy. The results of these deliberations were published as a supplement to the *Maternal and Child Health Journal*.[7] Simply stated, the numerous visits that a woman makes to a physician or healthcare provider prior to pregnancy should all be viewed as opportunities to advise and counsel her about proper health-seeking behaviours that optimize pregnancy outcome. Of the many potential issues that might be discussed, problems of overweight and obesity are high on the list. Having such programmes in place allows the risks associated with obesity or increased body mass index (BMI) to be repeatedly discussed and affords an opportunity for weight reduction prior to conception.

Interpregnancy weight gain

Multiparous women should be made aware before they conceive again that even modest weight gain between pregnancies is associated with increased risk of adverse outcome. One population-based study of over 150 000 women in Sweden showed that an increase in BMI of 3 units or more over an average of 2 years was followed by an increased risk of pre-eclampsia (adjusted OR [odds ratio] 1.78, 95% confidence interval [CI] 1.52–2.08), gestational hypertension (1.76, 1.39–2.23), gestational diabetes (2.09, 1.68–2.61), caesarean delivery (1.32, 1.22–1.44), stillbirth (1.63, 1.20–2.21), and large-for-gestational-age birth (1.87, 1.72–2.04). There was a linear association between the complications and the amount of weight gained. The risks affected both overweight women and those with normal BMI for both pregnancies.[8]

First visit in pregnancy

Both the ACOG (American College of Obstetricians and Gynecologists) in the USA[9] and NICE (National Institute for Health and Clinical Excellence) guidelines in the UK[10] recommend that all women should have their height and weight measured at the first antenatal appointment, and the woman's BMI should be calculated (weight [kg]/height [m][2]). In the UK, referral from the community to a consultant obstetrician is advised if the BMI is greater than or equal to 35.[10] In the UK, repeat measurements during pregnancy are not recommended, because of purported lack of evidence of benefit and the risk of causing 'unnecessary anxiety'. The only situation where repeated measurements are advised by NICE are if there are concerns about the woman's nutrition. In the USA, on the other hand, weight (but not height) is obtained at every visit for normal pregnancy as well as in the context of abnormal pregnancy conditions such as pre-eclampsia, where sudden increases in weight can indicate fluid retention. Practical preparations for delivery may necessitate repeated weighing of very obese women and special hospital preparation (see Chapters 9, 15, and 16).

The ACOG guidelines on obesity in pregnancy recommend that nutrition consultation should be offered to all obese women. They should also be advised to follow an exercise programme. These should continue after pregnancy and prior to planning another pregnancy.[9]

Weight gain during pregnancy

In 1990 the Institute of Medicine (IOM)[11] published guidelines for the recommended amount of weight gain in pregnancy according to prepregnancy BMI. The guidelines advised that women of normal weight should gain 11.5–16 kg (25–35 lb) during pregnancy. Overweight (BMI 25–29.9) women should gain 7–11.5 kg (15–25 lb). Obese women (BMI greater than 30) are advised to gain 6.8 kg (approximately 15 lb). No higher limit is specified in the IOM guidelines.[11]

These guidelines are now almost 20 years old and the growing concern about obesity suggests the need for revisions based on the evidence compiled in the years since the original publication. Other chapters in this volume also echo this concern.

One cohort study published in 1998, for example, comparing morbidly obese women with those of normal weight, found that weight gains of more than 25 lb (11.5 kg) were correlated with delivery of a large-for-gestational-age (LGA) neonate, and thus recommended that such gains should be avoided.[12] Several other studies published between 1996 and 2004 have shown that reduced gestational weight gain lowers the incidence of both LGA births and caesarean sections.[13–15] An observational study of more than 120 000 obese women in Missouri published in 2007 showed that reduced gestational weight gains were associated with lower incidence of pre-eclampsia.[16] A population-based cohort study of nearly 300 000 Swedish women, also published in 2007, examined maternal and fetal outcomes and suggested that the optimal weight gain according to prepregnancy BMI was less that recommended by the IOM – less than 20 lb (<9 kg) for a BMI 25–29.9 and less than 13 lb (<6 kg) for a BMI of 30 or more.[17] It must be remembered, however, that the 20-lb (9 kg) ceiling on weight gain for normal women that was so prevalent in the mid-twentieth century was a hold-over from the famous Prochownick diet of the late nineteenth century as a means to reduce fetal weight because of the widespread prevalence of rickets at that time.

The IOM guidelines also recommend that all obese women should receive an individual dietary assessment and nutritional counselling.[11] However, overweight and obese women find optimal weight gain targets difficult to achieve. The CDC Pediatric and Pregnancy Nutrition Surveillance System, for example, showed that, in 2006, 59.1% of the 133 760 overweight women studied gained more weight than defined as ideal by the IOM guidelines.[5] Worse, 43.2% of all women gained more weight in pregnancy than considered ideal.

Blood pressure

Blood pressure should be measured and recorded at the first and every subsequent antenatal visit. An appropriate-size cuff must be used. ACOG guidelines recommend use of a blood pressure cuff at least 1.5 times the upper arm circumference, or a cuff with a bladder that encircles at least 80% of the arm.[18] In the UK, PRECOG guidelines advise use of different cuff sizes according to the circumference of the upper arm (Table 8.3). Less error is caused by using too large a cuff than too small a cuff.[19] The arm circumference and cuff size used at the initial visit should be recorded in the woman's case notes for future reference.

TABLE 8.3 Cuff sizes for measurement of blood pressure[19]

Arm circumference	Appropriate cuff	Cuff size
Up to 33 cm	Standard	13 × 23 cm
Between 33 and 41 cm	Large	15 × 33 cm
41 cm or more	Thigh cuff	18 × 36 cm

Screening for diabetes

In the USA in 2005, nearly 21 million people had diabetes, 17 million of whom had type 2. The development of type 2 diabetes is clearly and indubitably associated with weight gain.[20] A recent review of the prevalence of gestational diabetes mellitus (GDM) showed that the incidence of both prepregnancy diabetes and GDM is increasing; the prevalence of GDM reflects the prevalence of type 2 diabetes within a population.[21] Prevalence rates of GDM range from 2% in Sweden to 4.9–12.8% in high-risk populations such as northern Californian Hispanics and Asians.[21] A study of birth certificate data from Minnesota shows prepregnancy and GDM rates increasing from 2.6 to 4.9 and from 25.6 to 34.8 per 1000 live births, respectively, over a 10-year period (1993–2003).

Screening at the time of the initial visit will identify those with undetected type 2 diabetes. ACOG guidelines advise that all women should be screened for GDM, whether by patient history, clinical risk factors, or a laboratory screening test to determine blood glucose levels.[23] The ACHOIS study demonstrated clear benefits of treatment of gestational diabetes.[24] Women with raised BMI are in a high-risk category and should have laboratory-based screening. ACOG guidelines advise a 50-g, 1-h oral glucose challenge at 24–28 weeks' gestation.[23]

Those women who develop GDM should be carefully counselled about their future. Their risk of developing GDM in a future pregnancy is reduced if they lose weight prior to the onset of that pregnancy. In one study, a loss of 10 lb (4.5 kg) gave a relative risk of 0.63 (95% CI 0.38–1.02), whereas a gain of 10 lb increased the risk of GDM to 1.47 (1.05–2.04).[25] More than half of women with GDM will go on to develop type 2 diabetes in later life.[23] The risk is increased in those who are obese.[20] The postnatal period is an ideal time to offer advice about weight loss to reduce the long-term consequences of overweight and obesity (see also Chapters 10 and 14).

Attitudes to overweight and obesity

Public perception of obesity is generally extremely negative; many see people with a weight problem as 'greedy' in terms of their food consumption or 'lazy' in terms of their unwillingness to engage in exercise. However, as other chapters of this volume so amply detail, obesity is a complex problem that is poorly understood by patients, their healthcare providers, and society in general, and one that is not easily solved.

Even the process of discussing obesity with women at the time of their surgery visit can be difficult. Healthcare professionals want to avoid appearing judgemental, or being criticized for making remarks that are considered too personal. Little published advice or information is available on how to address the issue. In the UK, the National Obesity Forum[26] has some general advice, suggesting that it is important to do the following:

- Acknowledge the extent and complexity of the issues surrounding obesity; e.g., that it is not just a condition of individuals who are in some way inadequate
- Initiate the discussion, as women may be reluctant to raise the issue themselves
- Recognize that most, if not all, women who are overweight are aware of their weight problem.

In the USA, the NAAFA (National Association to Advance Fat Acceptance) notes that many overweight patients have had negative experiences with healthcare providers. They provide advice for healthcare professionals about dealing with those for whom increased weight is an issue, as well as practical advice, from provision of armless, waiting-room chairs to stools to help reach the treatment couch.[27]

At the end of the discussion, it is imperative that women be aware of the effect that their BMI may have on their pregnancy. Plans for any increased investigation or pregnancy surveillance should be discussed and supported by written information.

Ongoing antenatal care

Hypertension and pre-eclampsia

Women with an elevated BMI need to be seen more frequently during pregnancy, in particular to monitor complications such as hypertension and pre-eclampsia because of their increased risk.[28,29] There is little consensus on the frequency of antenatal visits in such women. The PRECOG guidelines[19] suggest that for women with BMI greater than 35 and no other risk factor, visits should be at least every 3 weeks at 24–32 weeks' gestation and then at least every 2 weeks after 32 weeks. In the USA, weekly visits generally begin at 36 weeks' gestation, and many practitioners are not reluctant to see problem patients on a weekly basis even earlier.

Women who are significantly overweight are at increased risk of manifestations of the metabolic syndrome – hypertension, proteinuria, dyslipidaemia, and diabetes. As such, they may present with illnesses previously thought to affect an older age group, such as sleep apnoea, non-alcoholic fatty liver disease, and chronic cardiac and renal dysfunction. Sleep apnoea in particular can be diagnosed early in pregnancy or even preconceptually by appropriate sleep studies if the caregiver suspects its existence and questions the patient's sleeping partner. In a recent review of the management of the obese woman in pregnancy,

Catalano[29] suggests that such patients should be considered for assessment of cardiac and renal function. Pre-eclampsia and chronic hypertension can be difficult to distinguish in late pregnancy, and early baseline assessment of renal function and the quantification of proteinuria may help in diagnosis and management later on. Baseline liver function tests may also be useful, because their rise may be a manifestation of non-alcoholic fatty liver disease rather than severe pre-eclampsia.[29]

The Confidential Enquiries into Maternal Deaths in the UK 1994–6 emphasised the importance of educating all pregnant women about the symptoms of pre-eclampsia and the need to seek urgent advice.[30] This is particularly relevant to a high-risk group such as overweight women.

Venous thromboembolism

Venous thromboembolism (VTE) in pregnancy is a leading cause of maternal death in both the USA and the UK; in the USA, it accounts for 11% of maternal deaths.[31] In one population-based, case–control study of Danish women, a BMI of over 30 increased the risk of both pulmonary embolism (PE) (OR 14.9 [95% CI 3.0–74.8]) and deep venous thrombosis (DVT) (OR 4.4 [95% CI 1.6–11.9]).[32] A study of over 287 000 women in London, UK, showed a prevalence of thromboembolism of 0.04% in normal-weight, 0.07% in overweight, and 0.08% in obese women.[2] A national study of PE in the UK showed an adjusted OR of 2.93 (95% CI 1.09–7.83) for women with BMI > 30.[33]

The ACOG guidelines on thromboembolism in pregnancy do not discuss obesity.[34] Guidelines from The Royal College of Obstetricians and Gynaecologists (RCOG), however, state that a BMI of > 30, either prepregnancy or in early pregnancy, is an additional risk factor for VTE in pregnancy.[35] A detailed history, to seek other risk factors, including personal and family history, should be sought. Those with three or more risk factors should be considered for antenatal thromboprophylaxis with low-molecular-weight heparin (LMWH). Using these guidelines, a woman who is obese would not qualify; however, if she had other pre-existing risks, or acquired risks such as immobility during pregnancy, then consideration should be given to heparin thromboprophylaxis. A woman who is extremely obese, on the other hand, should be considered at even higher risk. The guideline also states that clinical judgement should be exercised, and there may be circumstances in which one or two risk factors may be sufficient for the administration of LMWH; 'for example an extremely obese woman admitted to the antenatal ward' (an actual BMI is not stated). At a minimum, steps such as avoiding dehydration and immobility, and use of TED (thromboembolic deterrent) stockings should be employed if hospital admission is required (see Chapters 9, 10, and 16).

Even if a woman with a BMI > 30 has had a vaginal birth, she is still at risk of postnatal VTE. The RCOG guidelines suggest that this factor, in combination with any other risk factor for VTE, should prompt consideration of treatment with LMWH for 3–5 days post partum. Plans for postnatal thromboprophylaxis should be discussed with the woman and documented in her notes as part of antenatal management (but should remain flexible, as they may be influenced by factors such as mode of delivery, blood loss, or clotting abnormalities). A somewhat more conservative point of view is that of a recent consensus report from the USA, which stated that more studies are required to determine the impact of factors such as obesity on the risk of VTE, and the effectiveness of VTE-prevention strategies on such risks.[31]

Both prophylactic and treatment doses of LMWH vary with maternal weight, so care should be taken to ensure that an adequate does is prescribed.

Stillbirth

Women who are overweight are at increased risk of stillbirth. A study of a retrospective cohort of over 280 000 pregnancies in London, for example, showed an OR for in utero death of 1.10 (95% CI 0.94–1.28) in moderately obese women and 1.40 (1.14–1.71) in very obese women.[2] A cohort study of more than 24 000 Danish women showed that maternal obesity more than doubled the risk of stillbirth (OR 2.8, 95% CI 1.5–5.3) and neonatal death (OR 2.6, 1.2–5.8).[36] A US population study covering more than 1.5 million deliveries in the USA found that obese mothers were 40% more likely to experience stillbirth than non-obese gravidas (hazards ratio 1.4 [95% CI 1.3–1.5]). These authors also noted that the risk of stillbirth increased in a dose-related fashion with ascending obesity class (P < 0.01).[37] A recent meta-analysis of nine studies showed an unadjusted OR for stillbirth of 1.47 (95% CI 1.59–2.74) for obese women compared with women of normal weight.[38]

Reasons for this association are unclear. Possibilities include: increased rates of diabetes and hypertensive disorders in pregnancy, both of which are known risk factors for stillbirth; undiagnosed diabetes or glucose intolerance; the altered metabolic state known to exist in the obese; the inherent difficulty in feeling reduced fetal movements among obese women, which may reduce the opportunity for intervention to avoid stillbirth; and, finally, the predisposition of obese women to sleep-related disordered breathing[39] (the fetus is an end-organ and reduced oxygen levels may reduce uterine blood flow).

Fetal growth

An estimation of fetal size should be made at each antenatal visit. The NICE guidelines recommend measurement of the symphysiofundal height (SFH) in centimetres with a tape measure. Serial measurements should be plotted on a chart to help detect small- and large-for-dates babies.[10] Measurement of SFH is non-invasive and requires minimal equipment, training, and time. However, the solitary use of a tape measure (especially if the person doing the measurements is different each time) is notoriously inaccurate in the prediction of fetal growth, and many abnormal fetal growth patterns may be missed. Estimation of fetal size, lie, presentation, and growth based on abdominal palpation can be also be unreliable in obese women.[40] Serial growth scans can be considered but are not always reliable (see below).

Third trimester

The NICE guidelines state that fetal presentation should be assessed by abdominal palpation at or beyond 36 weeks' gestation, but this may be a daunting task, if not impossible, in the very obese or morbidly obese patient, where ultrasound has a real value. Suspected malpresentation should always be confirmed by ultrasound whether the woman is obese or not. Those with an uncomplicated, singleton, breech presentation should be offered external cephalic version (ECV).

Risks for delivery

Induction of labour

Induction rates are generally higher in overweight women.[2,3] While this is a truism, it should not be forgotten that induction is not a benign phenomenon; rather, it increases intervention rates in itself. A study of 5131 women, for example, showed an increase in the incidence of failed induction in both overweight women ($P < 0.001$) and women who had gained more than one unit of BMI during pregnancy ($P < 0.001$).[14] Under these circumstances, induction of overweight women for 'soft' indications should be avoided.

Caesarean section

Both elective and emergency caesarean section rates are higher in overweight women (Table 8.2).

Vaginal birth after caesarean (VBAC)

Obesity reduces the chances of successful VBAC after one lower-segment caesarean section. In a study of 1213 women whose first child had been delivered by lower-segment caesarean section, the success rate for VBAC was 77.2% overall. The success rates for BMI groups of < 19, 19–26, 26–29, and > 29 were 83.1%, 79.9%, 69.3%, and 68.2%, respectively ($P < 0.001$). Women who gained more than 40 lb (18 kg) during pregnancy had a VBAC success rate of 66.8%, while those who gained less than 40 lb had a success rate of 79.1% ($P < 0.001$).[41] In another study of 510 women attempting VBAC, a success rate of 54.6% was achieved in obese women compared with 70.5% in women of normal BMI ($P = 0.003$).[42] A cohort study of 122 mothers showed a 57% VBAC success rate in obese women.[43] A cohort of 69 women each with a prepregnancy weight of over 300 lb (135 kg) had a VBAC success rate of just 13%, compared with a success rate of 57.1% in 70 women of 200–300 lb (90–135 kg) and 81.8% in 70 women weighing less than 200 lb (90 kg) prepregnancy.[44] Such evidence is compelling, and these reduced success rates may influence any decision to opt for a VBAC versus the alternative of a repeat elective caesarean section.

Anaesthetic referral

Overweight women should be seen before labour by an obstetric anaesthetist, because the risk of intervention in labour is higher and they are more likely to have coexisting medical diseases. Anaesthetic complications (such as a difficult intubation) are more common,[45] and obesity is a risk factor for anaesthesia-related maternal mortality.[46] These issues need to be discussed, explained, and explored with the patient early on when the discussion is also addressing the appropriate unit in which the patient should deliver (see below) (see Chapter 16).

Place of delivery

Both the recent NICE guidance on intrapartum care[47] and the Confidential Enquiry into Maternal and Child Health (CEMACH)[48] recommended that women with a BMI > 35 should be booked for delivery in a consultant-led rather than a midwifery-led unit. In the USA, many large teaching units have special clinics for the obese. Access to experienced obstetricians and anaesthetists, as well as a fully equipped operating suite with operating table capable of withstanding the weight of the morbidly obese patient, is necessary.

Practical arrangements for delivery

The management of women who are significantly overweight involves risk assessment and planning for practical aspects of caring for the woman, in particular when she arrives in labour. The weight of such women needs to be monitored throughout pregnancy and communicated in advance to the labour/delivery unit. Appropriate equipment such as beds, chairs, hoists, operating tables, and surgical instruments (such as bariatric operative equipment[49]) should be on hand long before the expected date of confinement in the event that preterm labour ensues. Part or all of this equipment may need to be borrowed or hired, so it is essential to plan effectively during the antenatal period. Most modern operating tables will support a body weight of 130–160 kg, but newer tables supporting weights of up to 360 kg are now commercially available.[50] Standard hospital beds will support a weight of around 230 kg, but operating on a hospital bed is suboptimal in terms of surgical access and comfort for operating staff and assistants. Various surgical incisional approaches have been suggested for the morbidly obese patient, as well as techniques such as the use of drains and staples; much will depend on the experience of the surgeon in charge (see Chapter 15). All such issues should ideally be discussed with the patient pre-operatively.[50]

Ultrasound monitoring

Ultrasound is used in modern obstetric practice to date pregnancies, to screen for aneuploidy and other fetal anomalies, and to monitor fetal growth and well-being. Although there have been significant technological advances in the quality of ultrasound machines, transabdominal ultrasound remains more difficult to perform in obese women. The excess adipose tissue attenuates the ultrasound signal. In order to penetrate the tissue and obtain an adequate depth of field, a lower-frequency signal is required, and this produces an image with lower resolution.[51]

Screening for aneuploidy

There are a multitude of screening tests for aneuploidy (mainly focusing on the detection of trisomy 21). In the UK, the National Screening Committee states that all women should be offered a screening test with a detection rate of at least 75% for a 3% invasive testing rate. In the USA, the ACOG guidelines advise that all women should be offered aneuploidy screening before 20 weeks' gestation, regardless of maternal age.[52] Screening tests involve blood tests in isolation (serum screening) or in combination with ultrasound and measurement of nuchal translucency.

Nuchal translucency scanning to detect aneuploidy was first described in the early 1990s. It is now well established that an increased nuchal translucency measurement can be an early presenting feature of fetal chromosomal, genetic, and structural anomalies.[52] The scan can be difficult to perform; specialized training, along with ongoing education and audit, is required to ensure that the scan is performed to a high standard.[53] Very little is written about how technically easy or difficult the scan is to perform in obese women. In one study, a nuchal scan was attempted in 1368 women attending for a routine first-trimester dating scan in 1992–3. The mean BMI of the group was 22.9. The nuchal scan was successfully completed in 82% of patients. The commonest reasons given for the inability to achieve the nuchal scan were fetal position and maternal obesity, although no numbers are given.[54]

Improved accuracy in the detection of fetal aneuploidy can be achieved by combining the measurement of nuchal translucency with serum analytes.[52] Maternal weight affects the levels of both first- and second-trimester serum markers detected in maternal blood. Increased maternal weight leads to lower levels of markers. The markers are fetally or placentally derived, and thus tend to be more diluted in larger women with increased blood volumes.[55] In the context of screening for Down's syndrome, dilution will increase the risk of false-positive results unless the results take into account the maternal weight. With maternal serum PAPP-A (pregnancy-associated plasma protein A) and free β-hCG (β-human chorionic gonadotraphin), a twofold variation in individual risk has been demonstrated depending on the mother's weight.[56] Maternal weight is routinely incorporated into screening programmes; it needs to be recorded accurately and documented on the request card when sending samples to the laboratory.

Congenital abnormality

Women who are overweight are at increased risk of having a baby with a congenital abnormality. This has been demonstrated in several studies (Table 8.4). The reasons for this circumstance are not entirely clear; the possible causes include: type 2 diabetes undiagnosed at conception; lower serum folate levels in overweight women, leading to an increased risk of neural tube defects NTDs; inadequate preconceptional folate intake; and decreased detection of fetal anomalies in obese women, leading to the continuation of pregnancies that otherwise have been terminated.

A case–control study of mothers enrolled in the National Birth Defects prevention Study across eight US states examined the relationships between maternal weight and the risk of structural birth defects.[57] The investigators found that overweight and obese mothers were at significantly increased risk of babies with spina bifida (adjusted OR [AOR] with BMI $\geq$ 30 2.10 [95% CI 1.63–2.71]), heart defects (1.40 [1.24–1.59]), anorectal atresia (1.46 [1.10–1.95]), hypospadias (1.33 [1.03–1.72]), limb reduction defects (1.36 [1.05–1.77]), diaphragmatic hernia (1.42 [1.03–1.98], and omphalocoele (1.63 [1.07–2.47].[57] However, the risk of gastroschisis was decreased (0.19 [0.10–0.34]), whereas there was no significant increase in the incidence of facial clefting. This is in contrast to another study of 1686 cases of cleft lip with or without cleft palate, which showed a slight increase in risk in obese (BMI > 29) women (AOR 1.30 [1.11–1.53]).[58] Other studies have found similar increases in the risk of spina bifida; obesity approximately doubles the risk of an NTD.[59] The increased risk of heart defects was also similar in other studies to the rates found in the latter study.[59]

Obese women are thus at risk of having babies with NTDs, cardiac anomalies, or omphalocoele. As these are similar anomalies to those seen in the offspring of mothers with diabetes, one cannot help but surmise that undiagnosed diabetes may be an important cause of congenital anomaly, a concept that the literature has not brought forward in the past.

TABLE 8.4 Maternal obesity and risk of congenital abnormality

	Reference
Neural tube defects	57, 59–61
Heart defects	57, 59, 62–64
Anorectal atresia	57
Hypospadias	57
Limb reduction defects	57
Congenital diaphragmatic hernia (CDH)	57
Omphalocoele	57, 59
Multiple anomalies	59
Orofacial clefting	58, 64
Talipes	64

NTDs are associated with folic acid deficiencies. Periconceptual supplementation with folic acid is well established as a way of reducing the incidence of NTDs, as obese women have lower serum folate concentrations. Some countries have introduced the fortification of flour with folic acid. However, one study has shown no evidence of benefit in terms of a reduction in the incidence of NTDs after introduction of this policy in Canada.[60]

Folic acid should be taken by all women periconceptually from 2–3 months prior to conception to reduce the incidence of NTDs (see Chapter 12). Consideration should also be given to starting obese women on higher doses of folic acid than the standard 400-µg dose, given their increased risk of NTDs, although the benefit of this in non-diabetic obese women has not been established.[9]

The ACOG advises that NTD screening should be offered in the second trimester to women who elect only first-trimester screening for aneuploidy.[52] This is especially relevant to obese women in whom ultrasound imaging of the fetus may be suboptimal.

Fetal imaging

Performing a transabdominal ultrasound scan is technically more difficult in a woman with elevated BMI. Technical alterations in the ultrasound machine, such as lowering frequency, may help optimize visualization. Scanning suprapubically or with the woman lying on her side may target areas where there is less adipose tissue.

One study scanning women at 28 weeks' gestation showed impaired visualization of fetal anatomy at a maternal BMI above the 90th percentile, when visualization fell by 14.5%.[65] The most difficult structures to see were the fetal heart and spine. Another study of over 11 000 patients showed that visualization of fetal anatomy was suboptimal in over 37% of obese patients compared with 18.7% of women of normal weight ($P < 0.0001$).[66] Problems remain even with advancing ultrasound technology. Deferring examination until a later week of gestation may be of some benefit; one study found fewer suboptimal views of the cardiac outflow tracts if the examination was performed after 18 weeks' gestation.[67] Repeating the examination may also help.[68] An experienced sonographer should perform the examination.

Transvaginal ultrasound has the advantage of bypassing maternal abdominal adipose tissue and can be used to examine the fetus; this is particularly helpful at earlier gestations (i.e., the first trimester). After this time, however, certain aspects of the fetus (such as the brain) may be amenable to transvaginal examination, dependent on fetal position. One study examined 25 consecutive obese women in whom fetal imaging had been deemed unsatisfactory when performed by the conventional transabdominal route – 19 because the fetal heart could not be seen properly. The umbilicus was filled with gel and a transvaginal probe used to visualize the fetus via the umbilicus. By this approach, the fetal heart was successfully visualized in 18 of the 19 cases, and a full examination became possible in all but one of the cases.[69]

The use of three-dimensional and four-dimensional ultrasound does not overcome the disadvantages of maternal obesity. The quality of a three-dimensional rendering is critically dependent on the quality of the two-dimensional image.[70] At the same time, magnetic resonance imaging (MRI) can be used as an adjunct to ultrasound, although it is unlikely to replace ultrasound as a routine diagnostic technique, not least because of the time taken to obtain images, its high cost, and the need to have expensive machines in referral centres to obtain the test. MRI is not affected by maternal obesity and may be helpful in situations where the possibility of an anomaly has been raised as the result of an ultrasound scan. It is particularly useful for suspected fetal central nervous system anomalies or in imaging non-fetal problems, such as ovarian cysts and fibroids,[70] both of which may be more difficult to visualize in the obese woman.

Fetal growth

Maternal obesity is an independent risk factor for fetal macrosomia. Obese women are more difficult to palpate abdominally. Overweight women are often referred for a scan for suspected 'large for dates'. However, ultrasound is not entirely accurate in detecting large babies. Although accuracy may be improving with advanced technology, one recent study of 1177 women in New Zealand showed an error in estimating fetal weight of more than 10% in one in four women.[71] Ultrasound tended to underestimate the weight of large infants (20% were estimated to be over 10% below and 6% over 10% above the actual birth weight). Ultrasound had the opposite effect in small-for-gestational age fetuses; it tended to overestimate those with birth weights less than 2500 g. It underestimated the weight of babies of diabetic mothers, whether they were large for dates or of normal weight.[71] Inaccuracy was also found in a systematic review of 11 studies of the estimation of fetal weight with ultrasound.[72] Among the non-diabetic women, ultrasound estimation of fetal weight detected only 60% of infants weighing more than 4000 g and just half those weighing more than 4500 g. The authors concluded that ultrasound did not reliably predict fetal macrosomia.[71] The implication of a 10% degree of error is that, if the ultrasound gives an estimated fetal weight of 4000 kg, the actual weight may be 3600–4400 g. This accuracy is not enough to be clinically useful. The ACOG has produced guidelines on the management of fetal macrosomia, concluding that the diagnosis of macrosomia is imprecise and that, when it is suspected, the use of ultrasound is no better than clinical palpation (level A recommendation).[73]

Both the ACOG in the USA and the NICE in the UK advise against induction of labour for suspected fetal macrosomia because of lack of evidence of benefit in terms of improved maternal or neonatal outcomes.[73,74] While accepting the imprecision of the diagnosis of macrosomia, the ACOG guidelines also suggest that prophylactic caesarean section may be considered with an estimated fetal weight of more than 5000 g in non-diabetic women and 4500 g in women with diabetes (level C recommendation).[73]

Future studies

The UK Obstetric Surveillance System (UKOSS) was established in 2005 and is run by the National Perinatal Epidemiology Unit (NPEU). It is a system that aims to study rare disorders of pregnancy on a national scale. It is currently conducting a survey of extreme obesity[75] to include women with a weight of more than 140 kg or BMI of more than 50 at any point during pregnancy, or a weight estimated to be in either of the above categories but which exceeds the capacity of the hospital scales. The aims are to establish the prevalence of extreme obesity in the UK, including the prevalence among different socioeconomic and ethnic groups. It will study the risk of adverse outcome associated with such obesity, and any adverse outcomes associated with inadequate weight capacity equipment. The study will run for 12 months.

Many observational studies now exist, examining the issue of obesity in pregnancy. However, there are as yet few interventional trials of the effect of weight reduction in obese women either before or during pregnancy.[40] There is no doubt that many issues surrounding obesity need to be addressed before pregnancy. However, pregnancy is a time when women meet healthcare professionals on a regular basis, perhaps for the first time in their adult lives, and, as such, this may be an opportunity at least to begin to gain control of this issue. Evidence of the benefit of intervention with regard to diet, exercise, and weight gain in pregnancy will help define these aims.

In the Confidential Enquiry into Maternal Deaths in the UK 2000–2, 78 (35%) women who died had a BMI of 30 or more.[76] In the 2003–5 report, more than half the women who died from direct or indirect causes were overweight or obese. The authors commented that 'obese pregnant women with a body mass index >30 are far more likely to die'. They stated that a national guideline for the management of the obese pregnant woman was urgently required.[48]

Conclusions

Pregnancy in a woman who is overweight is by definition a high-risk pregnancy. Management of that pregnancy therefore needs to be tailored to the needs of the woman in a way that is safe and acceptable for her as well as her baby. A suggested outline is presented in Table 8.5.

TABLE 8.5 Summary of suggestions for antenatal care for overweight and obese women

Prepregnancy	• Weight reduction • Folic acid (?increased dose) • Screen for type 2 diabetes
First visit	• Record height and weight and calculate BMI • Appropriate-size cuff for blood pressure measurement • If BMI > 35, refer to anaesthetist • Record weight when sending screening tests • Baseline investigations if morbidly obese • Decide appropriate pattern of antenatal care and place of delivery • Refer for nutrition consultation
Anomaly scan	• Experienced sonographer • Explain limitations of scan • Consider TVS/MRI if anomalies suspected
Ongoing care	• Discuss risks • Increase surveillance for PET, GDM, VTE
3rd trimester	• Screen for GDM • Monitor for PET, as a minimum as per PRECOG guidelines • Low threshold for scan if fetal presentation uncertain • Monitor weight and ensure equipment available at place of delivery
Preparation for labour	• Avoid IOL for 'soft' indications • Ensure obstetrician/anaesthetist/delivery suite aware • Discuss increased risks of intervention and management plans for possible operative delivery • Plan postnatal thromboprophylaxis

BMI, body mass index; GDM, gestational diabetes mellitus; IOL, induction of labour; MRI, magnetic resonance imaging; PET, pre-eclampsia; TVS, transvaginal sonography; VTE, venous thromboembolism.

References

1. Weiss JL, Malone FD, Emig D, et al. Obesity, obstetric complications and cesarean delivery rate – a population-based screening study. *Am J Obstet Gynecol* 2004;**190**:1091–7.
2. Sebire NJ, Jolly M, Harris JP, et al. Maternal obesity and pregnancy outcome: a study of 287 213 pregnancies in London. *Int J Obes Relat Metab Disord* 2001;**25**:1175–82.
3. Bhattacharya S, Campbell DM, Liston WA, Bhattacharya S. Effect of body mass index on pregnancy outcomes in nulliparous women delivering singleton babies. *BMC Public Health* 2007;**7**:168.
4. Callaway LK, Prins JB, Chang AM, McIntyre HD. The prevalence and impact of overweight and obesity in an Australian obstetric population. *Med J Aust* 2006;**184**:56–9.
5. Centers for Disease Control and Prevention. The Pediatric Nutrition Surveillance System (PedNSS) and the Pregnancy Surveillance System (PNSS). Atlanta: CDC, 2008. Available at: www.cdc.gov/pednss.
6. Riley L. *A call to action: obesity and pregnancy. Women's Health Policy Brief*. Massachusetts Physicians Organization, 2006.
7. Atrash HK, Keith LG, eds. Preconception care: science, practice, challenges and opportunities. *J Matern Child Health* 2006;**10**(Suppl 1):1–207.
8. Villamor E, Cnattingius S. Interpregnancy weight change and risk of adverse pregnancy outcomes: a population-based study. *Lancet* 2006;**368**:1164–70.
9. American College of Obstetricians and Gynecologists. Obesity in Pregnancy. ACOG Committee Opinion No. 315. *Obstet Gynecol* 2005;**106**:671–5.
10. National Institute for Health and Clinical Effectiveness. *Antenatal care*. London: NICE. Available at: www.nice.org.uk.
11. Committee on Nutritional Status During Pregnancy and Lactation, Institute of Medicine. *Nutrition during pregnancy: Part I – Weight gain; Part II – Nutrient supplements. Executive Summary*. Washington DC: National Academy Press, 1990.
12. Bianco AT, Smilen SW, Davis Y, et al. Pregnancy outcome and weight gain recommendations for the morbidly obese woman. *Obstet Gynecol* 1998;**91**: 97–102.
13. Edwards LE, Hellerstedt WL, Alton IR, et al. Pregnancy complications and birth outcomes in obese and normal-weight women: effects of gestational weight change. *Obstet Gynecol* 1996;**87**:389–94.
14. Kabiru W, Raynor BD. Obstetric outcomes associated with increase in BMI category during pregnancy. *Am J Obstet Gynecol* 2004;**191**:928–32.
15. Ogunyemi D, Hullett S, Leeper J, Risk A. Prepregnancy body mass index, weight gain during pregnancy, and perinatal outcome in a rural black population. *J Matern Fetal Med* 1998;**7**:190–3.
16. Kiel DW, Dodson EA, Artal R, et al. Gestational weight gain and pregnancy outcomes in obese women: how much is enough? *Obstet Gynecol* 2007;**110**: 752–8.

17. Cedergren MI. Optimal gestational weight gain for body mass index categories. *Obstet Gynecol* 2007;**110**:759–64.
18. ACOG Practice Bulletin no. 33. Diagnosis and management of preeclampsia and eclampsia. *Obstet Gynecol* 2002;**99**:159–70.
19. PRECOG guidelines. Available at: www.apec.org.uk.
20. Reece EA. Perspectives on obesity, pregnancy and birth outcomes in the United States: the scope of the problem. *Am J Obstet Gynecol* 2008;**198**:23–7.
21. Hunt KJ, Schuller KL. The increasing prevalence of diabetes in pregnancy. *Obstet Gynecol Clin North Am* 2007;**34**:173–99.
22. Devlin HM, Desai J, Holzman GS, Gilbertson DT. Trends and disparities among diabetes-complicated births in Minnesota, 1993–2003. *Am J Public Health* 2008;**98**:59–62.
23. ACOG Practice Bulletin no. 30. Gestational diabetes. *Obstet Gynecol* 2001;**98**:525–38.
24. Crowther CA, Hiller JE, Moss JR, et al. Australian Carbohydrate Intolerance Study in Pregnant Women (ACHOIS) Trial Group. *N Engl J Med* 2005;**352**:2477–86.
25. Glazer NL, Hendrickson AF, Schellenbaum GD, Mueller BA. Weight change and the risk of gestational diabetes in obese women. *Epidemiology* 2004;**15**: 733–7.
26. National Obesity Forum. Available at: www.nationalobesityforum.co.uk.
27. National Association to Advance Fat Acceptance. Guidelines for health care providers in dealing with fat patients. Oakland: NAAFA. Available at: www.naafa.org.
28. Duckitt K, Harrington D. Risk factors for pre-eclampsia at antenatal booking: systematic review of controlled studies. *BMJ* 2005;**330**:565.
29. Catalano PM. Management of obesity in pregnancy. *Obstet Gynecol* 2007;**109**:419–33.
30. Lewis G, ed. *Why Mothers Die. Report on Confidential Enquiries into Maternal Deaths in the United Kingdom 1994–6.* London: Stationery Office.
31. Duhl AJ, Paidas MJ, Ural SH, et al. Antithrombotic therapy and pregnancy: consensus report and recommendations for prevention and treatment of venous thromboembolism and adverse pregnancy outcomes. *Am J Obstet Gynecol* 2007;**197**:457–69.
32. Larsen TB, Sorensen HT, Gislum M, Johnsen SP. Maternal smoking, obesity, and risk of venous thromboembolism during pregnancy and the puerperium: a population-based nested case-control study. *Thromb Res* 2007;**120**:505–9.
33. Knight M, UKOSS. Antenatal pulmonary embolism: risk factors, management and outsomes. *Br J Obstet Gynaecol* 2008;**115**:453–61.
34. ACOG guideline no. 19. Thromboembolism in pregnancy. *Obstet Gynecol* 2000;**96**(2) (reaffirmed 2005).
35. Royal College of Obstetricians and Gynaecologists. *Thromboprophylaxis during pregnancy, labour and after vaginal delivery.* RCOG Guideline No. 37. London: RCOG, 2004. Available at: www.rcog.org.uk.

36. Kristensen J, Vestergaard M, Wisborg K, et al. Pre-pregnancy weight and the risk of stillbirth and neonatal death. *Br J Obstet Gynaecol* 2005;**112**:403–8.

37. Salihu HM, Dunlop A-L, Alio AP, et al. Extreme obesity and risk of stillbirth among black and white gravidas. *Obstet Gynecol* 2007;**110**:552–7.

38. Chu SY, Kim SY, Lau J, et al. Maternal obesity and risk of stillbirth: a meta analysis. *Am J Obstet Gynecol* 2007;**197**:223–8.

39. Maasilta P, Bachour A, Teramo K, et al. Sleep-related disordered breathing during pregnancy in obese women. *Chest* 2001;**120**:1448–54.

40. Krishnamoorthy U, Schram CMH, Hill SR. Maternal obesity in pregnancy: is it time for meaningful research to inform preventive and management strategies? *Br J Obstet Gynaecol* 2006;**113**:1134–40.

41. Juhasz G, Gyamfi C, Gyamfi P, et al. Effect of body mass index and excessive weight gain on success of vaginal birth after cesarean delivery. *Obstet Gynecol* 2005;**106**:741–6.

42. Durnwald CP, Ehrenberg HM, Mercer BM. The impact of maternal obesity and weight gain on vaginal birth after cesarean section success. *Am J Obstet Gynecol* 2004;**191**:954–7.

43. Edwards RK, Harnsberger DS, Johnson IM, et al. Deciding on route of delivery for obese women with a prior cesarean delivery. *Am J Obstet Gynecol* 2003;**189**:385–9.

44. Carroll CS, Magann EF, Chauhan SP, et al. Vaginal birth after cesarean section versus elective repeat cesarean delivery: weight-based outcomes. *Am J Obstet Gynecol* 2003;**188**:1516–20.

45. Fernando R, Price CM. Regional anaesthesia for labour. In: Collis R, Plaat F, Urquhart J, eds. *Textbook of Obstetric Anaesthesia*. Cambridge: Greenwich Medical Media, 2002: 71–98.

46. Saravanakumar K, Rao SG, Cooper GM. The challenges of obesity and obstetric anaesthesia. *Curr Opin Obstet Gynecol* 2006;**18**:631–5.

47. National Institute for Health and Clinical Excellence. *Intrapartum Care: Care of healthy women and their babies during childbirth*. NICE clinical guideline 55. London: NICE, 2007. Available at: www.nice.org.uk.

48. Lewis G, ed. *The Confidential Enquiry into Maternal and Child Health (CEMACH). Saving Mothers' Lives: Reviewing Maternal Deaths to Make Motherhood Safer – 2003–2005*. The Seventh Report on Confidential Enquiries into Maternal Deaths in the United Kingdom. London: CEMACH, 2007.

49. Porreco RP, Adelberg AM, Lindsay LG, Holdt DG. Cesarean birth in the morbidly obese woman: a report of 3 cases. *J Reprod Med* 2007;**52**:231–4.

50. Alexander CI, Liston WA. Operating on the obese woman – a review. *Br J Obstet Gynaecol* 2006;**113**:1167–72.

51. Ramsay JE, Greer I, Sattar N. Obesity and reproduction. *BMJ* 2006;**333**: 1159–62.

52. ACOG Practice Bulletin no. 77. Screening for fetal chromosomal abnormalities. *Obstet Gynecol* 2007;**109**:217–26.

53. Nicolaides KH. The $11–13^{+6}$ weeks scan. London: Fetal Medicine Foundation, 2004. Available at: www.fetalmedicine.com.

54. Roberts LJ, Bewley S, Mackinson A-M, Rodeck CH. First trimester nuchal translucency: problems with screening the general population. I. *Br J Obstet Gynaecol* 1995;**102**:381–5.

55. Watt HC, Wald NJ. Alternative methods of maternal weight adjustment in maternal serum screening for Down's syndrome and neural tube defects. *Prenat Diagn* 1998;**18**:842–5.

56. Spencer K, Bindra R, Nicolaides KH. Maternal weight correction of maternal serum PAPP-A and free beta-hCG MoM when screening for trisomy 21 in the first trimester of pregnancy. *Prenat Diagn* 2003;**23**:851–5.

57. Waller DK, Shaw GM, Rasmussen SA, et al. National Birth Defects Prevention Study. Prepregnancy obesity as a risk factor for structural birth defects. *Arch Pediatr Adolesc Med* 2007;**161**:745–50.

58. Cedergren M, Kallen B. Maternal obesity and the risk for orofacial clefts in the offspring. *Cleft Palate Craniofac J* 2005;**42**:367–71.

59. Watkins ML, Rasmussen SA, Honein MA, et al. Maternal obesity and risk for birth defects. *Pediatrics* 2003;**111**:1152–8.

60. Ray JG, Wyatt PR, Vermeulen MJ, et al. Greater maternal weight and the ongoing risk of neural tube defects after folic acid flour fortification. *Obstet Gynecol* 2005;**105**:261–5.

61. Anderson JL, Walker DK, Canfield MA, et al. Maternal obesity, gestational diabetes, and central nervous system birth defects. *Epidemiology* 2005;**16**:87–92.

62. Cedergren MI, Kallen BA. Maternal obesity and infant heart defects. *Obes Res* 2003;**11**:1065–71.

63. Watkins ML, Botto LD. Maternal prepregnancy weight and congenital heart defects in offspring. *Epidemiology* 2001;**12**:439–46.

64. Moore LL, Singer MR, Bradlee ML, et al. A prospective study of the risk of congenital defects associated with maternal obesity and diabetes mellitus. *Epidemiology* 2000;**11**:689–94.

65. Wolfe HM, Sokol RJ, Martier SM, Zador IE. Maternal obesity: a potential source of error in sonographic prenatal diagnosis. *Obstet Gynecol* 1990;**76**:339–42.

66. Hendler I, Blackwell SC, Treadwell MC, et al. Does advanced ultrasound equipment improve the adequacy of ultrasound visualization of fetal cardiac structures in the obese gravid woman? *Am J Obstet Gynecol* 2004;**190**:1616–19.

67. Hendler I, Blackwell SC, Bujold E, et al. The impact of maternal obesity on mid-trimester sonographic visualization of fetal cardiac and cranio-spinal structures. *Int J Obstet Relat Metab Disord* 2004;**28**:1607–11.

68. Hendler I, Blackwell SC, Bujold E, et al. Suboptimal second-trimester ultrasonographic visualization of the fetal heart in obese women: should we repeat the examination? *J Ultrasound Med* 2005;**24**:1205–9.

69. Rosenberg JC, Guzman ER, Vintzileos AM, Knuppel RA. Transumbilical placement of the vaginal probe in obese pregnant women. *Obstet Gynecol* 1995;**85**:132–4.

70. Angtuaco TL. Three- and four-dimensional ultrasound and magnetic resonance imaging in pregnancy. In: Reece EA, Hobbins JC, eds. *Clinical Obstetrics*, 3rd edn. Oxford: Blackwell, 2007: 526–60.

71. Colman A, Maharaj D, Hutton J, Tuohy J. Reliability of ultrasound estimation of fetal weight in term singleton pregnancies. *N Z Med J* 2006;**119**:U2146.

72. Dudley NJ. A systematic review of the ultrasound estimation of fetal weight. *Ultrasound Obstet Gynecol* 2005;**25**:80–9.

73. ACOG Practice Bulletin no. 22. Fetal macrosomia. *Obstet Gynecol* 2000;**96**(5) (reaffirmed 2005).

74. National Institue for Health and Clinical Evidence. Induction of labour. NICE guidelines, 2001. Available at: www.nice.org.uk.

75. UKOSS. Extreme obesity. Available at: www.npeu.ox.ac.uk/ukoss/current-surveilance/eo.

76. Lewis G, ed. *Why Mothers Die 2000–2002 – The Sixth Report of Confidential Enquiries into Maternal Deaths in the United Kingdom*. London: RCOG Press. Available at: www.cemach.org.uk.

9 Intrapartum care

Leslie Iffy and Lisa N Gittens–Williams

Introduction

Excessive maternal body mass presents an obstetric challenge from the time of conception until the end of the puerperium. In early gestation, obesity entails an increased risk of spontaneous pregnancy loss. It is also conducive to fetal malformations, including neural tube defects, congenital heart disease, and omphalocele.[1] During midgestation, chronic hypertension and pre-eclampsia, both of which predispose to preterm delivery, are frequent complications. Sleep apnea, impaired respiratory capacity, and coexisting cardiac, gastrointestinal, and biliary diseases are also frequent.

The obstetrician encounters management difficulties throughout the pregnancy, including inability to obtain adequate blood samples because of body habitus, difficulty in assessing fetal position and weight, and poor ability to generate adequate ultrasound images of the uterine contents, a circumstance that hinders prenatal diagnosis of congenital fetal anomalies.[1] As a result of these inherent and continuing challenges, the management of obese patients requires both close observance of traditional principles of midwifery[2-4] and skillful application of modern technology. This chapter discusses obesity-related risk factors, preparation for delivery, intrapartum monitoring, delivery, and management of complications.

Obesity-related risk factors

The identification of specific risk factors during the antenatal period is of critical importance to intrapartum care. Pregestational counseling of obese women offers the clinician an opportunity to avert adverse pregnancy outcome. Along with assessment of comorbidities, such as diabetes, hypertension, and heart disease, markedly overweight women contemplating childbearing should have their body mass index (BMI) calculated and should be made aware of the benefits of exercise and weight reduction. Ideally, nutritional counseling, including the importance of preconception folic acid supplementation, should start at this time.

Information about pregnancy following antiobesity surgery may be a matter of interest for some women.[5] Preconceptual weight loss in obese women improves the outlook for the child to be born[6] (see also Chapters 7 and 13).

The identification of specific pregnancy-related risk factors begins at the first antenatal visit and continues until the final postpartum checkup:

A. Because obese mothers are predisposed to diabetes,[7] glucose screening should begin at the first prenatal visit. It should then be repeated between weeks 24 and 28 of gestation and whenever glucosuria or suspicion of large-for-gestational-age (LGA) fetal status signals its possible development. Failure to achieve glycemic control with oral agents may occur in mothers with a diagnosis of gestational diabetes. If insulin is needed, higher than usual doses are often required, as relative insulin resistance is common in this group. The need for higher doses and poor peripheral absorption may also necessitate the use of a concentrated insulin.

B. Both chronic and pregnancy-induced hypertension are frequent among obese women (see Chapter 5). As they often occur together with diabetes,[8] the development of one may herald the presence of the other. Because diabetes is conducive to fetal macrosomia, and hypertension predisposes to intrauterine growth restriction (IUGR), their effects upon the fetus are unpredictable. Thus, most obese gravidas suffering from hypertension need sonographic assessment of the fetal growth at approximately 2-week intervals.

C. Morbid obesity adversely affects inspiratory capacity, expiratory reserve volume, vital capacity, and total lung capacity.[9] As such, it is conducive to hypoxemia. During the antenatal course, obese gravidas should be evaluated for sleep apnea, and pulmonary function should be assessed when indicated. Because the mother's oxygen requirement increases in labor, particularly during the second stage, clinical manifestations of inadequate oxygenation are frequent. Because the physiologic mechanism of labor causes reduced fetal oxygenation,[10] manifestations of fetal hypoxia are likely to precede maternal symptoms. Prior to the onset of active labor, obese women should be assessed for oxygen saturation in order to establish a baseline for later reference.

D. The maintenance of adequate oxygenation imposes an extra burden upon the blood circulation of overweight gravidas. Of necessity, the factors mentioned under items B and C increase the workload of the heart. The relative frequency of coronary artery disease among obese individuals also needs to be considered when the maternal circulatory status is assessed.[11] Electrocardiogram and maternal echocardiogram should be obtained during the antenatal visits or prior to the induction of labor in case of a planned delivery.

E. Obesity is associated with increased stomach volume and acidity of secretions.[12] This may create problems throughout the pregnancy, which may be further exacerbated intrapartum, if medications obscure the mother's sensorium. In this situation, the horizontal position predisposes the parturient to aspiration of gastric contents.

F. Pregnancy is conducive to thromboembolic disorders. Confinement to bed augments the risk, and early postpartum or postoperative mobilization is essential. Prophylactic administration of heparin is recommended for all morbidly obese mothers delivered by cesarean section. This medication should also be considered whenever the patient requires long periods of immobilization.

G. Obese women are susceptible to infections, including those of the urinary tract.[13] This circumstance underlines the importance of rigid aseptic techniques in obstetric units.[14,15] Avoidance of elective rupture of the fetal membranes during and, more importantly, before labor, reduction of the number of pelvic examinations, meticulous operative technique, and the administration of perioperative antibiotics all contribute to the elimination of the risk of infection.

H. Conduction and general anesthesia both involve increased technical difficulties in obese gravidas[9] (see Chapter 16). Unpredictable drug tolerance presents additional problems. It is therefore advisable to involve the anesthetist in the evaluation of the parturient well before the administration of anesthesia becomes necessary. Antenatal consultation allows early identification of airway problems and patients at risk of difficult intubation or problematic regional anesthesia. Although routine use of conduction anesthesia is not recommended, as it may impair uterine function during the second stage of labor and hinder the recognition of obstetric emergencies, it may be preferable to general anesthesia in certain clinical situations. If difficulty with regional anesthesia is anticipated, secondary to body habitus, and general anesthesia is felt to entail undue risks, an epidural catheter may be placed, without administration of medication, in an early stage of the labor to avoid placement failure in an emergency situation.

I. The high prevalence of macrosomic fetuses among obese mothers is associated with numerous problems. Relative fetopelvic disproportion is conducive to protraction and arrest disorders in labor.[2] Obese patients are more likely than normal-weight women to require use of oxytocin and prostaglandin, and artificial rupture of the membranes. The administration of uterine stimulants leads to (a) use of extraction instruments, (b) abdominal delivery, (c) fetal compromise in labor, (d) shoulder dystocia at delivery, and (e) maternal injuries during the birthing process or from cesarean section.[16,17]

J. Obesity is conducive to postmaturity. Apart from its intrinsic risks, prolonged gestation necessitates induction of labor, inviting those complications enumerated earlier.[13]

K. Excessive maternal weight hinders external fetal heart-rate monitoring and tocography, both antepartum and intrapartum. Poor-quality tracings frequently invite the use of invasive techniques, including scalp electrodes and intrauterine pressure catheters, and cesarean delivery. Although these devices may improve fetal monitoring, they exponentially augment the risk of maternal and fetal infection.

L. Because of respiratory difficulties, obese women do not easily tolerate the lithotomy, Trendelenburg, and McRoberts positions. This circumstance may interfere with the implementation of techniques utilized in case of shoulder dystocia at birth[17-19] and even of those used for normal vaginal deliveries or instrumental extractions.[4] Excessive maternal weight and ensuing decreased mobility may delay maternal transfer to the operating room when urgent surgical intervention is required.

M. Intrapartum, maternal obesity puts the attendant at disadvantage and this disadvantage increases exponentially with increasing body weight. Recognition of obstetric complications, such as uterine rupture, prolapse of the umbilical cord, and abruption of the placenta, may be delayed because of the difficulty involved with palpating the uterus and because the external monitors may inadequately or incorrectly record uterine contractions and fetal heart-rate patterns.

N. Obesity predisposes to postpartum hemorrhage. Ensuing hypovolemia, often superimposed upon an already impaired circulatory equilibrium, may quickly lead to circulatory failure. Body habitus also hinders assessment of uterine contractility after delivery and makes transabdominal uterine massage ineffective. In addition, respiratory compromise may obscure signs of shock, hypovolemia, pulmonary embolism, and amniotic fluid embolism.

The fetus shares its mother's predicament resulting from the risk factors described above. Brachial plexus and central nervous system (CNS) injuries are frequent during the birthing process.[19-21] Neonatal hypoglycemia occurs often. Infants of obese women have more birth injuries, feeding difficulties, and incubator requirements than infants of women of normal BMI.[13] They are also more likely than other newborns to become obese by 2 years of age.[1] Moreover, they have an increased risk of death in the first year of life[20] and are predisposed to a variety of health problems in infancy, childhood, and even adult life.[21]

The risk factors described above may present in a variety of combinations with various degrees of severity. Their identification may challenge the knowledge and skill of the physician and others who provide antenatal care. Yet, it is incumbent on the antenatal care team to formulate a management plan, based upon the pros and cons of vaginal versus abdominal delivery, and to carry out the formulated plan expediently. Paramount to the decision-making process is understanding of the respective risk factors by both the obstetrician and the mother.[21]

Preparation for delivery

Opinions vary whether the current rates of cesarean section – 29% in the USA[18] and even higher in South America – are justifiable. While the subject is often disputable, morbid obesity is a point in favor, rather than against, abdominal delivery. Some risk factors serve as indications for cesarean section by themselves. Although the risk of operative and postoperative morbidity is markedly lower when the cesarean section is elective than when it is performed after prolonged labor, obese women may have been the prime victims of doctors' at times overzealous endeavor to reduce cesarean section rates. In spite of the fact that vaginal deliveries of macrosomic fetuses carry serious fetal[22-24] and even maternal risk,[16,17] well-respected professional societies both in America[25] and in Europe[26] still recommend vaginal delivery of fetuses with estimated weights as high as 4500 g for diabetic and 5000 g for nondiabetic gravidas. It has been estimated recently that adherence to these guidelines in the North American environment may expose an unborn child to a risk as high as 5% of irreversible neurologic birth injury[21] and even to a higher risk if delivery is effected by forceps or Ventouse.[27] In the last analysis, the decision with regard to the method of delivery must rest upon awareness of the respective maternal and fetal risk. The mother is entitled to realistic information to allow her to decide what degree of risk she is willing to assume for herself and expose her unborn child to during the birthing process.[21,28]

Some authors have proposed to factor maternal height into the fetal weight equation, noting that short mothers are less likely than taller mothers to give birth to large babies. This seems to be a sound recommendation. The same consideration probably applies to maternal obesity, another factor known to affect the likelihood of successful vaginal delivery. Trial of labor represents an option rather than a routine choice for morbidly obese women. In the face of major risks, and particularly in case of major fetal macrosomia, the limits of its significance depending on a wide array of modifying factors,[16–19,21] elective abdominal delivery may carry the lowest risk to the fetus and sometimes even to the mother.

Antepartum and intrapartum care represent a continuum. The latter involves judicious implementation of a plan formulated on the basis of identification and objective interpretation of all risk factors. Before the onset or indicated induction of labor, the physician should formulate a realistic picture of the unborn child's and the mother's tolerance of the stress involved in the labor process. Executing this plan with an open mind and with readiness to change course if necessary is the task of the true accoucheur. Thus, it is axiomatic that well-coordinated individual or teamwork based on a thorough knowledge of all risks cannot be replaced by calling upon a junior or even senior physician who happens to cover the service at a particular time to take over the care of an unknown parturient on short notice, sometimes only a few hours before an anticipated delivery. The importance of avoiding capricious actions, based upon drop-of-the-hat 'medical judgment', cannot be overemphasized.

When the balance of considerations favor an attempt at vaginal delivery, the gravida should be advised to proceed to the hospital without delay if uterine contractions occur at 5-min intervals and even earlier if she is multiparous. Suspicion of rupture of the membranes calls for immediate hospitalization. In this situation, the advantage deriving from the patient's timely arrival may be cancelled, however, if, before the onset of 'active' labor,[2] an uninitiated intern performs a manual pelvic examination on arrival, a by no means infrequent violation of good standards of practice. Development of chorioamnionitis is almost predictable under such circumstances.[15,29,30] As another potential disadvantage, early hospitalization may create a situation where, either as a routine procedure or on account of momentary bed utilization logistics, a physician elects to 'speed up' the labor process, a frequent reason for the unduly liberal use of oxytocin in contemporary practice.

An important aspect of Emanuel Friedman's work concerning normal labor was the appreciation that, unlike 'active' labor, the latent phase imposes no significant stress upon the fetus.[2] The more recent information, namely that induction and augmentation of labor with oxytocin are conducive to shoulder dystocia and its sequelae,[19,31] serves as another warning against its use in the absence of indication. The contention that 'active management of labor' increases the safety of the birthing process in obese women is not supported by the authors' experience.[32] It is not recommended, therefore, for the routine management of obese parturients.

Upon arrival in the labor suite, fetal presentation should be confirmed by ultrasound if possible, since obesity is often associated with malpresentation. Provision of nursing care on a one-to-one basis is advisable during parturition. Whereas attempted vaginal delivery after cesarean section is not contraindicated by maternal obesity,[33] obese patients were almost 50% less likely to succeed than underweight patients (odds ratio or OR 0.53, 95% confidence interval or 95% CI 0.29–0.98; $P < 0.043$). Similarly, patients who gained more than 10lb (18 kg) during their pregnancy were almost 40% less likely to have a successful vaginal birth than those who gained less than this (OR 0.63, 95% CI 0.42–0.97; $P < 0.034$).

Those making relevant decisions must pay attention to the fact that the rate of success in such women is lower than average and intrapartum surveillance is more problematic than usual.

Intrapartum monitoring

The rules governing electronic surveillance are equally applicable to slim and obese parturients. However, external monitoring may be difficult and burdensome for the nursing personnel in charge. The physician, in turn, may feel insecure when the heart-rate patterns are interrupted by uninterpretable, 'Chinese letter' tracings for prolonged periods of time. The answer to this problem, far too often, unfortunately, is rupture of the membranes in the absence of a real indication and placement of a scalp electrode on the head of the fetus. Apart from the loss of mechanical protection, as explained by Pascal's law of fluid-containing spaces,[34] the result is introduction of infectious microorganisms, with consequences that have been described at length in retrospect,[14,15,29,30] but remain far too often unconsidered prospectively. The modest advantages deriving from internal fetal heart-rate monitoring seldom balance its inherent risks in markedly obese women. If the quality of the tracings is poor or not interpretable, a strict protocol for intermittent auscultation is an acceptable alternative. The latter method of surveillance can be facilitated by the use of ultrasound to locate the fetal heart.

Paradoxically, the benefit of the scalp electrode is widely ignored in a specific clinical situation, when its dangers are minimal. It is believed by some practitioners that, after the expulsion of the head from the birth canal, the fetal condition deteriorates rapidly. Evidence to the contrary[4,19,35] having failed to convince some practitioners, the placement of a scalp electrode on the already delivered head can reassure the anxious doctor about the condition of the child, thus removing

33. Juhasz G, Gyamfi C, Gyamfi P, et al. Effect of body mass index and excessive weight gain on success of vaginal birth after cesarean delivery. *Obstet Gynecol* 2005;**106**:741–6.

34. Mergoni A. La legge di Pascal e il torchio pelvico nel meccanismo fisiologico del parto. *Minerva Ginecol* 1988;**40**:199–214.

35. Stallings SP, Edwards RK, Johnson JWC. Correlation of head-to-body delivery intervals in shoulder dystocia and umbilical artery acidosis. *Am J Obstet Gynecol* 2001;**185**:268–7.

36. Bryant RD, Danforth DN. Conduct of normal labor. In: Danforth DN, ed. *Textbook of Obstetrics and Gynecology*, 2nd edn. New York: Harper & Row, 1971: 561–84.

37. Greenhill JP. *Obstetrics*, 11th edn. Philadelphia: WB Saunders, 1955: 278.

38. Allen R, Sorab J, Gonik B. Risk factors of shoulder dystocia: an engineering study of clinician-applied forces. *Obstet Gynecol* 1991;**77**:352–5.

39. Frisoli G, Leo MV, Sama JC. Postpartum hemorrhage. In: Iffy L, Apuzzio JJ, Vintzileos AM, eds. *Operative Obstetrics*, 2nd edn. New York: McGrew-Hill, 1992: 352–69.

40. Allen RH, Rosenbaum TC, Ghidini A, et al. Correlating head-to-body delivery intervals with neonatal depression in vaginal births that result in permanent brachial plexus injury. *Am J Obstet Gynecol* 2002;**187**:839–42.

41. Beall MH, Spong CY, Ross MG. Randomizing controlled trial of prophylactic maneuvers to reduce head-to-body delivery time in patients at risk of shoulder shoulder dystocia. *Obstet Gynecol* 2003;**102**:31–5.

42. Wood C, Ng KH, Hounslow D, Benning H. The influence of differences of birth times upon fetal condition in normal deliveries. *J Obstet Gynaecol Br Commonw* 1973;**80**:289–94.

43. Wood C, Ng KH, Hounslow D, Benning H. Time – an important variable in normal delivery. *J Obstet Gynaecol Br Commonw* 1973;**80**:295–300.

44. Hope P, Breslin S, Lamont L, et al. Fatal shoulder dystocia: a review of 56 cases reported to the Confidential Enquiry into Stillbirths and Deaths in Infancy. *Br J Obstet Gynaecol* 1998;**105**:1256–61.

45. Roseveas SK, Stirrat GM. *Handbook of Obstetric Management*. Oxford: Blackwell Science, 1996: 251.

46. Szabo I, Gocze P. Koros vajudas es szules. In: Papp Z, ed. *A Szuleszet-Nogyogyaszat Tankonyve*, 3rd edn. Budapest: Semmelweis, 2007: 273–337.

47. Iffy L, Apuzzio J, Ganesh V. A randomized controlled trial of prophylactic maneuvers to reduce head-to-body delivery time in patients at risk for shoulder dystocia. *Am J Obstet Gynecol* 2003;**102**:1089–90.

48. Apuzzio JJ, Salamon CG. Cesarean section. In: Apuzzio JJ, Vintzileos AM, Iffy L, eds. *Operative Obstetrics*, 3rd edn. London: Taylor & Francis, 2006: 365–86.

49. Ende N, Portuondo N, Iffy L. The time of clamping the umbilical cord. *Hungarian J Obstet Gynaecol* 2006;**69**:5–8.

50. Yiyang JL, Qunxi C, Weiling W. Closure vs. non-closure of the peritoneum at cesarean delivery. *Int J Gynaecol Obstet* 2006;**94**:103–7.

51. Lynch CB, Keith LG, Campbell WH. Internal iliac (hypogastric) artery ligation. In: Lynch CB, Keith L, Lalonde A, Karoshi M, eds. *A Textbook of Postpartum Haemorrhage*. Kirkmahoe, UK: Sapiens Publishing, 2006: 299–307.

52. Sukalich S, Mingione MJ, Glantz JC. Obstetric outcomes in overweight and obese adolescents. *Am J Obstet Gynecol* 2006;**190**:1335–40.

10 Postpartum care

Kirsten Duckitt

Introduction

The postpartum period is the time after birth during which the woman, her baby, and the wider family of origin begin their new life together. Care from medical professionals during this period, which is usually defined as the time from birth until 6 weeks postpartum, revolves about recognizing any deviation from the expected recovery after birth and about providing support and information about infant feeding as well as the return to the normal nonpregnant state. Because much of the input is directed toward the baby, mothers often look backward and reflect that their health was largely ignored. Common maternal health issues include physical morbidity, consisting of backache, breastfeeding problems, perineal pain, stress incontinence, and mental health problems that may extend to postnatal depression. Nearly half of 11 701 women who gave birth at one maternity unit in the UK reported onset of one or more new health problems since giving birth which lasted for over 6 weeks.[1] Researchers from Scotland found that 76% of over 1200 women questioned experienced at least one new health problem with onset at some time between discharge from the postnatal ward and 8 weeks postpartum.[2] Studies in other developed countries show similar findings.[3,4]

The majority of postpartum care provision takes place outside the hospital setting and crosses acute and primary healthcare sectors. In the UK, most of this care is provided by midwives, maternity care assistants, health visitors, and general practitioners. In other countries, such as the USA and Canada, public health nurses, obstetricians, and family practitioners take care of the mother, with the baby being looked after by the family doctor or a pediatrician. In either instance, most new mothers only spend 1–3 days in the hospital, and this circumstance makes standardization of care and collection of data challenging. This chapter concentrates on medical issues and providing care during the postpartum period in the obese mother. Common medical problems in the initial postpartum period are considered first, followed by the effect of obesity on breastfeeding and then weight retention and weight loss.

Postpartum hemorrhage

Although several often-quoted population or case–control studies on postpartum hemorrhage (PPH) and serious maternal morbidity[5–6] do not include obesity as a variable, perhaps because of lack of recorded data, there are now sufficient data to show a positive association between obesity and risk of PPH.

Stones et al[7] retrospectively looked at 37 497 women who delivered in 1988 in north-west London. Of these, 498 had PPH, defined as blood loss of >1000 ml. Obesity increased the risk of PPH by 60% (odds ratio or OR 1.64, 95% confidence interval or 95% CI 1.24–2.17). In the same population, but using pooled data for the years 1989–97, Sebire et al[8] found that out of 287 213 women with singleton pregnancies, the risk of major PPH increased as the BMI at the initial antenatal visit increased, with an OR for BMI 25–30 of 1.17 (95% CI 1.07–1.27) and an OR for BMI > 30 of 1.44 (95% CI 1.30–1.80). Kiran et al[9] found a similar relationship. The population studied was 60 167 primigravid women with singleton pregnancies in the Cardiff area of Wales in 1990–9. Compared with a BMI at the initial antenatal visit of 20–30, the women with a BMI over 30 had an increased likelihood of losing over 500 ml of blood at delivery (OR 1.5, 95% CI 1.2–1.8). In Australia, Doherty et al[10] analyzed 2827 women with singleton pregnancies who had prepregnancy BMI data available. The adjusted OR for BMI of 25–30 and PPH was 1.55 (95% CI 1.17–2.06), whereas BMI of > 30 gave an adjusted OR of 1.71 (95% CI 1.20–2.44). Bhattacharya et al,[11] in their analysis of all nulliparous women delivering singletons in Aberdeen, Scotland, between 1976 and 2005, also found that the rates of PPH increased linearly with rising BMI. Adjusted ORs for BMI 25–29.9 and BMI 30–34.5 were 1.1 (95% CI 1.0–1.2) and 1.5 (95% CI 1.3–1.7), respectively.

One hypothesis for this association comes from Zhang et al,[12] who propose that the myometrium of obese women does not contract optimally, thus leading to poor contractions in labor and after delivery with resultant PPH. They conducted in vitro studies with myometrium obtained from women having elective cesarean sections, finding that myometrium obtained from obese women contracted with less force and less frequently than that obtained from normal-weight women. Alterations in the intracellular calcium ion concentrations were also seen, and they postulated that this could be caused by the elevated cholesterol levels found in obese women.[13] The association between obesity and PPH means that clinicians have to be vigilant, anticipate PPH in such women, and manage the third stage appropriately, with early recourse to ergometrine and oxytocin infusion if required and timely cross-matching of blood (see Chapter 9).

In the light of the above evidence, it is not surprising that obesity also increases the risk of postpartum anemia. Bodnar et al[14] found that the adjusted relative risk (RR) of postpartum anemia increased as BMI increased from 24 to 38. Women with BMI of 28 had 1.8 times the postpartum risk of anemia of a woman with a BMI of 20 (95% CI 1.3–2.5), and obese women with BMI of 36 had 2.8 times the risk (95% CI 1.7–4.7). As the authors suggest that postpartum anemia can lead to relative immunodeficiency with an increase in infection and can also lead to inactivity and depression, assessing for anemia and instituting appropriate postpartum iron supplementation are vital in obese women (see Chapter 12).

Postpartum sepsis

A large population study of 287 213 women showed that obesity is associated with a greater risk of all types of postpartum infections (Table 10.1).Even with elective cesarean sections when prophylactic antibiotics are used, an increased risk of infectious morbidity exists.[13] In a population-based, observational study of 60 167 deliveries in Wales, Kiran et al[9] compared women with initial visit BMI of 20–30 with those with BMI >30. These authors found an increased risk of postpartum urinary tract infection (OR 1.9, 95% CI 1.9–3.4), but not of wound or uterine infection. However, this may be a result of including the BMI 25–30 group along with the BMI 20–25 group, thus diluting any difference. In their cohort study of 2827 women with singleton pregnancies, Doherty et al[10] found an increased risk of maternal infection in the obese group (BMI > 30), but not in the overweight group (BMI 25–30) (adjusted OR 2.03, 95% CI 1.09–3.79).

No randomized controlled trials (RCTs) have compared vertical with transverse skin incisions for cesarean section in obese women. However, in a retrospective study of 239 women with BMI greater than 35 undergoing primary cesarean delivery,[15] the overall incidence of wound complications, including infection and dehiscence, was 12.1%. A vertical skin incision was associated with a significantly higher wound infection rate than a transverse skin incision, even when

TABLE 10.1   Postpartum sepsis[8]

	OR (95% CI) using BMI 20–25 as reference
Genital tract infection	
BMI 25–30	1.24 (1.09–1.41)
BMI > 30	1.30 (1.07–1.56)
Wound infection	
BMI 25–30	1.27 (1.09–1.48)
BMI>30	2.24 (1.91–2.64)
UTI	
BMI 25–30	1.17 (1.04–1.33)
BMI > 30	1.39 (1.18–1.63)
PUO	
BMI 25–30	1.19 (1.08–1.32)
BMI > 30	1.29 (1.13–1.48)

Adjusted for ethnic group, parity, age, history of hypertension, history of gestational or pre-existing diabetes, elective and emergency cesarean section.

BMI, body mass index; CI, confidence interval; OR, odds ratio; PUO, pyrexion of unknown origin; UTI, urinary tract infection.

prophylactic antibiotics and other strategies, such
subcutaneous sutures, were used. A meta-analysis of
of the subcutaneous space, compared with nonclos
wound disruption when the subcutaneous layer i
95% CI 0.48, 0.91).[16] This finding has a number r
suggests that cesarean wounds always require
women.

Pre-eclampsia/eclampsia

Prepregnancy obesity or obesity noted at the first antenatal visit is a risk facto.
pre-eclampsia/eclampsia. One meta-analysis shows that raised prepregnancy
BMI doubles the risk of pre-eclampsia (six cohort studies, RR 2.47, 95% CI 1.66–
3.67), and raised BMI at the initial prenatal visit raises the risk of pre-eclampsia
by about 50% (one cohort study, RR 2.12, 95% CI 1.56–2.88).[17] Another systematic
overview shows that the risk of pre-eclampsia doubles for every 5–7 increase in
prepregnancy BMI.[18]

Women who develop pregnancy-induced hypertension before birth obviously
need monitoring postpartum, when pre-eclampsia and eclampsia can arise anew.
No studies have assessed whether the risk factors described above change when
only postpartum pre-eclampsia and eclampsia are considered, although this is
unlikely. The incidence of postpartum eclampsia varies with different studies and
different populations. Two UK prospective studies show rates of 32%[19] and 44%[20]
of eclampsia occurring postpartum. A US retrospective study found that 27%
(97/334 over a 15-year period) of all eclampsia cases occurred postpartum, with
54 of these cases occurring between 48 h and 4 weeks postpartum.[21] Chames et
al[22] found that, out of 29 women with postpartum eclampsia, 23 had late-onset
postpartum eclampsia (> 48 h). These women were more likely to have headaches,
visual symptoms, and at least one symptom of pre-eclampsia compared with
women whose eclampsia manifested itself before delivery or in the early
postpartum period. Vigilance for postpartum pre-eclampsia and eclampsia is
required in obese women even if neither was present antenatally.

Thromboembolic disease (VTE)

Venous thromboembolism (VTE) remains a main direct cause of maternal death
in the UK[23] as well as in Canada[24] and the USA.[25] In pooled data from the Center
for Disease Control and Prevention's National Pregnancy Mortality Surveillance
System from 1991 to 1999, pulmonary embolism (PE) was the most common
cause of pregnancy-related death when both live births and all pregnancy
outcomes were considered. PE accounted for 20% of the maternal mortality,
higher than both maternal hemorrhage (17%) and pregnancy-associated
hypertension (16%).[26] It can occur at any time in pregnancy, but the puerperium
is the time of highest risk.[27] Pregnancy alone increases the risk of VTE by a factor
of 3–5, and obesity in pregnancy increases this risk further by a factor of about 4
(OR 4.4, 95% CI 3.4–5.7).[26] In a retrospective study of 287 213 pregnant women

ton pregnancies in north-west London, UK, the prevalence of mbolism was 0.04% in normal-weight, 0.07% in overweight, and 0.08% e women.[8]

thromboprophylaxis at the time of cesarean section has become more mmon, about half of the maternal deaths due to postpartum PE in the UK in oth the 2000–2 and 2003–5 triennia occurred after vaginal delivery.[23,28] Of the eight women who died from VTE in the puerperium in the most recent triennia, three were overweight or obese, three were morbidly obese, and two did not have their weight recorded. None of the three morbidly obese women received thromboprophylaxis. Most VTEs that cause death are from PE, but cerebral vein thrombosis is almost always fatal and seems to have the same risk factors as PE, including obesity.[25] Appropriate thromboprophylaxis should prevent cerebral vein thrombosis too.

Continued vigilance for VTE should not be limited to the immediate postpartum period, as 12 out of the 14 deaths from PE in the 6 weeks after delivery occurred after the first postpartum week. A high index of clinical suspicion is required in order to detect PE. It may often be preceded by calf or femoral DVT, but these, too, can be difficult to diagnose. It is PE, however, that has the highest risk of death. The British Thoracic Society suggests a model for assessing clinical probability of PE. If the patient has clinical features compatible with PE, that is, breathlessness and/or tachypnea, with or without pleuritic chest pain and/or hemoptysis, then two other factors should be sought: (a) the absence of another reasonable clinical explanation and (b) the presence of a major risk factor. If (a) and (b) are both true, there is a high probability of PE.[29]

The Royal College of Obstetricians and Gynaecologists' guideline on thromboprophylaxis during pregnancy and labor, and after vaginal delivery,[30] recommends that, as obesity (BMI over 30 or weight over 90 kg) is an important independent risk factor for postpartum VTE, even after vaginal delivery, the combination of obesity with any other risk factor for VTE (Table 10.2) should lead to thromboprophylaxis with low-molecular-weight heparin (LMWH) for 3–5 days postpartum. The guideline goes on to say that postpartum thrombo-prophylaxis should be given as soon as possible after delivery, provided that there is no PPH. Those with PPH should be fitted with thromboembolic deterrent stockings. If the woman has been given regional analgesia, LMWH should be withheld until 4 h after insertion or removal of the epidural catheter (or 6 h if either insertion or removal was traumatic). The first postpartum dose can be given after insertion but before removal of the epidural catheter. The risk of VTE reduces when women are mobile postpartum but does not disappear. The course of thromboprophylaxis should be finished even if the woman is discharged home before completion. The use of LMWH is not contraindicated with breastfeeding.[31]

The dose of LMWH should be adjusted according to body weight. For women over 90 kg (200 lb) needing postpartum thromboprophylaxis, the dose required for three commonly used types of LMWH is as follows: enoxaparin 40 mg, 12-hourly; dalteparin 5000 units, 12-hourly; tinzaparin 4500 units, 12-hourly.

TABLE 10.2[30] Risk factors for venous thromboembolism (VTE) in pregnancy and the puerperium[a]

Pre-existing	New onset or transient[b]
Previous VTE	Surgical procedure in pregnancy or
Thrombophilia	puerperium, e.g., evacuation of
Congenital	retained products of conception,
antithrombin deficiency	postpartum sterilization
Protein C deficiency	Hyperemesis
Protein S deficiency	Dehydration
Factor V Leiden	Ovarian hyperstimulation syndrome
Prothrombin gene variant	Severe infection, such as
Acquired (antiphospholipid syndrome)	pyelonephritis
lupus anticoagulant	Immobility (> 4 days' bed rest)
Anticardiolipin antibodies	Pre-eclampsia
Age over 35 years	Excessive blood loss
Obesity (BMI > 30 kg/m^2) either	Long-haul travel
prepregnancy or in early pregnancy	Prolonged labour[c]
Parity > 4	Midcavity instrumental delivery[c]
Gross varicose veins	Immobility after delivery
Paraplegia	
Sickle cell disease	
Inflammatory disorders such as	
inflammatory bowel disease	
Some medical disorders, such as	
nephrotic syndrome, certain cardiac	
diseases	
Myeloproliferative disorders, such as	
essential thrombocythemia,	
polycythemia vera	

[a]Although these are all accepted as thromboembolic risk factors, few data support the degree of increased risk associated with many of them.
[b]These risk factors are potentially reversible and may develop at later stages in gestation than the initial risk assessment or may resolve; an ongoing individual risk assessment is important.
[c]Risk factors specific to postpartum VTE only.

Breastfeeding

The WHO recommends that babies be exclusively breastfed for at least 6 months,[32] yet routinely collected data on infant feeding persistently show low uptake and duration of breastfeeding.[33] In the year 2000, in England and Wales, breastfeeding rates at 1 week postpartum were only 57% among the 71% of women who initially breastfed, despite this being the period of the most intense input from health professionals who provide postnatal care.[34] At 6 weeks, only 43% of all women were breastfeeding, and, of the women who had initiated breastfeeding, only 65% were still doing so. Among women participating in this survey, only 21% were still breastfeeding at 6 months.[36]

Several studies have shown an association between poor lactation performance, in terms of both reduced breastfeeding initiation rates and shorter duration of breastfeeding, and obesity. These studies have been reviewed by Lovelady[35] (Table 10.3). There may be many causes of this relationship if it does exist; physical difficulties because of large breasts, concern about body image, low self-esteem, and a different hormonal environment may all contribute. As obesity is commonly associated with emergency cesarean sections and possibly more stress during labor and delivery, these consequences may also be involved in poorer lactation performance.[36] Rasmussen and Kjolhede[37] found that the prolactin response to suckling in the first 48 h is delayed in overweight/obese women, perhaps leading to delayed lactogenesis and premature cessation of breastfeeding. It is not certain whether this is a hormonally mediated phenomenon or a result of poor positioning and latching due to obesity. It is clear, however, that breastfeeding failure leads to higher rates of formula feeding, greater rates of childhood obesity, and perpetuation of the cycle of obesity from generation to generation.[38] Under these circumstances, obese women should have access to dedicated lactation support in the first few days after delivery with support afterward until breastfeeding is well established.

Postpartum weight loss

The weight retained after pregnancy is defined as the difference between postpartum and prepregnancy weight.[39] Advising women on weight loss after childbirth is important, because postpartum retention of the weight can lead to subsequent obesity that becomes a significant risk factor for diabetes, hypertension, and heart disease.

Although the *average* weight gain per pregnancy is relatively small, 0.5 –4.0 kg,[40–45] there seems to be a subset of women who are particularly at risk of gaining large amounts of weight with each pregnancy.[41,42] Some 14–25% of women retain more than 4.5 kg after pregnancy.[42–44,47,49] These women are particularly at risk of doing so again in subsequent pregnancies.[46] Low socioeconomic class, high prepregnancy BMI, and high parity are all risk factors,[43,51] but excessive weight gain in pregnancy seems to be the greatest contributing factor to excessive postpartum weight retention.[44,46,49] The postpartum check or other opportunistic visits in the postnatal period, such as for baby immunization, represent important encounters where maternal weight can be measured and advice about weight loss provided.

TABLE 10.3 Studies illustrating relationship between breastfeeding and obesity (adapted from Lovelady[35])

Study	Population	Findings
Baker 2004[56]	3768 women in Denmark. No ethnic unformation provided	Obese women (BMI > 30) breastfed for significantly shorter time than normal-weight women (BMI 20–25) (27.3 ± 15.7 vs 31.3± 14.6 weeks)
Dewey 2003[36]	280 women; 78% non-Hispanic white, 11% Hispanic, 8% Asian, 3% black	Women with BMI > 27 were 2.5 times more likely than normal-weight women to have delayed onset of lactation. Infants were three times more likely to have suboptimal feeding behavior on day 7
Donath 2000[57]	1991 women in Australia. No ethnic information provided	Lower rates of breastfeeding initiation among obese (BMI > 30) than normal-weight (BMI > 20–25) women (82.3% vs 89.2%). Obese women breastfed for shorter length of time than normal-weight women (22.7 vs 28.7 weeks)
Hilson 2004[58]	151 women in rural USA, mostly white	Prepregnant BMI and primiparity were each associated with later onset of lactogenesis, but only primiparity remained significant when both were considered simultaneously. Only obese (BMI ≥ 29) women were at significantly higher risk of earlier discontinuation of breastfeeding than underweight/normal-weight women (RR 2.03, 95% CI 1.07–4.5)
Kúgyelka 2004[59]	1227 urban American women; 48% Hispanic, 52% black	Obese (BMI ≥ 29) Hispanic women were more likely than normal-weight women to feed formula and breast milk versus exclusive breastfeeding before discharge (OR 1.9, 95% CI 1.2–3.1), and more likely to discontinue exclusive breastfeeding (RR 1.5, 95% CI 1.1–2.0) or breastfeeding to any extent (RR 1.6, 95% CI 1.1–2.1). No association between breastfeeding and obesity in black women
Sebire 2001[8]	287 213 women in London, UK. Approximately 70% white, 12% Indian, with the remainder black, Asian, or other	Breastfeeding at discharge significantly less likely in overweight (BMI 25–29.9, OR 0.86, 95% CI 0.84–0.88) or obese (BMI 30, OR 0.58, 95% CI 0.56–0.60) than normal-weight (BMI 20–24.9) women

What strategies are most effective for losing weight after pregnancy?

It may be possible to restrict excessive weight gain in pregnancy in certain subgroups of women with behavioral interventions geared at reminding them what their ideal weight gain should be. However, these interventions do not work in all women, particularly women who are already obese prior to pregnancy.[45,46] Women who return to their prepregnancy weight by about 6 months have a lower risk of being overweight 10 years later.

A Cochrane Review[47] found six RCTs that looked at interventions for losing weight in postpartum women who were either obese or overweight, or had gained excessive weight during pregnancy. One trial looked at exercise alone, one trial looked at diet alone, and four trials looked at diet plus exercise compared with usual care. However, only 245 women were included in all these trials. The combined findings of these trials showed that diet alone and diet plus exercise led to more weight loss than usual care. Exercise alone did not lead to greater weight loss compared with no intervention. In view of the low number of included women, the review concluded that larger trials are needed, particularly with regard to breastfeeding women.

A literature review on exercise in the postpartum period[48] found similar results with respect to exercise alone without calorie restriction in the postpartum period. The author concluded that moderate exercise without specific calorie restriction does not promote greater weight or fat loss, nor does it seem to affect breastfeeding in lactating mothers. However, the author did suggest that postpartum exercise may have other health benefits such as improving aerobic fitness, high-density lipoprotein-cholesterol levels, insulin sensitivity, and psychological well-being, which in turn could reduce postpartum depression.

In a large, prospective study on weight gain during pregnancy conducted on 1423 postpartum women in Stockholm, Ohlin et al[49] found that women with regular breakfast and lunch habits were more likely to return to their prepregnancy weight, whereas breastfeeding had only a small effect on weight loss after pregnancy when eating habits were taken into consideration. Postpartum weight retention was more affected by lifestyle changes during and after pregnancy than by factors before pregnancy. A recently reported prospective cohort study of 902 postpartum women[50] found that women who watched less than 2 h of television per day, walked for at least 30 min, and consumed *trans*-fat below the median had an OR of 0.23 (95% CI 0.08–0.66) of retaining at least 5 kg at 12 months postpartum. Results from the same cohort study (Project Viva) reported on 940 postpartum women who had their amount of sleep assessed at 6 months postpartum.[51] Sleeping for no more than 5 h/day at 6 months postpartum led to a threefold risk of retaining at least 5 kg at 1 year postpartum compared with mothers getting 7 h of sleep or more (unadjusted OR 3.08, 95% CI 1.76–5.38). The authors suggest that interventions to prevent postpartum obesity should consider strategies to attain optimal maternal sleep duration.

In order not to retain a substantial amount of weight after pregnancy (> 5 kg), women should exercise, with at least 30 min of walking daily, restrict TV time to less than 2 h, have a diet containing less than average amounts of *trans*-fats, eat regular breakfast and lunch, sleep more than 7 h in a 24-h period, and consider dieting.

Postpartum depression

Although the relationship between obesity and depression in women is well documented,[52,53] very few studies have looked at the relationship between obesity and postpartum depression. In a small study of 67 women, Carter et al[54] looked at the interrelationship of BMI, eating attitudes, depression, and anxiety during and after pregnancy. Although they concluded that there was a relationship between BMI and depressive symptoms, only 17 of the included women had a BMI over 27. Lacoursiere et al[55] looked at the association between BMI and self-reported indices of depression in the postpartum period in 3439 women in Utah, USA. Obese women reported significantly greater rates of depression than normal-weight women (30.8% vs 22.8%; $P < 0.001$). This correlation merits further study.

Conclusion

Obesity is a risk factor for many untoward postpartum events. Vigilance, appropriate prophylaxis, and aggressive management are required. Clinicians must remember that the postpartum period is an ideal time to discuss weight loss so that weight retention from one pregnancy is not carried forward into the next.

References

1. MacArthur C, Lewis M, Knox EG. *Health After Childbirth. An Investigation of Long-Term Health Problems After Childbirth in 11701 Women.* London: HMSO, 1991.
2. Glazener CM, Abdalla M, Stroud P, et al. Postnatal maternal morbidity: extent, causes, prevention and treatment. *Br J Obstet Gynaecol* 1995;**102**;282–7.
3. Brown S, Lumley J. Maternal health after childbirth: results of an Australian population based survey. *Br J Obstet Gynaecol* 1998;**105**:156–61.
4. Saurel-Cubizolles MJ, Romito P, Lelong N, Ancel PY. Women's health after childbirth: a longitudinal study in France and Italy. *Br J Obstet Gynaecol* 2000;**107**:1202–9.
5. Hall MH, Halliwell R, Carr-Hill R. Concomitant and repeated happenings of complications of the third stage of labour. *Br J Obstet Gynaecol* 1985;**92**:732–8.
6. Waterstone M, Bewley S, Wolfe C. Incidence and predictors of severe obstetric morbidity: case-control study. *BMJ* 2001;**322**:1089–94.
7. Stones RW, Paterson CM, Saunders NJ. Risk factors for major obstetric haemorrhage. *Eur J Obstet Gynecol Reprod Biol* 1993;**48**:15–18.
8. Sebire NJ, Jolly M, Harris JP, et al. Maternal obesity and pregnancy outcome: a study of 287,213 pregnancies in London. *Int J Obes Relat Metab Disord* 2001;**25**:1175–82.

9. Kiran TSU, Hemmadi S, Bethel J, Evans J. Outcome of pregnancy in a woman with an increased body mass index. *Br J Obstet Gynaecol* 2005;**112**:768–72.

10. Doherty DA, Magann EF, Francis J, et al. Pre-pregnancy body mass index and pregnancy outcomes. *Int J Gynaecol Obstet* 2006;**95**:242–7.

11. Bhattacharya S, Campbell DM, Liston WA, Bhattacharya S. Effect of body mass index on pregnancy outcomes in nulliparous women delivering singleton babies. *BMC Public Health* 2007;**7**:168. Available at: www. biomedcentral.com/1471 2458/7/168.

12. Zhang J, Bricker L, Wray S, Quenby S. Poor uterine contractility in obese women. *Br J Obstet Gynaecol* 2007;**114**:343–8.

13. Myles TD, Gooch J, Santolaya J. Obesity as an independent risk factor for infectious morbidity in patients who undergo caesarean delivery. *Obstet Gynecol* 2002;**100**:959–64.

14. Bodnar LM, Siega-Riz AM, Cogswell ME. High prepregnancy BMI increases the risk of postpartum anemia. *Obes Res* 2004;**12**:941–8.

15. Wall PD, Deucy EE, Glantz JC, Pressman EK. Vertical incisions and wound complications in the obese parturient. *Obstet Gynecol* 2003;**102**:952–6.

16. Chelmow D, Rodriguez EJ, Sabatini MM. Suture closure of subcutaneous fat and wound disruption after cesarean delivery: a meta-analysis. *Obstet Gynecol* 2004;**103**:974–80.

17. Duckitt K, Harrington D. Risk factors for pre-eclampsia at antenatal booking: systematic review of controlled studies. *BMJ* 2005:**330**:565–7.

18. O'Brien TE, Ray JG, Chan WS. Maternal body mass index and the risk of preeclampsia: a systematic overview. *Epidemiology* 2003;**14**:368–74.

19. Tuffnell DJ, Jankowicz D, Lindow SW, et al and Yorkshire Obstetric Critical Care Group. Outcomes of severe pre-eclampsia/eclampsia in Yorkshire 1999/2003. *Br J Obstet Gynaecol* 2005;**112**:875–80.

20. Douglas KA, Redman CW. Eclampsia in the United Kingdom. *BMJ* 1994;**309**:1395–400.

21. Lubarsky SL, Barton JR, Friedman SA, et al. Late postpartum eclampsia revisited. *Obstet Gynecol* 1994;**83**:502–5.

22. Chames MC, Livingston JC, Ivester TS, et al. Late postpartum eclampsia: a preventable disease? *Am J Obstet Gynecol* 2002;**186**:1174–7.

23. Lewis G, ed. *The Confidential Enquiry into Maternal and Child Health (CEMACH). Saving Mothers' Lives: Reviewing Maternal Deaths to Make Motherhood Safer – 2003–2005*. The Seventh Report on Confidential Enquiries into Maternal Deaths in the United Kingdom. London: CEMACH, 2007.

24. Health Canada. *Special Report on Maternal Mortality and Severe Morbidity in Canada – Enhanced Surveillance: The Path to Prevention*. Ottawa: Minister of Public Works and Government Services Canada, 2004.

25. Chang J, Elam-Evans LD, Berg CJ, et al. Pregnancy-related mortality surveillance – United States, 1991–1999. *MMWR Surveill Summ* 2003;**52**:1–8.

26. James AH, Jamison MG, Brancazio LR, Myers ER. Venous thromboembolism during pregnancy and the postpartum period: incidence, risk factors, and mortality. *Am J Obstet Gynecol* 2006;**194**:1311–15.

27. Ray JG, Chan WA. Deep vein thrombosis during pregnancy and the puerperium: a meta-analysis of the period of risk and the leg of presentation. *Obstet Gynecol Surv* 1999;**54**:265–71.

28. Lewis G, ed. Confidential Enquiries into Maternal and Child Health. *Why Mothers Die*. The Sixth Report of the United Kingdom Confidential Enquiries into Maternal Deaths in the United Kingdom. London: RCOG Press, 2004. Available at: www.cemach.org.uk.

29. British Thoracic Society Standards of Care Committee Pulmonary Embolism Guideline Development Group. British Thoracic Society guidelines for the management of suspected acute pulmonary embolism. *Thorax* 2003;**58**:470–84.

30. Royal College of Obstetricians and Gynaecologists Green Top Guideline no. 37. *Thromboprophylaxis during pregnancy, labour and after vaginal delivery*. London: RCOG, 2004. Available at: www.rcog.org.uk.

31. Nelson-Piercy C. Hazards of heparin: allergy, heparin-induced thrombocytopenia and osteoporosis. *Baillière's Clin Obstet Gynaecol* 1997;**11**: 489–509.

32. World Health Organization. *Global Strategy for Infant and Young Child Feeding*. Geneva: World Health Organization, 2003.

33. Renfrew MJ, Dyson L, Wallace L, et al. *Effectiveness of Public Health Interventions to Promote the Duration of Breastfeeding: Systematic Review*. London: National Institute for Health and Clinical Excellence, 2005.

34. Hamlyn B, Brooker S, Oleinikova K, Wands S. *Infant Feeding 2000*: a survey conducted on behalf of the Department of Health, the Scottish Executive, the National Assembly for Wales and the Department of Health Social Services and Public Health in Northern Ireland. London: Stationery Office, 2002.

35. Lovelady CA. Is maternal obesity a cause of poor lactation performance? *Nutr Rev* 2005;**63**:352–5.

36. Dewey KG, Nommsen-Rivers LA, Heinig MJ, Cohen RJ. Risk factors for suboptimal infant breastfeeding behavior, delayed onset of lactation, and excess neonatal weight loss. *Pediatrics* 2003;**112**:607–19.

37. Rasmussen KM, Kjolhede CL. Prepregnant overweight and obesity diminish the prolactin response to suckling in the first week postpartum. *Pediatrics* 2004;**113**:e465–71.

38. Li C, Kaur H, Choi WS, et al. Additive interactions of maternal pre-pregnancy BMI and breastfeeding on childhood overweight. *Obes Res* 2005;**13**:362–71.

39. Institute of Medicine. *Nutrition during pregnancy*. Washington, DC: National Academy Press, 1990.

40. Ohlin A, Rossner S. Maternal body weight development after pregnancy. *Int J Obes* 1990;**14**:159–73.

41. Rossner S. Pregnancy, weight cycling and weight gain in obesity. *Int J Obes Relat Metab Disord* 1992;**16**:145–7.

42. Rossner S, Ohlin A. Pregnancy as a risk factor for obesity: lessons from the Stockholm Pregnancy and Weight Development Study. *Obes Res* 1995;**3**(Suppl 2):267S–75S.

43. Crowell DT. Weight change in postpartum period. A review of the literature. *J Nurse Midwifery* 1995;**40**:418–23.

44. Gunderson EP, Abrams B. Epidemiology of gestational weight gain and body weight changes after pregnancy. *Epidemiol Rev* 1999;**21**:261–75.

45. Polley BA, Wing RR, Sims CJ. Randomized controlled trial to prevent excessive weight gain in pregnant women. *Int J Obes Relat Metab Disord* 2002;**26**:1494–502.

46. Olson CM, Strawderman MS, Reed RG. Efficacy of an intervention to prevent excessive gestational weight gain. *Am J Obstet Gynecol* 2004;**191**:530–6.

47. Amorim AR, Linne YM, Lourenco PMC. Diet or exercise, or both, for weight reduction in women after childbirth. Cochrane Review. *Cochrane Database Syst Rev* 2007(3):CD005627.

48. Larson-Meyer DE. Effect of postpartum exercise on mothers and their offspring: a review of the literature. *Obes Res* 2002;**10**:841–53.

49. Ohlin A, Rossner S. Factors related to body weight changes during and after pregnancy: the Stockholm Pregnancy and Weight Development Study. *Obes Res* 1996;**4**:271–6.

50. Oken E, Taveras EM, Popoola FA, et al. Television, walking, and diet: associations with postpartum weight retention. *Am J Prev Med* 2007;**32**:305–11.

51. Gunderson EP, Rifas-Shiman SL, Oken E, et al. Association of fewer hours of sleep at 6 months postpartum with substantial weight retention at 1 year postpartum. *Am J Epidemiol* 2008;**167**:178–87.

52. Onyike CU, Crum RM, Lee HB, et al. Is obesity associated with major depression? Results from the Third National Health and Nutrition Examination Survey. *Am J Epidemiol* 2003;**158**:1199–47.

53. Roberts RE, Deleger S, Strawbridge WJ, Kaplan GA. Prospective association between obesity and depression: evidence from the Alameda County Study. *Int J Obes Relat Metab Disord* 2003;**27**:514–21.

54. Carter AS, Baker CW, Brownell KD. Body mass index, eating attitudes, and symptoms of depression and anxiety in pregnancy and the postpartum period. *Psychosom Med* 2000;**62**:264–70.

55. LaCoursiere DY, Baksh L, Bloebaum L, Varner MW. Maternal body mass index and self-reported postpartum depressive symptoms. *Matern Child Health J* 2006;**10**:385–90.

56. Baker JL, Michaelsen KF, Rasmussen KM, Sorensen TIA. Maternal prepregnant body mass index, duration of breastfeeding, and timing of complementary food introduction are associated with infant weight gain. *Am J Clin Nutr* 2004;**80**:1579–88.

57. Donath SM, Amir LH. Does maternal obesity adversely affect breastfeeding initiation and duration? *J Paediatr Child Health* 2000;**36**:482–6.

58. Hilson JA, Rasmussen KM, Kjolhede CL. High prepregnant body mass index is associated with poor lactation outcomes among white, rural women independent of psychosocial and demographic correlates. *J Hum Lact* 2004;**20**:18–29.

59. Kugyelka JG, Rasmussen KM, Frogillo EA. Maternal obesity is negatively associated with breastfeeding success among Hispanic but not Black women. *J Nutr* 2004; **134**:1746–53.

11 Obesity and contraception

Ailsa E Gebbie

Introduction

There is a complex association between a woman's weight and her use of contraception. Contraception is very widely used, and concern about weight has the potential to influence strongly patterns of usage. The most popular methods of contraception in the USA, the UK, and Australia are the combined oral contraceptive pill and the male condom[1-3] (Table 11.1). Women are quick to attribute the cause of any weight gain to their contraception, particularly if it is a hormonal method. Fear of gaining weight from hormonal methods can lead to poor compliance and early discontinuation. As the epidemic of obesity affects around one-third of women in the USA with similar numbers in Europe, many obese women will clearly be in the reproductive age range with a need for accurate contraceptive advice and safe prescribing.

Whenever contraception is prescribed, there is always a degree of balancing the small risks of the method against the consequences of pregnancy if effective contraception is withheld. On the other hand, when prescribing contraception for the obese woman, it is important to acknowledge that continuing a pregnancy or having an unplanned pregnancy terminated can both pose their own significant risks. Additionally, if an obese woman commences contraception in the postpartum period, particular care must be taken to ensure that the chosen method is safe and effective at this particular stage of her reproductive life.

The three main issues with contraception to consider in an obese woman are as follows:

- the efficacy of the method in obese women
- the safety profile of the method in obese women
- the potential of the method to cause weight gain.

These three issues are discussed in the context of the individual methods.

TABLE 11.1 Number of women 15–44 years of age and percentage distribution by current contraceptive method according to age in the USA, 2002

Contraceptive status and method	Age in years						
	15–44	15–19	20–24	25–29	30–34	35–39	40–44
Number in thousands							
Women aged 15–44 years[1]	61561	9834	9840	9249	10273	10823	11512
Percentage distribution							
Total	100.0	100.0	100.0	100.0	100.0	100.0	100.0
Using contraception							
Female sterilization	16.7	–	2.2	10.3	19.0	29.2	34.7
Male sterilization	5.7	–	0.5	2.8	6.4	10.0	12.7
Pill	19.0	16.7	31.8	25.6	21.8	13.2	7.6
Implant, Lunelle, or contraceptive patch	0.8	0.4	0.9	1.7	0.9	0.5	0.2
3-month injectable (Depo-Provera)	3.3	4.4	6.1	4.4	2.9	1.5	1.1
Intrauterine device (IUD)	1.3	0.1	1.1	2.5	2.2	1.0	0.8
Diaphragm	0.2	–	0.1	0.3	0.1	–	0.4
Condom	11.1	8.5	14.0	14.0	11.8	11.1	8.0
Periodic abstinence – calendar rhythm	0.7	–	0.8	0.3	0.9	1.1	1.2
Periodic abstinence – natural family planning	0.2	–	–	0.4	0.2	0.3	0.4
Withdrawal	2.5	0.8	3.1	5.3	2.6	2.4	1.0
Other methods[2]	0.6	0.6	0.2	0.4	0.4	0.5	1.1
Not using contraception							
Surgically sterile, female (noncontraceptive)	1.5	–	0.0	0.4	0.9	2.1	4.9
Non-surgically sterile, female or male	1.6	0.7	0.7	0.9	1.4	1.2	4.4
Pregnant or postpartum	5.3	3.5	9.5	8.4	6.9	3.8	0.8
Seeking pregnancy	4.2	1.2	2.8	5.5	7.0	5.1	3.3
Other non-use Never had intercourse	10.9	49.5	11.4	2.7	1.5	1.6	1.1

TABLE 11.1 (continued)

Contraceptive status and method	Age in years						
	15–44	15–19	20–24	25–29	30–34	35–39	40–44
Other non-use (continued)							
No intercourse in 3 months before interview	7.2	6.7	6.6	6.2	6.1	7.5	9.7
Had intercourse in 3 months before interview	7.4	6.9	8.4	8.0	7.0	7.7	6.7
All other non-use	0.0	–	–	–	–	0.1	0.1

Reproduced from the National Center for Health Statistics. Fertility, Family Planning, and Reproductive Health of U.S. Women: Data from the 2002 National Survey of Family Growth. Series 23, no. 25.[1]

TABLE 11.2 Current use of contraception by women using at least one method by age in the UK

Current use of contraception	Age in years							
	16–19	20–24	25–29	30–34	35–39	40–44	45–49	Total
Pill*	48	64	55	48	28	17	11	35
Male condom	63	39	37	28	26	20	16	30
Withdrawal	5	2	5	8	1	6	4	4
Intrauterine device	7	2	5	6	4	6	7	6
Injection	3	11	6	5	2	3	1	4
Implant	4	5	4	2	1	–	–	2
Periodic abstinence	2	4	3	4	5	3	3	3
Diaphragm/cap	–	–	–	1	1	–	3	1
Hormonal intrauterine system	1	1	2	2	6	1	1	2
Female condoms	–	–	–	–	–	1	–	0
Emergency contraception	5	0	2	0	0	0	0	1
Female sterilization	–	2	4	5	11	18	29	12
Vasectomy	–	–	1	8	20	30	28	15
Base	80	112	126	136	153	165	178	951

* Includes women who did not know which type of pill they were taking. Adapted from *Contraception and Sexual Health*, 2007.[2] Source: National Statistics website: www.statistics.gov.uk.

Combined hormonal contraception

The combined oral contraceptive pill (COC) was first approved for use in the USA in 1959 and in the UK 2 years later. Very rapidly, it became a highly popular method of contraception, and it is estimated that 200 million women have taken the combined pill since it first became available. Approximately 12 million women currently use the combined pill in the USA (3 million in the UK).[1,2] Combined hormonal contraceptive patches and rings are now marketed in many countries, but these non-oral routes of administration have been much less widely studied. It is likely that they share many of the characteristics of the oral method.

Efficacy

The current data are suggestive, but not conclusive, of a trend of slightly higher failure rates of COC in the presence of obesity. However, even if a small association does exist, it is unlikely that this would affect clinical practice, as the effectiveness of the method would still remain high.

The UK Oxford Family Planning Association study found no effect of body weight on efficacy of COC, although the numbers involved were small.[4] Although strong effects of age and parity on failure rates were found, no influence of body weight on risk of accidental pregnancy was found. The failure rates per 100 woman-years adjusted for age and parity were 0.21 (95% CI 0.15–0.30) in women weighing 51–57 kg and 0.21 (95% CI 0.04–0.61) in women weighing over 77 kg. In contrast, data from North America consistently suggest an association between weight and failure rates. One retrospective cohort analysis of 755 women found that those in the highest body-weight quartile (> 70.5 kg) had a significantly increased risk of pregnancy while taking COC (relative risk [RR] 1.6, 95% CI 1.1–2.4) compared with women of lower weight.[5] Women weighing over 70.5 kg had a failure rate of 5.6 per 100 person-years of COC use compared with a mean of 3.1 per 100 person-years in the lower three quartiles. In addition, higher elevations of risk associated with the highest weight quartile were seen among the very low-dose COC users. Similar results have been reported in users of the combined contraceptive patch.[6] Several recent studies show a trend of higher weight and increased risk of COC failure. After adjustment for factors such as education, income, and ethnicity, however, the results are attenuated and are no longer statistically significant.[7]

The potential biological mechanism whereby weight could lower COC efficacy is unknown. Metabolism of steroid hormones could be disordered, and one small study found a non-significant reduction in serum ethinyl estradiol concentrations in women in the highest weight quartile.[8] In obese women, there may simply be dilution of steroid hormones in a larger blood volume or greater absorption of hormones into a higher fat volume.

Safety

The World Health Organization (WHO) has published medical eligibility criteria (MEC) for contraceptive use, which include guidance relating to weight. For users of COC, BMI ≥ 30 kg/m^2 is a category 2 condition, i.e., the method can generally be used, but more careful follow-up may be required.[9] In the UK medical eligibility criteria, advice is more specific, as detailed in Table 11.3.[10] In addition, this varies slightly with the advice from the *British National Formulary* (BNF), which recommends an upper limit of 39 as an absolute contraindication to the combined pill, and 30 if there is any other risk factor for venous thromboembolism (VTE).[11]

Increased risk of VTE is the main safety concern for obese women using COC. In the general population, the baseline incidence of VTE in young women is very low, ranging from 7 per 100 000 to 10 per 100 000, but rises to 6–34 per 100 000 among woman aged 40–44 years.[12] COC increases risk of VTE across the board in all users by three- to sixfold and is highest in the first year of use.[13–15] Obesity alone also increases VTE risk significantly, and studies have shown an increasing gradient of risk as BMI increases. Results from the UK Mediplus Database and General Practice Research Database show that BMI > 25 was positively associated with an increased risk of VTE in COC users, Those with BMI > 35 had over three times the VTE risk of those with BMI 20–24.[16] Another study from the Netherlands showed a 10-fold increased risk in women with BMI > 25 taking COC compared with women of low weight.[17]

Risk of arterial disease in obese women taking COC is much harder to quantify. The WHO has extensively reviewed cardiovascular disease and steroid hormone contraception, although there are no specific data relating to weight.[18] Incidence and mortality rates from arterial disease in women of reproductive age are very low, and any increase attributable to use of COC is similarly very small if users do not smoke or have risk factors for cardiovascular disease, particularly hypertension.

TABLE 11.3 Use of combined hormonal contraception and obesity – UK medical eligibility criteria (UKMEC)[10]

BMI	UKMEC category	Definition of category
< 29	1	No restriction on using combined oral contraceptive pill (COC)
30–34	2	Advantages of using COC generally outweigh the theoretical or proven risks
35–39	3	Theoretical or proven risks of COC usually outweigh the advantages
≥ 40	4	Using COC represents an unacceptable health risk

Clinical judgement should therefore be exercised in prescribing COC to obese women who have other risk factors for arterial disease, such as hypertension, diabetes, or a strong family history, or who smoke. The BNF recommends that the combined pill be used with caution if a single risk factor exists, and that COC is contraindicated if there is a combination of two or more cardiovascular risk factors.[11]

Effect on weight

Various mechanisms have been postulated to explain why the combined pill could cause weight gain.[19] This could be through stimulation of the renin-angiotensin–mechanism, increased fluid retention, alteration of carbohydrate metabolism, or increased appetite. There is a general consensus that the older, higher-dose pills could theoretically be associated with weight gain, although this is much less likely with the low-dose preparations.[20] As over 80% of women in the USA use oral contraceptives for an average of 5 years, any effect of this method on real or perceived weight gain has the potential to exert a strong influence on continuation rates of the pill.[1]

In a National Opinion Poll in the 1990s of 1753 randomly selected British women, 73.1% of respondents thought that weight gain was a disadvantage of COC, and this was the commonest disadvantage cited in the study.[21] This compared with 45.1% of women who thought that headaches were an issue, 45% who were concerned about cardiovascular disease, and 41% who thought oral contraceptives had cancer risk. In a German survey of 1466 women, a considerable number perceived side effects during use of COC, 21% of current users and 31% of past users reporting weight gain (median increase of 5 kg, range 1–20 kg).[22] Similarly, in a cohort of Swedish women aged 19 years, 20% gave weight gain as the reason for cessation of use of COC.[23]

In the available trials that have examined the association between weight and use of COC, weight was rarely a primary outcome. As a result, most trials did not use rigorous methods for measuring weight. All women tend to gain weight with time, and most studies lacked a contemporaneous control group to assess the effect of this. A Cochrane Group has reviewed the effect of COC on weight. In summary, they found that there was no major effect on weight, although the available evidence was insufficient for total certainty.[24] Moreover, most comparisons of different combinations of hormones in combined preparations showed no substantial difference in weight gain or in discontinuations due to weight.[24] These data are generally very reassuring and should empower healthcare providers to inform women that weight gain should not be viewed as a direct consequence of taking COC, a highly effective method of contraception.

Practical prescribing of COC in obese women

Postpartum women
COC is not recommended in a woman breastfeeding immediately following birth. The Faculty of Sexual and Reproductive Healthcare guidance in the UK

is that breastfeeding women can use the combined pill from 6 months post partum without restriction.[10] However, from 6 weeks to 6 months, it is classed as UKMEC category 2/3 (2 = benefits usually outweigh risks, 3 = risks usually outweigh benefits) depending on the frequency of breastfeeds.[10] In non-breastfeeding women, COC is generally commenced at 21 days. Use of COC before 21 days is classed as UKMEC category 3. There is no specific evidence to alter this advice in the presence of obesity, but clinical judgement may dictate that obese women avoid use of COC in the postpartum period when risk of VTE is increased physiologically, particularly in the presence of other cardiovascular risk factors.

Choice of COC preparation

This is generally not influenced by obesity. In the UK, most women are routinely prescribed the older, cheaper, second-generation preparations, which have the lowest risk of VTE.[25] The preparation containing ethinyl estradiol plus cyproterone acetate (Dianette UK, Diane-35 USA) possibly has the highest risk of VTE and therefore should be prescribed with greatest caution in obese women.[26] In practical terms, this can be difficult, as women who benefit most from Dianette because of a history of polycystic ovarian syndrome often have more risk factors for cardiovascular disease including obesity. Specialist advice should be obtained, and a few women will be able to switch from Dianette to a preparation with lower VTE risk once their androgenic symptoms are suppressed.

Progestogen-only pill

The progestogen-only pill (POP) has never had a high market share in the USA or the UK, although it can have particular advantages for older women or those with cardiovascular risk factors. A more potent POP containing desogestrel (Cerazette) was introduced relatively recently, and it is more effective than traditional low-dose POP, as it inhibits ovulation in all cycles.

Efficacy

The Oxford Family Planning Association (FPA) contraceptive study in the UK did not find evidence that unplanned pregnancies occurred more often in overweight women who were taking the POP.[27] This study may not have had the power to detect a difference related to weight, however, as the overall number of accidental pregnancies was small. One small, in vitro study showed a lack of effect of the POP on cervical mucus from overweight women, giving indirect evidence of a lesser contraceptive action.[28] This is a continuing area of controversy, and, although it has been concluded that there is no real evidence that POPs are less effective in women weighing over 70 kg, double-dose POP is frequently recommended in the obese population and is unlikely to be harmful.[29] In women weighing over 70 kg with inherently lower fertility (such as women in their 40s or breastfeeding), it is not necessary to give double-dose POP. The desogestrel-containing POP Cerazette does not need to be administered in double dose to women weighing over 70 kg.

Safety

The POP is an extremely safe method of contraception and, in common with all progestogen-only methods of contraception, there are no restrictions on prescribing POP to women who are overweight.[10] No evidence comes from the scientific literature to suggest that obese women who use POP are at any greater adverse health risk than non-obese women.

Effect on weight

The Oxford FPA study found that around 6–8% of women who discontinued POP because of side effects did so because of perceived weight gain. This compared with around 60% of discontinuations for menstrual disturbance and was on a similar scale to the discontinuations for weight gain in women using COC in the same study.[27] No evidence exists to support the concept that women who are already obese at the time of initiation of POP will be specifically at increased risk of further weight gain.

Implanon

Implanon (releasing etonorgestral) is a single subdermal rod inserted into the upper arm under local anaesthetic; it lasts for 3 years. It offers extremely high efficacy and convenience, and is generally very well tolerated. For many years after its introduction, no genuine Implanon failures were reported in the literature, although a few have now appeared.[30]

Efficacy

No data in the literature suggest that the contraceptive effect of Implanon is affected by a woman's weight.[31] In contrast, there has been evidence of an effect on efficacy related to weight with the six-rod implant Norplant (releasing levonorgestral), which has now been largely superseded by Implanon in most countries. Pooled data with Norplant show a 5-year cumulative pregnancy rate above 7 per 100 users for women weighing more than 70 kg compared with 0.2 per 100 users weighing less than 50 kg.[32] A subsequent change in the capsule of Norplant to a softer formulation appeared to make it more effective in women of all weights.[33]

Safety

The recommendation in the UK is that there is no restriction on a woman of any weight using Implanon for contraception.[10] In common with other low-dose, progestogen-only contraceptive methods, the paucity of data prevent any assessment of the risk of cardiovascular disease with Implanon and whether this is affected by factors such as obesity.[13]

Effect on weight

Changes in weight in Implanon users have been examined in recent studies. In one review, about 60% of women had gained at least 1 kg by 24 months of using Implanon, and 37% had gained at least 3 kg. Analysis by initial body weight suggested that a weight gain of 3 kg or more was slightly more likely in women whose initial weight was less than 50 kg (48%) than in those who weighed more than 50 kg (38%).[34] Body weight increases gradually in almost all women of reproductive age, so it is difficult to attribute this change in weight solely to use of an implant. In a recent study looking at side effects of Implanon, weight gain was perceived to be a problem in only 4 out of 102 women and was a much less common complaint than bleeding disturbance or mood change.[35]

Injectables

Depot-medroxyprogesterone acetate (Depo-Provera) is a highly effective contraceptive method that has been in use worldwide for over 40 years. It is administered by intramuscular injection every 12 weeks.

Efficacy

Lower efficacy related to weight has not been reported in users of Depo-Provera. Pharmacokinetic studies show suppression of ovulation in women of all BMIs with both standard Depo-Provera and the newer, lower-dose, subcutaneous formulation.[36]

Safety

The UKMEC have no restriction related to weight in women wishing to use Depo-Provera for contraception.[10] The WHO's large, multinational, case–control study assessed the risk of cardiovascular disease with injectable progestogen-only contraceptives and found that it was not associated with any significant increase in risk of arterial disease or VTE.[13] The combined risk of stroke, myocardial infarction, and VTE in Depo-Provera users was not increased compared with non-users (OR 1.02, 95% CI 0.68–1.54). This gives reassurance that Depo-Provera can be used safely in women who are obese and in the presence of other risk factors for cardiovascular disease.

Effect on weight

Weight gain is a common concern for women starting to use Depo-Provera. Clearly, the individual response of any woman may vary and, in addition, ethnicity and social background probably play a very significant role in weight issues. Many, but not all, studies confirm that weight gain is more common with Depo-

Provera than with other methods of hormonal contraception. In one study, 12% of discontinuations of Depo-Provera were due to weight gain, compared with 20% for menstrual disturbances.[37] Another study reported a discontinuation rate of 5.7% due to weight in Depo-Provera users compared with 2.5% of combined pill users and 0.1% of users of intrauterine devices (IUDs).[38] When Depo-Provera users were compared retrospectively with IUD users in terms of measured weight gain, the Depo-Provera users gained 4.3 kg during 5 years of use compared with 1.8 kg in the IUD group.[39] In addition, the extra fat accumulated by Depo-Provera users appears to be largely of central distribution, which has long-term, potential metabolic and vascular implications.[40] The Faculty of Sexual and Reproductive Healthcare in the UK acknowledge that weight gain does limit the acceptability of Depo-Provera in western countries and more than 70% of women will gain weight.[41]

The veracity of the statement that obese women are likely to gain proportionately more weight during use of Depo-Provera than slim women is questionable due to limited and poor-quality evidence. One study suggested an increase in weight in overweight adolescent Depo-Provera users compared with normal-weight Depo-Provera users and overweight COC users (average gain in first year of use 13.6 lb versus 7.4 lb (3.4 kg) versus 6.9 lb (3.1 kg), respectively).[42] Another study found no statistically significant weight differential between Depo-Provera users who weighed greater or less than 200 lb (average weight gain 4.2 lb versus 4.4 lb, respectively, after 2 years of use).[43]

Finally, overweight and obese women tend to have slightly fewer bleeding disturbances when using Depo-Provera for contraception. One retrospective cohort study found the total percentages of women without excessive bleeding to be 94%, 96%, and 90% in obese, overweight, and normal weight users, respectively.[44] These small differences were not statistically different and are unlikely to affect clinical prescribing.

Practical prescribing of progestogen-only methods of contraception

Post partum

All progestogen-only methods can be commenced post partum in women whether they are breastfeeding or not. The only slight caveat in the UKMEC is that Depo-Provera is category 2 (benefits usually outweigh risks) in breastfeeding women up to 6 weeks post partum, although the other methods are category 1 (no restriction for use).[10] This advice is not altered in any way in relation to the presence of obesity, and progestogen-only methods are a recommendable choice for many postpartum women.

Choice of progestogen-only method

This is entirely related to individual choice with respect to acceptability of delivery system, duration of use, and effect on menstrual bleeding pattern. Women over

70 kg may find the daily regimen of double-dose POP cumbersome and opt for a long-acting method of contraception for greater convenience.

Intrauterine contraception

Intrauterine contraception comprises the copper IUD and the levonorgestrel-releasing intrauterine system (IUS). Both are highly effective methods and may be recommended for obese women despite the occasional practical difficulties in terms of gaining clear access to the cervix if the vaginal walls are extremely lax. This can be overcome by an experienced operator with a selection of specula and other vaginal instruments. It is important that clinics offer a suitable bariatric couch for the safety and comfort of any obese woman.

Efficacy

Intrauterine methods of contraception are no less effective in obese than in non-obese women.

Safety

Obese women experience no particular safety issues relating to use of intrauterine contraception. An IUD or IUS can be inserted postpartum 4 weeks following delivery.[10] Moreover, because obese women have an elevated risk of endometrial neoplasia, the use of the IUS may be a beneficial choice for these women.[45]

Effect on weight

A retrospective cohort study of users of copper IUDs over 7 years showed that women did gain weight with time, albeit entirely in keeping with the trend of normal weight gain with age.[46] Long-term follow-up of IUS users over a mean of 12.2 (range 9.8–13.3) years showed an average increase in weight of 5.7 kg (range 11–23 kg).[47] Again, this is entirely consistent with normal weight gain due to age and lifestyle. In IUS users, weight gain is perceived as a much less common side effect than bleeding problems.[48]

Barrier methods

Barrier methods comprise condoms and female barriers (diaphragm and cervical cap). No contraindication to any of these methods exists based on weight alone, and no method contributes in any way to weight gain. Obesity does not affect the efficacy of barrier methods. In the UK, the Faculty of Sexual and Reproductive Healthcare recommends that women be reassessed for diaphragm or cervical cap size in the event of weight change of 3 kg or more.[49]

Sterilization

On a global scale, female sterilisation is an extremely popular method of contraception. However, compared with the decades following the introduction of laparoscopy into clinical practice, the number of women being sterilized in recent years has declined substantially[1] (Figures 11.1 and 11.2). Many possible factors can explain this change. However, high on the list is the fact are that long-acting reversible contraceptive methods, such as the IUS, have become more widely used and are viewed as safe and effective alternatives for all groups of women.[50] In addition, women are delaying childbearing and do not wish to have a permanent form of contraception.

Efficacy and safety

Most female sterilization procedures are undertaken laparoscopically under general anaesthesia. Not surprisingly, obese women are more likely to have a technical failure of a laparoscopic procedure resulting in the operation being uncompleted, or completed by changing to a different surgical approach. In one multicentre comparative study, 22% of obese women (defined as over 120% more than the desirable weight) had a technical failure of the procedure compared with 4% of controls.[51] Instrument problems were common, the trochar often being too short to reach the peritoneal cavity. The US Collaborative Review of Sterilization Group found that obesity (defined as BMI > 30) was an independent

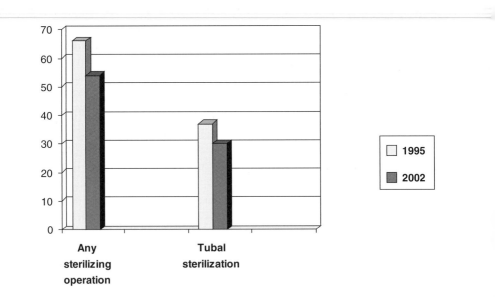

FIGURE 11.1 Percentage of married women aged 40–44 years who have ever had a sterilizing operation and percentage who have ever had tubal sterilization – 1995 and 2002 in the USA[1]

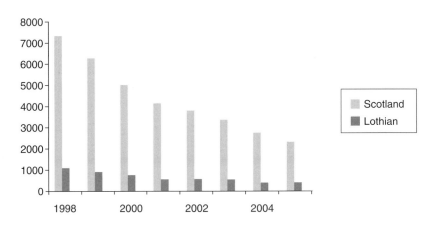

FIGURE 11.2 Female sterilization rates in Scotland and Lothian region 1998–2004. Adapted from Information Services Division, Scotland.[55]

predictor of one or more peri- or postoperative complications (OR 1.7, 95% CI 1.4–2.6) and on a similar scale to the same complications in women with previous abdominal or pelvic surgery (OR 2, 95% CI 1.4–2.9).[52] In addition, general anaesthesia itself carries more risk in an obese woman, with a high likelihood of difficult intubation or failed venous cannulation. ESSURE, a new technique that involves placing hysteroscopically guided microcoils into the fallopian tubes under local anaesthesia, may be a better option for the morbidly obese woman and this is currently under trial in several countries.[53]

Effect on weight

The term 'post-sterilization syndrome' has been coined to describe a variety of symptoms that women attributed to being sterilized; it includes menstrual dysfunction, premenstrual syndrome, psychosexual issues, and weight gain. A review of the literature concluded that sterilization is not associated with increased risk of any of these problems except where women are sterilized at a young age and the symptoms may be a manifestation of regret.[54]

Summary

Table 11.4 gives a summary of the effects on weight of the varying contraceptive methods.

TABLE 11.4 Summary of effects of contraceptive methods on weight

Contraceptive method	Summary of effect on weight
Combined hormonal contraception	No major effect on weight with modern low-dose preparations, although evidence inconclusive. No evidence of substantial variation between different preparations
Progestogen-only pill	No effect
Implant	No effect
Injectables	Weight gain greater than that of non-users; 70% of users likely to gain weight. Trend of greater weight gain in women who are already obese but data mixed
Barrier methods	No effect
Intrauterine contraception	No effect
Female sterilization	No effect

References

1. National Center for Health Statistics. *Fertility, Family Planning, and Reproductive Health of US Women: Data from the 2002 National Survey of Family Growth*. Series 23, no. 25. Available at: www.cdc.gov/nchs/data/series/sr_23/sr23_025.pdf.
2. Lader D. *Contraception and Sexual Health*. A report on research using the National Statistics Omnibus Survey produced on behalf of the Information Centre for health and social care. Omnibus Survey Report no. 3. Office for National Statistics, UK, 2007. Available at: www.statistics.gov.uk/downloads/theme_health/contraception2006-07.pdf.
3. Yusuf F, Siedlecky S. Patterns of contraceptive use in Australia: analysis of the 2001 National Health Survey. *J Biosoc Sci* 2007;**39**:735–44.
4. Vessey MP. Oral contraceptive failures and body weight. Findings in a large cohort study. *J Fam Plann* 2001;**27**:90–1.
5. Holt V, Cushing-Haugen KL, Daling JR. Body weight and risk of oral contraceptive failure. *Obstet Gynecol* 2002;**99**:820–7.
6. Zieman M, Guillebaud J, Weisberg E, et al. Contraceptive efficacy and cycle control with the Ortho Evra™/Evra™ transdermal system: the analysis of pooled data. *Fertil Steril* 2002;**77**:S13–18.
7. Brunner Huber LR, Hogue CJ, Stein AD, et al. Body mass index and risk for oral contraceptive failure: a case-cohort study in South Carolina. *Ann Epidemiol* 2006;**16**:637–43.
8. Stadel BV, Sternthal PM, Schlesselman JJ, et al. Variation of ethinyl estradiol blood levels among healthy women using oral contraceptives. *Fertil Steril* 1980;**33**:257–60.

9. World Health Organization. *Medical Eligibility Criteria for Contraceptive Use*, 3rd edn. Geneva: World Health Organization, 2004. Available at: www.who. int/reproductive-health/publications/mec/index.htm.

10. Faculty of Family Planning and Reproductive Health Care. UK Medical Eligibility Criteria 2005/06. Available at: www.ffprhc.org.uk.

11. Joint Formulary Committee. British National Formulary 55. London: Pharmaceutical Press, 2008.

12. Curtis K, Marchbanks PA. Hormonal contraception and cardiovascular safety. In: Glasier A, Wellings K, Critchley H (eds), *Contraception and Contraceptive Use*. London: RCOG Press, 2005.

13. WHO Scientific Group on Cardiovascular Disease and Steroid Hormone Contraception. *WHO Technical Report Series 877*. Geneva: World Health Organization, 1997.

14. Jick H, Kaye JA, Vasilikis-Scaramozza C, Jick SS. Risk of venous thromboembolism among users of third generation oral contraceptives compared with users of oral contraceptives with levonorgestrel before and after 1995: cohort and case-control analysis. *BMJ* 2000;**321**:119–15.

15. Lewis MA, Spitzer WO, Heinemann LA, et al. Third generation oral contraceptives and risk of myocardial infarction: an international case-control study. Transnational Research Group on Oral Contraceptives and the Health of Young Women. *BMJ* 1996;**312**:88–90.

16. Nightingale AL, Lawrenson RA, Simpson TJ, et al. The effects of age, body mass index, smoking and general health on the risk of venous thromboembolism in users of combined oral contraceptives. *Eur J Contracept Reprod Health Care* 2000;**5**:265–74.

17. Abdollahi M, Cushman M, Rosendaal FR. Obesity: risk of venous thrombosis and the interaction with coagulation factor levels and oral contraceptive use. *Thromb Haemost* 2003;**89**:493–8.

18. WHO Scientific Group on Cardiovascular Disease and Steroid Hormone Contraception. Who Technical Report Series 877. Geneva: World Health Organization, 1998.

19. Gupta S. Weight gain on the combined pill – is it real? *Hum Reprod Update* 2000;**6**:427–31.

20. Neel EV, Litt IF, Jay MS. Side effects and compliance with low and conventional dose COCs among adolescents. *J Adolesc Healthcare* 1987;**8**:327–9.

21. Oddens BJ, Visser AP, Vemer HM, et al. Contraceptive use and attitudes in Great Britain. *Contraception* 1994;**49**:3–86.

22. Oddens BJ. Women's satisfaction with birth control: a population survey of physical and psychological effects of oral contraceptives, intrauterine devices, condoms, natural family planning, and sterilisation among 1466 women. *Contraception* 1999;**59**:277–86.

23. Larsson G, Blohm F, Sundell G, et al. A longitudinal study of birth control and pregnancy outcome among women in a Swedish population. *Contraception* 1997;**56**:9–16.

24. Gallo MF, Lopez LM, Grimes DA, et al. Combination contraceptives: effects on weight. *Cochrane Database Syst Rev* 2006; **1**:CD003987.

25. Hennessy S, Berlin JA, Kinman JL, et al. Risk of venous thromboembolism from oral contraceptives containing gestodene and desogestrel versus levonorgestrel: a meta-analysis and formal sensitivity analysis. *Contraception* 2001;**64**:25–33.

26. Vasilikis-Scarmozza C, Jick H. Risk of venous thromboembolism with cyproterone or levonorgestrel contraceptives. *Lancet* 2001;**358**:1427–9.

27. Vessey MP, Lawless M, Yeats D, McPherson K. Progestogen-only oral contraception. Findings in a large prospective study with special reference to effectiveness. *Br J Fam Plann* 1985;**10**:117–21.

28. Kovacs GT, Kendricks J, Summerball C, et al. A pre-coital pill? A preliminary in vitro study. *Br J Fam Plann* 2000;**26**:165–6.

29. De Souza A, Brechin S, Penney G. The members' enquiry service: frequently asked questions. *J Fam Plann Reprod Health Care* 2003;**29**:160–1.

30. Meirik O, Fraser IS, d'Arcangues C. Implantable contraceptives for women. *Hum Reprod Update* 2003;**9**:49–59.

31. Croxatto HB, Urbancsek J, Massai R, et al. A multicentre efficacy and safety study of the single contraceptive implant Implanon. *Hum Reprod* 1999;**14**: 976–81.

32. Sivin I. International experience with Norplant and Norplant-2 contraception. *Stud Fam Plann* 1988;**19**:81–94.

33. Sivin I, Mishell D, Darney P, et al. Levonorgestrel capsule implants in the United States: a 5 year study. *Obstet Gynecol* 1998;**92**:337–44.

34. Edwards JE, Moore A. Implanon – a review of clinical studies. *Br J Fam Plann* 1999;**24**:3–16.

35. Raj K, Gupta S, Cotter S. Experience with Implanon in a north-east London family planning clinic. *Eur J Contracep Reprod Health Care* 2004;**9**:39–46.

36. Jain J, Dutton C, Nicosia A, et al. Pharmacokinetics, ovulation suppression and return to ovulation following a lower dose subcutaneous formulation of Depo-Provera. *Contraception* 2004;**70**:11–18.

37. Paul C, Skegg DCG, Williams S. Depot medroxyprogesterone acetate; patterns of use and reasons for discontinuation. *Contraception* 1997;**56**: 209–14.

38. Colli E, Tong D, Penhallegon R, Parazzini F. Reasons for contraceptive discontinuation in women 20–39 years old in New Zealand. *Contraception* 1999;**59**:227–31.

39. Bahamondes L, Del Castillo S, Tabares G, et al. Comparison of weight increase in users of depo-medroxyprogesterone acetate and copper IUD up to 5 years. *Contraception* 2001;**64**:223–5.

40. Clark MK, Dillon JS, Sowers M, Nichols S. Weight, fat mass, and central distribution of fat increase when women use depot-medroxyprogesterone acetate for contraception. *Int J Obes* 2005;**29**:1252–8.

41. Bigrigg A, Evans M, Gbolade B, et al. Depo-Provera. Position paper on clinical use, effectiveness and side effects. *Br J Fam Plann* 1999;**25**:69–76.

42. Mangan SA, Larsen PG, Hudson S. Overweight teens at increased risk for weight gain while using depot medroxyprogesterone acetate. *J Pediatr Adolesc Gynecol* 2002;**15**:79–82.

43. Leiman G. Depo-medroxyprogesterone acetate as a contraceptive agent: its effect on weight and blood pressure. *Am J Obstet Gynecol* 1972;**114**:97–102.

44. Connor PD, Tavernier LA, Thomas SM, et al. Determining risk between Depo-Provera use and increased uterine bleeding in obese and overweight women. *J Am Board Fam Pract* 2002;**15**:7–10.

45. American College of Obstetricians and Gynecologists Committee on Practice Bulletins – Gynecology. ACOG Practice Bulletin, no. 73. Use of hormonal contraception in women with coexisting medical conditions. *Obstet Gynecol* 2006;**107**:1453–72.

46. Hassan DF, Petta CA, Aldrighi JM, et al. Weight variation in a cohort of women using copper IUD for contraception. *Contraception* 2003;**68**:27–30.

47. Ronnerdag M, Odlind V. Health effects of long-term use of the intrauterine levonorgestrel-releasing system. A follow-up study over 12 years of continuous use. *Acta Obstet Gynaecol Scand* 1999;**78**:716–21.

48. Varma R, Sinha D, Gupta JK. Non-contraceptive uses of levonorgestrel-releasing hormone system (LNG-IUS) – a systematic enquiry and overview. *Eur J Obstet Gynecol* 2006;**124**:9–28.

49. Clinical Effectiveness Unit of the Faculty of Family Planning. *Female barrier methods*. London: Faculty of Family Planning, 2007. Available at: www.ffprhc. org.uk.

50. National Institute for Health and Clinical Excellence. *Long acting reversible contraception: the effective and appropriate use of long-acting reversible contraception*. London: NICE, 2005. Available at: www.nice.org.uk/pdf/CG030fullguideline.pdf.

51. Chi I, Mumford SD, Laufe LE. Technical failures in tubal ring sterilisation. *Am J Obstet Gynecol* 1980;**138**:307–12.

52. Jamieson DJ, Hillis SD, Duerr A, et al. Complications of interval laparoscopic tubal sterilization: findings from the United States Collaborative Review of Sterilization. *Obstet Gynecol* 2000;**96**:997–1002.

53. Duffy S, Marsh F, Rogerson L, et al. Female sterilisation: a cohort controlled comparative study of ESSURE versus laparoscopic sterilisation. *BJOG* 2005; **112**:1522–8.

54. Glasier A. Sterilisation. In: Glasier A, Gebbie A, eds. *Handbook of Family Planning and Reproductive Health Care*, 5th edn. London: Churchill Livingstone, Elsevier, 2008.

55. Adapted from data from Information Services, Scotland. Available at: www. scotland.gov.uk/resource/doc/924/0044637.pdf and www.scotland.gov.uk/ resource/doc/35596/0012575.pdf.

12 Diet and anti-obesity drugs

Manny Noakes and Jane Scott

Introduction

The increasing rate of obesity in women of childbearing age presents a concern for two reasons. First, there is an increased likelihood that women entering pregnancy with a high BMI will gain and retain more weight in subsequent pregnancies and, second, the effects of maternal obesity on the fetus and the propensity of the child also to become obese later are now well documented.[1] Under these circumstances, the optimal nutritional management of women of childbearing age before conception, as well as during and after pregnancy, may provide opportunities to improve health outcomes for the mother and her child.

Diet

Preconception

Obesity in young women impairs fertility via ovulatory disturbance consequent to insulin resistance.[2] Modest weight losses of 5–10% in obese women through diet and physical activity improve insulin resistance, menstrual cyclicity, and the hormonal milieu conducive to fertilization.[3] Hyperandrogenism and insulin sensitivity are improved significantly within the first 4 weeks of calorie restriction, and this is unrelated to the magnitude of weight loss.[4] When the effects of diet composition on outcomes have been assessed under equal calorie conditions, no differential effects of weight loss have been observed with high-protein, moderate-carbohydrate diets or high-carbohydrate, moderate-protein diets with a 7.5% weight loss over 12 weeks.[5] However, the high-protein, moderate-carbohydrate diet was associated with significant reduction in depression and improvement in self-esteem, whereas no change in either of these factors was observed with the high-carbohydrate diet.[6] Weight loss by meal replacements effectively results in short-term weight loss of 5.6 ± 2.4 kg in 8 weeks in overweight women with polycystic ovary syndrome (PCOS), a common disorder in women of reproductive age. Weight loss was sustained to 6 months by either a carbohydrate-restriction approach (< 120 g/day) or a fat-restriction (< 50 g/day) regimen.[7]

Crosignani[8] studied 33 anovulatory overweight patients with PCOS over 6 months on a 1200-kcal/day diet and physical exercise. Three-quarters of the participants lost at least 5% of their body weight. Ovarian morphology changed during the diet, with a significant reduction in ovarian volume and in the number of microfollicles per ovary. Among the 27 patients with oligo-amenorrhoea, 18 resumed regular cycles, and 15 had spontaneous ovulation; 10 spontaneous pregnancies occurred in patients who lost at least 5% of their weight.

In a review of the management of subfertility in obese women with PCOS,[9] weight loss of over 5% of pretreatment weight restored menstrual regularity in 89% of the women, of whom 30% achieved spontaneous pregnancy. Approximately 75–80% of anovulatory PCOS women respond to clomiphene citrate and 35–50% achieve pregnancy. For clomiphene citrate-resistant PCOS women (20–25%), clomiphene citrate plus metformin (1.5 g/day) for 3–6 months results in a 70% chance of restoration of regular menses and ovulation, along with a 23% chance of pregnancy.

Not all women who lose weight respond with improvements in reproductive function. Recently, anti-müllerian hormone (AMH), an inhibitor of follicle recruitment and maturation, which is increased in women with PCOS, has been shown to predict menstrual response to weight loss in PCOS. Moran et al[10] demonstrated that women who experienced improved menstrual cyclicity had lower AMH levels at baseline.

For obese women, bariatric surgery presents an approach associated with substantial weight loss (see Chapter 13). Such an approach may be advantageous as a means of assisting fertility as well as reducing risks to mother and fetus normally associated with obesity in pregnancy. However, the operation itself is not without risk, the nature of which may depend on procedure (gastric bypass versus banding). With the former, nutrient deficiencies are common,[11] with deficiencies in vitamins A, C, D, B_1, B_2, B_6, and B_{12} among those commonly reported at 12 months after surgery. Studies suggest that, while previous bariatric surgery may be an independent risk factor for caesarean delivery, the operation appears not to be associated with adverse perinatal outcomes.[12,13] Indeed, in those undergoing laparoscopic adjustable gastric banding, the incidence of adverse obstetric outcomes was lower than in obese women who did not have the procedure.[13] However, because the numbers of participants in studies to date have been small, a prudent approach would be to limit pregnancy to at least 2 years after bariatric surgery.[14]

Obesity also appears to be associated with deficiencies in several nutrients. Iron deficiency and the hypoferraemia observed in obesity appear to be explained both by true iron deficiency and by inflammatory-mediated functional iron deficiency.[15] Vitamin D deficiency has also been noted to be more prevalent in obesity.[16] Folate nutrition is important in both normal-weight and overweight women of reproductive age; the US Institute of Medicine (IOM) recommends 400 μg/day during pregnancy.[17] Subsequent studies have indicated that folate should commence 3 months prior to conception.[18] This has been shown to prevent up to 50–60% of neural tube defects; 4000 μg/day is recommended for those at high risk (by virtue of a previous neural tube defect pregnancy outcome).[19] Mandatory folate fortification of cereal grain products (140 μg/100 g) in the USA ensued when it became evident that such recommendations were not adequately implemented. More recently, an extensive Cochrane Review sponsored by the Society of Obstetricians and Gynaecologists of Canada[20] has recommended that women of reproductive age follow a diet of folate-rich foods and daily supplementation with a multivitamin with folic acid (400–1000 μg) for at least 2–3 months before conception and throughout pregnancy and the postpartum period (4–6 weeks and as long as breastfeeding continues). For women with a past history of congenital abnormality, high-dose folic acid (5000 μg) plus multivitamins is recommended to prevent recurrence of a congenital anomaly and should begin at least 3 months before conception and continue until 10–12 weeks after conception.[20] The Canadian guidelines also recommend that patients with health risks, such as epilepsy, type 1 diabetes, obesity with body mass index (BMI) over 35, and family history of neural tube defects, require increased dietary intake of folate-rich foods and daily supplementation with multivitamins and 5000 μg folic acid, also beginning at least 3 months before conception and continuing until 10–12 weeks after conception[20] From 12 weeks after conception and continuing throughout pregnancy and the postpartum period (4–6 weeks or as long as breastfeeding continues), supplementation should consist of a multivitamin with folic acid (400–1000 μg).

Clearly, for optimal reproductive health in overweight or obese women, preconception is the ideal time for lifestyle intervention, weight management, and appropriate nutritional guidelines. However, a survey of Canadian family physicians and obstetrician–gynaecologists[21] showed that fewer than 50% discussed weight management with women of childbearing age who were not pregnant. The survey authors suggest that there are missed opportunities in preconception screening to identify women with suboptimal reproductive health status who are at risk of adverse conception, pregnancy, and birth outcomes On the other hand, in a cross-sectional survey of 900 practising members of the American College of Obstetricians and Gynecologists (ACOG),[22] 80% reported counselling patients about weight control and 84% about physical activity 'most of the time' or 'often', although only 44% believed that they could help their patients lose weight.

Antenatal

Calorie intake and weight gain

Once an obese woman has become pregnant, weight gain during that pregnancy is associated with differential outcomes. Jain et al[23] retrospectively assessed the independent effect of prepregnancy obesity and weight gain of more than 34 lb (15 kg), showing an increased rate of caesarean section in primiparous and multiparous women, macrosomia, and a lower rate of breastfeeding at 10 weeks postpartum. This is consistent with the recommendations of the IOM[17] regarding the importance of optimal BMI at the start of pregnancy and modified weight gain in those with high BMI at conception in order to achieve better pregnancy outcomes in obese and overweight women. The recommended total weight gain for pregnant women with a BMI of > 26–29 is 7–11.5 kg, whereas the recommendation for obese women (BMI > 29) is only 6.8 kg. A recent Swedish study[24] found that decreased risk of adverse obstetric and neonatal outcomes was associated with the lower gestational weight gain recommended, particularly among obese women. This study showed that the optimal gestational weight gain in women was less than 9 kg for BMI 25–29.9 and less than 6 kg for BMI of 30 or more. Weight gain recommendations are shown in Table 12.1.

Despite the existence and relevance of these guidelines, among overweight women with prepregnancy BMI of 26.1–29.0, a survey in the San Francisco Bay area (USA) found that 24.1% of these women reported being advised on a target weight gain above the IOM guidelines compared with 4.3% of normal-weight women who became pregnant ($P < 0.001$).[25]

A Cochrane Review of the maternal outcomes of using calorie/protein restriction to limit weight gain in overweight women during pregnancy[26] cites three trials totalling 384 women that showed no effect on either (proteinuric) pre-eclampsia or pregnancy-induced hypertension (with or without proteinuria), although the small number of trials and participants provided inadequate statistical power to exclude a small effect. Effects of protein/calorie restriction on birth weight were also equivocal with heterogeneous results. Some of this heterogeneity may be related to the degree of calorie restriction. Knopp[27] compared 33% and 50% calorie restriction in women with gestational diabetes and showed that both interventions provided similar improvements in glycaemia but only the 50% restriction resulted in ketonuria. Plasma ketones have been causally related to increase the risk of fetal malformations largely because growth retardation has been observed in in vitro studies with at least 20-fold higher concentrations of ketones than in human studies. One study compared ketone levels in pregnant women with or without type 1 diabetes and found that first-trimester plasma ketones were significantly higher in diabetic than non-diabetic pregnant women and that ketone levels were inversely related to birth weight. However, ketone levels were lower, not higher, in mothers who had a malformed infant or pregnancy loss.[28] The role of plasma ketones induced by severe caloric or carbohydrate restriction in pregnant women with and without diabetes warrants further study.

Randomized trials attempting to limit weight gain in pregnancy have had mixed success in preventing excessive weight gain during pregnancy. Polley[29] was able to achieve this in normal-weight women, but not in overweight women,

TABLE 12.1 Comparison of gestational weight gain recommendations

Institute of Medicine[17] (1990)	Gestational weight gain (kg)	Cedergren[24] (2007)	Gestational weight gain (kg)
Low (BMI < 19.8)	12.5–18	BMI < 20	4–10
Normal (BMI 19.8–26)	11.5–16.0	BMI 20.0–24.9	2–10
High (BMI > 26–29)	7.0–11.5	BMI 25.0–29.9	< 9
Obese (BMI > 29)	At least 6.8	BMI ≥ 30	< 6

whereas Kinnunen[30] was able to achieve dietary change but unable to prevent excessive gestational weight gain. On the other hand, Crowther et al[31] found that, in predominantly overweight pregnant women, treatment of gestational diabetes with diet, blood glucose monitoring, and insulin as required was associated with lower frequency of pre-eclampsia, fourfold reduction in serious perinatal morbidity, and improvement in health-related quality of life. In this study, the intervention group gained significantly less weight than the control group (8.1±0.3 vs 9.8±0.4 kg; $P = 0.01$). A lifestyle intervention programme to restrict weight gain in women with gestational diabetes found that those who gained weight had a higher percentage of macrosomic infants than those who either lost weight or had no weight change during pregnancy.[32] For women with PCOS, metformin during pregnancy was associated with a 10-fold reduction in gestational diabetes (31–3%).[33] However, it is known that metformin crosses the placenta;[34] hence, its routine use has been cautioned against[35,36] (discussed more extensively in Chapters 6 and 14).

Contradictory observational data are emerging on the relationship of glycaemic index (GI)[37] and glycaemic load[38] of the diet before or during pregnancy on pregnancy outcomes. A randomized controlled trial of a high- and low-GI diet during pregnancy in 62 Australian women[39] showed that, compared with the low-GI group, women in the high-GI group gave birth to infants who were significantly heavier (+236 g), and had higher birth percentile (69 vs 48), ponderal index (2.74 vs 2.62), and prevalence of large for gestational age (33.3% vs 3.1%). Further studies are needed to confirm these observations.

Supplements

Apart from total calorie intake and weight gain guidelines during pregnancy, nutritional requirements need additional consideration. For the general population of pregnant women, the IOM recommends supplements of 30 mg ferrous iron during the second and third trimesters.[17] Similarly, the IOM recommends a folate supplement of 300 μg/day when there are doubts about the adequacy of dietary folate. Women who do not consume fruit or juice, or wholegrain or fortified cereals, and eat green vegetables infrequently are likely to have low folate intake. Such individuals may also have dietary intakes inadequate in several critical nutrients, as would women in high-risk categories such as those carrying more than one fetus, heavy cigarette smokers, and alcohol and drug abusers. For such individuals, the IOM recommends a daily multivitamin-mineral preparation containing the following nutrients, beginning in the second trimester:

- iron 30 mg
- vitamin B_6 2 mg
- zinc 15 mg
- folate 300 μg
- copper 2 mg
- vitamin C 50 mg

- calcium 250 mg
- vitamin D 5 μg.

In addition, vitamin D 10 μg (400 IU) daily is advised for complete vegetarians consuming no animal products at all and others with a low intake of vitamin D-fortified milk. Calcium 600 mg daily is advised for women under age 25 whose daily dietary calcium intake is less than 600 mg. Vitamin B_{12} 2 μg daily is advised for vegetarians not consuming dairy or eggs products. When therapeutic levels of iron (> 30 mg/day) are given to treat anaemia, supplementation with approximately 15 mg zinc and 2 mg copper is recommended because the iron may interfere with the absorption and utilization of these trace elements. It is important to remember that these recommendations were published in 1990 and that the mid-1980s science that informed them has been updated in many areas. For example, it is now generally recommended that 400 μg folic acid is the preferable dose.[20] Recent studies suggest that lower iron doses of 20 mg/day are effective in treating anaemia during pregnancy with fewer associated gastrointestinal side effects,[40] and that iron and calcium should not be given in the same preparation because the calcium interferes with the absorption of iron.[41] Vitamin D deficiency has also been observed in black and white pregnant women and neonates residing in the northern USA even if taking vitamin supplements.[42] Rise of prepregnancy BMI from 22 to 34 has also been associated with twofold (95% CI 1.2, 3.6) and 2.1-fold (1.2, 3.8) increases in the odds of midpregnancy and neonatal vitamin D deficiency,[42] and it is associated with increased risk of pre-eclampsia.[43] While it is recommended that women whose clothing severely restricts their access to sunlight should also be taking vitamin D, vitamin D deficiency is clearly widespread and may warrant routine assessment. Perhaps most importantly, the IOM recommends that supplementation begin in the second trimester, whereas more recent recommendations on supplementation recognize the importance of starting both folate and appropriate multivitamins in the preconception period and carrying on throughout the pregnancy and the interconception period.[20]

Iodine is another nutrient with an intake that may be inadequate, and its deficiency is widespread in many pregnant women in Europe. The American Thyroid Association has recommended that women planning a pregnancy should receive an iodine-containing supplement (approximately 150 μg/day) during pregnancy and lactation.[44] In Tasmania, Australia, although iodine fortification of bread has corrected iodine deficiency in children, the deficiency in pregnancy persists, and the authors call for mandatory universal salt iodization as the strategy to eliminate iodine deficiency in Australia.[45] Finally, meta-analyses by Goh et al on maternal consumption of folic acid-containing, prenatal multivitamins showed a significantly decreased risk of several congenital anomalies[46] and paediatric cancers,[47] not only neural tube defects. Consistent with this finding, maternal multiple micronutrient supplementation in Indonesia showed an explicit additional 14% reduction of fetal loss and infant death compared with supplementation with iron and folic acid alone, undernourished and anaemic women receiving most benefit.[48]

Postpartum

Failure to return to prepregnancy weight within 6 months postpartum is a predictor of long-term obesity.[49] However, only about one-third of women return to prepregnancy weight by 6 months postpartum,[50] and many women cite pregnancy as one of the events associated with the advent of weight gain in adulthood. One year after childbirth, women retain, on average, 0.5–4.0 kg, with as many as 25% retaining 4.5 kg or more.[50] This is particularly important in light of the evidence that a woman who retains an excessive amount of weight after pregnancy has a higher risk of doing so in subsequent pregnancies.[51]

Postpartum weight retention is a function of gestational weight gain, and women whose weight gain during pregnancy is within the IOM guidelines retain less weight postpartum in all categories of BMI.[52] Conversely, gestational weight gain above the recommended range is associated with postpartum weight retention. Women with the highest gestational weight gain and with body fat of $\geq 30\%$ have the highest likelihood of developing maternal obesity.[53] A study of Brazilian women showed that 35% of each kilogram of weight gained during pregnancy was retained after 9 months postpartum, even after adjustment for age, prepregnancy BMI, body fat, and years since first delivery.[53] In practice, many pregnant women gain weight well in excess of the IOM guidelines, two US studies noting that 42.8% of women with normal BMI[54] and 77% of obese women[55] gained more than the IOM guidelines.

Evidence from a large prospective study in the USA[56] fails to suggest that exclusive breastfeeding is associated with less weight retention. There is, however, a theoretical risk that weight reduction may compromise lactation, and it has been argued that lactating women should not attempt to lose weight until after 6 months postpartum, after which breast milk is no longer the sole source of nutrition for their infant.[52] As most Australian women (83%) initiate breastfeeding and almost half continue to 6 months postpartum,[57] the impact of postpartum weight loss on breastfeeding success should be carefully considered. Evidence from several studies suggests that dietary restriction that promotes modest weight loss has no effect on milk volume and concentration. For example, no adverse effect on lactation was seen among women who lost an average of 0.48 kg/week for 10 weeks.[58] Nor was a reduction of breast milk volume observed among women who consumed ≥ 6.28 MJ/day (1500 kcal/day), whereas women who consumed under 6.28 MJ/day experienced a decrease in milk volume.[59] A randomized controlled trial of short duration[60] found that an average weekly weight loss of 1.2 kg, associated with a daily calorie deficit of 35%, did not appear to compromise breastfeeding among a group of women with average BMI of 25.2 at baseline. Leermakers[61] showed that a behavioural weight loss intervention, delivered via correspondence, was effective at 6 months postpartum (–7.8 kg vs –4.9 kg). Lovelady et al[62] showed that weight loss of approximately 0.5 kg per week at 4–14 weeks postpartum in overweight women who were exclusively breastfeeding did not affect the growth of their infants. O'Toole[63] showed that a structured diet and exercise programme for 12 weeks postpartum was successful in 23 of 40 participants who achieved a mean 7.3-kg weight loss that persisted at 1 year; this was significantly different from the control group, who experienced no weight loss. Kinnunen,[64] in a study conducted through child health clinics in Finland, showed a fourfold odds ratio for returning to prepregnancy weight in the intervention (individual counselling on diet and physical activity) group compared with controls. Hence, there is growing evidence that programmes targeting postpartum weight management may assist in containing weight gain after childbirth.

Anti-obesity drugs

A number of pharmaceutic agents target obesity management, but, to date, their effectiveness compared with placebo is not striking. Bulking agents such as guar gum act to increase gastric distension and theoretically induce short-term satiety, although meta-analyses do not show a benefit compared with placebo.[65] Orlistat is a lipase inhibitor that acts in the small intestine by blocking absorption of some of the fat in foods eaten. This unabsorbed fat is then removed in stools from the body. Orlistat can impair the body's absorption of some fat-soluble vitamins and beta-carotene, requiring a daily multivitamin supplement containing vitamins A, D, E, K, and β-carotene. It is associated with an additional 2.9-kg weight loss at 1 year compared with placebo.[66] Side effects occur in a minority of individuals, including diarrhoea, abdominal pain, flatulence, nausea/vomiting, rectal discharge, and faecal incontinence.[67] It is contraindicated for use during pregnancy. Sibutramine is a serotonin–noradrenaline reuptake inhibitor. Weight loss at 1 year averages 4.2 kg compared with placebo.[66] Of 52 pregnant women who were exposed to sibutramine in the first trimester of pregnancy, seven cases of hypertensive complications have been reported, and no cases of congenital anomalies in neonates have been observed.[68] Nevertheless, more data are required, and sibutramine is currently contraindicated for use in pregnancy. Rimonabant is a selective cannabinoid-1 receptor antagonist that lowers weight at 1 year by an average of 4.7 kg relative to placebo. Meta-analyses have shown that rimonabant increases the risk of depressive episodes, suicide, and anxiety, although depressive symptoms are an exclusion criterion in these trials.[69] The safety of rimonabant remains a significant concern limiting its use, and it is clearly contraindicated during gestation or post partum.

Conclusions

Many 'teachable moments' exist to assist women of childbearing age to lose weight or limit weight gain. Before pregnancy would seem to be the optimum time for such preventive care, although this is more difficult given that many pregnancies are not planned. The monitoring of weight gain, as well as significant attention to nutritional status during pregnancy, is an additional opportunity for teaching, as are weight-management programmes that can be instituted as a component of postpartum care. All such approaches need to be tailored to the nutritional and psychological needs of women during their reproductive years, recognizing that each healthcare provider–patient contact moment is not an isolated event but an important part of a continuum of care. Finally, short- and long-term studies on programme cost-effectiveness in relevant target groups are warranted.

References

1. Boney CM, Verma A, Tucker R, Vohr BR. Metabolic syndrome in childhood: association with birth weight, maternal obesity, and gestational diabetes mellitus. *Pediatrics* 2005;**115**:e290–e6.
2. Azziz R, Carmina E, Dewailly D, et al. Position statement: criteria for defining polycystic ovary syndrome as a predominantly hyperandrogenic syndrome: an Androgen Excess Society guideline. *J Clin Endocrinol Metab* 2006; **91**:4237–45.
3. Norman RJ, Noakes M, Wu R, et al. Improving reproductive performance in overweight/obese women with effective weight management. *Hum Reprod Update* 2004;**10**:267–80.
4. Moran LJ, Brinkworth G, Noakes M, Norman RJ. Effects of lifestyle modification in polycystic ovarian syndrome. *Reprod Biomed Online* 2006;**12**:569–78.
5. Moran LJ, Noakes M, Clifton PM, et al. Dietary composition in restoring reproductive and metabolic physiology in overweight women with polycystic ovary syndrome. *J Clin Endocrinol Metab* 2003;**88**:812–19.
6. Galletly C, Moran L, Noakes M, et al. Psychological benefits of a high-protein, low-carbohydrate diet in obese women with polycystic ovary syndrome – a pilot study. *Appetite* 2007;**49**:590–3.
7. Moran LJ, Noakes M, Clifton PM, et al. Short-term meal replacements followed by dietary macronutrient restriction enhance weight loss in polycystic ovary syndrome. *Am J Clin Nutr* 2006;**84**:77–87.
8. Crosignani PG, Vegetti W, Colombo M, Ragni G. Resumption of fertility with diet in overweight women. *Reprod Biomed Online* 2002;**5**:60–4.
9. Saleh AM, Khalil HS. Review of nonsurgical and surgical treatment and the role of insulin-sensitizing agents in the management of infertile women with polycystic ovary syndrome. *Acta Obstet Gynecol Scand* 2004;**83**:614–21.
10. Moran LJ, Noakes M, Clifton PM, Norman RJ. The use of anti-Mullerian hormone in predicting menstrual response after weight loss in overweight women with polycystic ovary syndrome. *J Clin Endocrinol Metab* 2007;**92**:3796–3802.
11. Clements RH, Katasani VG, Palepu R, et al. Incidence of vitamin deficiency after laparoscopic Roux-en-Y gastric bypass in a university hospital setting. *Am Surg* 2006;**72**:1196–1202.
12. Sheiner E, Levy A, Silverberg D, et al. Pregnancy after bariatric surgery is not associated with adverse perinatal outcome. *Am J Obstet Gynecol* 2004;**190**:1335–40.
13. Ducarme G, Revaux A, Rodrigues A, et al. Obstetric outcome following laparoscopic adjustable gastric banding. *Int J Gynaecol Obstet* 2007;**98**:244–7.

14. Patel JA, Colella JJ, Esaka E, et al. Improvement in infertility and pregnancy outcomes after weight loss surgery. *Med Clin North Am* 2007;**91**:515–28, xiii.
15. Yanoff LB, Menzie CM, Denkinger B, et al. Inflammation and iron deficiency in the hypoferremia of obesity. *Int J Obes (Lond)* 2007;**31**:1412–19.
16. Bodnar LM, Catov JM, Roberts JM, Simhan HN. Prepregnancy obesity predicts poor vitamin D status in mothers and their neonates. *J Nutr* 2007;**137**:2437–42.
17. Institute of Medicine. *Nutrition During Pregnancy*. Washington DC: National Academy Press, 1990.
18. MRC Vitamin Study Research Group. Prevention of neural tube defects: results of the Medical Research Council Vitamin Study. *Lancet* 1991;**338**:131–7.
19. Wald NJ. Folic acid and the prevention of neural-tube defects. *N Engl J Med* 2004;**350**:101–3.
20. Wilson RD, Johnson JA, Wyatt P, et al. Pre-conceptional vitamin/folic acid supplementation 2007: the use of folic acid in combination with a multivitamin supplement for the prevention of neural tube defects and other congenital anomalies. *J Obstet Gynaecol Can* 2007;**29**:1003–26.
21. Tough SC, Clarke M, Hicks M, Cook J. Pre-conception practices among family physicians and obstetrician-gynaecologists: results from a national survey. *J Obstet Gynaecol Can* 2006;**28**:780–8.
22. Power ML, Cogswell ME, Schulkin J. Obesity prevention and treatment practices of U.S. obstetrician-gynecologists. *Obstet Gynecol* 2006;**108**:961–8.
23. Jain NJ, Denk CE, Kruse LK, Dandolu V. Maternal obesity: can pregnancy weight gain modify risk of selected adverse pregnancy outcomes? *Am J Perinatol* 2007;**24**:291–8.
24. Cedergren MI. Optimal gestational weight gain for body mass index categories. *Obstet Gynecol* 2007;**110**:759–64.
25. Stotland NE, Haas JS, Brawarsky P, et al. Body mass index, provider advice, and target gestational weight gain. *Obstet Gynecol* 2005;**105**:633–8.
26. Kramer MS. Effects of energy and protein intakes on pregnancy outcome: an overview of the research evidence from controlled clinical trials. *Am J Clin Nutr* 1993;**58**:627–35.
27. Knopp RH, Magee MS, Raisys V, Benedetti T. Metabolic effects of hypocaloric diets in management of gestational diabetes. *Diabetes* 1991;**40**(Suppl 2):165–71.
28. Jovanovic L, Metzger BE, Knopp RH, et al. The Diabetes in Early Pregnancy Study: beta-hydroxybutyrate levels in type 1 diabetic pregnancy compared with normal pregnancy. NICHD-Diabetes in Early Pregnancy Study Group (DIEP). National Institute of Child Health and Development. *Diabetes Care* 1998;**21**:1978–84.
29. Polley BA, Wing RR, Sims CJ. Randomized controlled trial to prevent excessive weight gain in pregnant women. *Int J Obes Relat Metab Disord* 2002;**26**:1494–1502.
30. Kinnunen TI, Pasanen M, Aittasalo M, et al. Preventing excessive weight gain during pregnancy – a controlled trial in primary health care. *Eur J Clin Nutr* 2007;**61**:884–91.

31. Crowther CA, Hiller JE, Moss JR, et al. Effect of treatment of gestational diabetes mellitus on pregnancy outcomes. *N Engl J Med* 2005;**352**:2477–86.

32. Artal R, Catanzaro RB, Gavard JA, et al. A lifestyle intervention of weight-gain restriction: diet and exercise in obese women with gestational diabetes mellitus. *Appl Physiol Nutr Metab* 2007;**32**:596–601.

33. Glueck CJ, Wang P, Goldenberg N, Sieve-Smith L. Pregnancy outcomes among women with polycystic ovary syndrome treated with metformin. *Hum Reprod* 2002;**17**:2858–64.

34. Hague WM, Davoren PM, Oliver J, Rowan J. Contraindications to use of metformin. Metformin may be useful in gestational diabetes. *BMJ* 2003;**326**:762.

35. Norman RJ, Wang JX, Hague W. Should we continue or stop insulin sensitizing drugs during pregnancy? *Curr Opin Obstet Gynecol* 2004;**16**:245–50.

36. Simmons D, Walters BN, Rowan JA, McIntyre HD. Metformin therapy and diabetes in pregnancy. *Med J Aust* 2004;**180**:462–4.

37. Scholl TO, Chen X, Khoo CS, Lenders C. The dietary glycaemic index during pregnancy: influence on infant birth weight, fetal growth, and biomarkers of carbohydrate metabolism. *Am J Epidemiol* 2004;**159**:467–4.

38. Zhang C, Liu S, Solomon CG, Hu FB. Dietary fiber intake, dietary glycaemic load, and the risk for gestational diabetes mellitus. *Diabetes Care* 2006;**29**:2223–30.

39. Moses RG, Luebcke M, Davis WS, et al. Effect of a low-glycemic-index diet during pregnancy on obstetric outcomes. *Am J Clin Nutr* 2006;**84**:807–12.

40. Zhou SJ, Gibson RA, Crowther CA, Makrides M. Should we lower the dose of iron when treating anaemia in pregnancy? A randomized dose-response trial. *Eur J Clin Nutr* advance online publication, 10 October 2007. DOI 10.1038/sj.ejcn.1602926.

41. Gleerup A, Rossander-Hulthen L, Gramatkovski E, Hallberg L. Iron absorption from the whole diet: comparison of the effect of two different distributions of daily calcium intake. *Am J Clin Nutr* 1995;**61**:97–104.

42. Bodnar LM, Simhan HN, Powers RW, et al. High prevalence of vitamin D insufficiency in black and white pregnant women residing in the northern United States and their neonates. *J Nutr* 2007;**137**:447–52.

43. Bodnar LM, Catov JM, Simhan HN, et al. Maternal vitamin D deficiency increases the risk of preeclampsia. *J Clin Endocrinol Metab* 2007;**92**:3517–22.

44. Becker DV, Braverman LE, Delange F, et al. Iodine supplementation for pregnancy and lactation – United States and Canada: recommendations of the American Thyroid Association. *Thyroid* 2006;**16**:949–51.

45. Burgess JR, Seal JA, Stilwell GM, et al. A case for universal salt iodisation to correct iodine deficiency in pregnancy: another salutary lesson from Tasmania. *Med J Aust* 2007;**186**:574–6.

46. Goh YI, Bollano E, Einarson TR, Koren G. Prenatal multivitamin supplementation and rates of congenital anomalies: a meta-analysis. *J Obstet Gynaecol Can* 2006;**28**:680–9.

47. Goh YI, Bollano E, Einarson TR, Koren G. Prenatal multivitamin supplementation and rates of pediatric cancers: a meta-analysis. *Clin Pharmacol Ther* 2007;**81**:685–91.

48. Shankar AH, Jahari AB, Sebayang SK, M, et al. Effect of maternal multiple micronutrient supplementation on fetal loss and infant death in Indonesia: a double-blind cluster-randomised trial. *Lancet* 2008;**371**:215–27.

49. Rooney BL, Schauberger CW. Excess pregnancy weight gain and long-term obesity: one decade later. *Obstet Gynecol* 2002;**100**:245–52.

50. Amorim AR, Linne YM, Lourenco PM. Diet or exercise, or both, for weight reduction in women after childbirth. *Cochrane Database Syst Rev* 2007;(3): CD005627.

51. Linne Y, Rossner S. Interrelationships between weight development and weight retention in subsequent pregnancies: the SPAWN study. *Acta Obstet Gynecol Scand* 2003;**82**:318–25.

52. Butte NF. Dieting and exercise in overweight, lactating women. *N Engl J Med* 2000;**342**:502–03.

53. Kac G, Benicio MH, Velasquez-Melendez G, et al. Gestational weight gain and prepregnancy weight influence postpartum weight retention in a cohort of Brazilian women. *J Nutr* 2004;**134**:661–6.

54. DeVader SR, Neeley HL, Myles TD, Leet TL. Evaluation of gestational weight gain guidelines for women with normal prepregnancy body mass index. *Obstet Gynecol* 2007;**110**:745–51.

55. Kiel DW, Dodson EA, Artal R, et al. Gestational weight gain and pregnancy outcomes in obese women: how much is enough? *Obstet Gynecol* 2007;**110**:752–8.

56. Sichieri R, Field AE, Rich-Edwards J, Willett WC. Prospective assessment of exclusive breastfeeding in relation to weight change in women. *Int J Obes Relat Metab Disord* 2003;**27**:815–20.

57. Australian Bureau of Statistics. *Breastfeeding in Australia, 2001 – 4810.0.55.001.* Canberra: Australian Bureau of Statistics, 2001.

58. Dusdieker LB, Booth BM, Seals BF, Ekwo EE. Investigation of a model for the initiation of breastfeeding in primigravida women. *Soc Sci Med* 1985;**20**:695–703.

59. Strode MA, Dewey KG, Lonnerdal B. Effects of short-term caloric restriction on lactational performance of well-nourished women. *Acta Paediatr Scand* 1986;**75**:222–9.

60. McCrory MA, Nommsen-Rivers LA, Mole PA, et al. Randomized trial of the short-term effects of dieting compared with dieting plus aerobic exercise on lactation performance. *Am J Clin Nutr* 1999;**69**:959–67.

61. Leermakers EA, Anglin K, Wing RR. Reducing postpartum weight retention through a correspondence intervention. *Int J Obes Relat Metab Disord* 1998;**22**:1103–9.

62. Lovelady CA, Garner KE, Moreno KL, Williams JP. The effect of weight loss in overweight, lactating women on the growth of their infants. *N Engl J Med* 2000;**342**:449–53.

63. O'Toole ML, Sawicki MA, Artal R. Structured diet and physical activity prevent postpartum weight retention. *J Womens Health (Larchmt)* 2003;**12**:991–8.
64. Kinnunen TI, Pasanen M, Aittasalo M, et al. Reducing postpartum weight retention – a pilot trial in primary health care. *Nutr J* 2007;**6**:21.
65. Pittler MH, Ernst E. Guar gum for body weight reduction: meta-analysis of randomized trials. *Am J Med* 2001;**110**:724–30.
66. Rucker D, Padwal R, Li SK, et al. Long term pharmacotherapy for obesity and overweight: updated meta-analysis. *BMJ* 2007; **335**:1194–9.
67. Acharya NV, Wilton LV, Shakir SA. Safety profile of orlistat: results of a prescription-event monitoring study. *Int J Obes (Lond)* 2006;**30**:1645–52.
68. De Santis M, Straface G, Cavaliere AF, et al Early first-trimester sibutramine exposure: pregnancy outcome and neonatal follow-up. *Drug Safety* 2006;**29**: 255–9.
69. Christensen R, Kristensen PK, Bartels EM, et al. Efficacy and safety of the weight-loss drug rimonabant: a meta-analysis of randomised trials. *Lancet* 2007;**370**:1706–13.

13 Surgical treatment of chronic overnutrition

John G Kral

Introduction

Complications of obese pregnancies are numerous and hazardous.[1] Gestational obesity threatens the mother, her fetus, the neonate, the child, and ultimately, the health of nations. US mortality statistics demonstrate that the maternal mortality rate, which had been below 10 deaths per 100 000 live births since 1977, rose to 12 in 2003 and 13 in 2004, the latest year for which figures are available. The rise is largely attributable to the increasing prevalence of obesity that has occurred at the same time.[2,3] The mortality rate is three times higher in black women, where obesity is significantly more prevalent than in white women.[4]

It follows that preventing and treating obesity in girls and young women is extremely important, but very difficult, as it places huge demands on education to achieve societal change. Obesity is more prevalent in women for biologic and sociological reasons and thus is more refractory to treatment: biologic, because of the greater body fat of females associated with the gonadal maturation process subserving reproductive capacity and increased fat accrual during pregnancy and menopause; sociological, owing to the traditional, cultural sedentariness of girls and women, who participate less in sports and exercise programs than males.[5,6] Many easily identifiable risk factors for female obesity appear to have simple remedies, but they are exceedingly hard to implement on any level.

Pathogenesis

Chronic overnutrition leads to obesity and diseases affecting all tissues and organ systems. The mechanism is a subcellular/cellular substrate–product disequilibrium caused by nutrients exceeding metabolic and/or storage capacity relative to oxygen supply. Increased maternal body fat and nutrient intake deliver excess substrate to the fetus (nutritional teratogenesis), whereas environmental factors such as quality and quantity of food supply, relationship to the father, neighborhood safety, and various other psychosocial stresses, including food insecurity,[7] induce excess maternal corticosteroid production, also delivered to the fetus (hormonal teratogenesis). Excess steroids in turn influence the maternal eating behavior that contributes to overnutrition and affects the fetus, shaping its metabolic pathways and eating behavior (Figure 13.1).

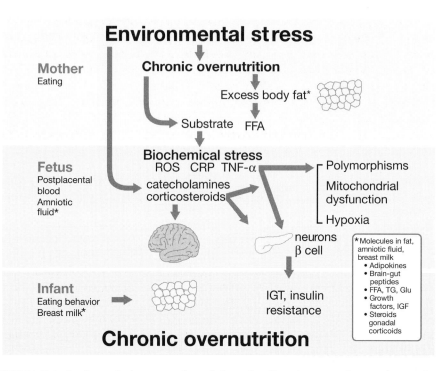

FIGURE 13.1 A schematic interpretation of the role of environmental stress in causing chronic overnutrition (obesity and insulin resistance, type 2 diabetes mellitus) during development. CRP, c-reactive protein; FFA, free fatty acids; Glu, glucose; IGF, insulin-like growth factor; IGT, impaired glucose tolerance; ROS, reactive oxygen species; TG, triglycerides; TNFα, tumor necrosis factor alpha.

At the same time, gestational *undernutrition*, with consequent intrauterine growth restriction (IUGR), preterm delivery, and small-for-gestational-age (SGA) offspring, is also linked to chronic overnutrition in the offspring, mainly from accelerated catch-up growth and weight gain from maternal overfeeding, impaired neurologic development, or normal compensatory neurobiologic survival mechanisms. Since maternal obesity in itself is a risk factor for preterm delivery, and IUGR and SGA offspring, these postnatal pathways to juvenile and ultimately adult obesity are similar. Interestingly, the metabolic effects of gestational overnutrition, such as hyperlipidemia and hyperinsulinemia, cause similar impairments of fetal neurogenesis as do excess steroids.

Prevention of overnutrition

Neither therapeutic nihilism nor genetic determinism should influence the efforts to curb the increase and spread of overnutrition. Belatedly, the medical profession and the public that it informs have realized the importance of obesity, prompting them to send messages to their elected officials.

Secondary prevention has had very limited success, although the numbers of reports of community-level efforts are increasing. The sharp rise in childhood obesity makes it unlikely that there would be any substantial decrease in the prevalence of obesity over the next two generations, even if broad-based remedies were implemented today.[8] Recent studies demonstrate risks associated with interpregnancy weight gain[9] and intrauterine 'metabolic imprinting',[10,11] and call for accelerated efforts at screening and management.[12] As yet, however, the success of most nonoperative treatments for overweight and obesity in achieving and maintaining weight loss is poor (see Chapters 3 and 12).[13]

The following is a description of the surgical treatment of obesity or so-called bariatric surgery, a practice that demonstrates the potential for primary prevention of obesity in families with a preponderance of genetic and environmental risk factors.

Indications for anti-obesity surgery

The safety and effectiveness of anti-obesity surgery in obese patients (defined as body mass index [BMI] greater than 30 kg/m²) is well documented.[14,15] The most important advantage of surgical treatment over all other modalities described to date is the magnitude and durability of weight loss, which results in decreases in mortality[16,17] and morbidity,[18] and improvements in health-related quality of life.[19]

Weight

When obesity surgery was introduced, it was approved only for patients with extreme (and unusual) obesity, corresponding to a doubling of the desirable weight for height (or 45.4 kg of excess weight) according to actuarial standards, subsequently expressed as BMI of 40 or more. These weight criteria were later expanded to include BMI in the range 35–40 in the presence of serious comorbidity. Since the introduction of less traumatic laparoscopic approaches, and with increased safety of anesthesia and perioperative management in the early 1990s, the relative weight at which these operations are performed has decreased.[14,15] This trend has been encouraged by the increased understanding of the serious morbidity of obesity, the burgeoning numbers of obese individuals, and the continued failures of other methods of treatment.

Minimum age?

The majority of patients in surgical series are women (~80%), more than half of whom are of reproductive age. Although obesity in women (not men) is inversely related to socioeconomic status, this is not the case in surgical populations. Women typically have fewer and less severe complications of obesity surgery than men. Whereas male sex, age, and duration of pre-existing chronic diseases (such as type 2 diabetes mellitus, hypertension, and cardiopulmonary failure) are the main risk factors for adverse perioperative outcomes, including death, it logically follows that *women at younger ages, before obesity comorbidities appear or progress, are less prone to complications and, therefore, are ideal candidates for obesity surgery.* The 90-day mortality rates for all patients in large registries of bariatric surgery are of the same magnitude as those reported for appendectomy. Of interest, the increased safety, in parallel with a dramatic increase in child and adolescent obesity, also has prompted exploration of the feasibility or utility of performing obesity surgery at ages younger than previously.[20,21] This point of view is strengthened by recognition that chronic overnutrition is established during childhood, and progressively becomes less tractable, as the eating disorder is exacerbated and exercising becomes difficult, causing a vicious circle. Obese adolescent girls, compared with those of normal weight, have a threefold increased risk of dying by middle age.[22]

Although bariatric surgery is increasingly performed in adolescents, very few data on long-term effects exist. In the absence of such information, it would be premature to operate at younger ages, even though severe obesity is spreading among schoolage children, who increasingly are exhibiting early onset of hypertension, diabetes, and psychosocial dysfunction.[23–25]At the same time, menarche is occurring at younger ages,[26,27] and the rate of unintended pregnancy among the very young is escalating, especially in socioeconomically challenged environments[28] (Table 13.1).

For most of human history, undernutrition has been the greatest problem. The prevailing hesitancy to restrict the nutrition of growing, physically, sexually, and mentally immature individuals, emanating from findings of laboratory experiments (chiefly in "semi-precocial" rodents) and epidemiologic studies of famine, and the traditional instincts of mothers, has prevented determination of evidence-based 'minimum daily requirements', optimal for human growth and development, especially in obese individuals. Similarly, there are no data on 'maximum dietary requirements', although laboratory research clearly documents deleterious effects of excess substrate. However, one seminal study has described energy balance during human pregnancies.[29]

Since many women of childbearing age have undergone bariatric operations with the potential to limit intrauterine nutrition during the most vulnerable period of human growth, information on the outcomes of such pregnancies and the ultimate development of the resultant offspring might be relevant to assessing risks of performing such surgery at younger ages.[30]

TABLE 13.1 Maternal characteristics and prevalence of unintended pregnancies among 8886 women in an inner-city population (New York City 1998–2001)[28]

	Percentage of population	Prevalence of unintended pregnancies (%)
Age 10–19 years	27	90
Black	62	85
No insurance	62	80
≥3 prior pregnancies	26	82

Current obesity operations

The most common of the generic types of operations are the following:

1. Adjustable gastric banding, a *gastric* restrictive procedure, which is achieved laparoscopically by placing a proximal adjustable circumgastric band which shrinks gastric reservoir capacity (to 20 ml) and reduces the rate of flow through the constricting band (Figure 13.2A)
2. Gastric bypass, a *diversionary* operation, which reduces the size of the proximal stomach but also diverts undigested food and liquids, bypassing most of the stomach, directly into a segment of small intestine, which also bypasses varying lengths of the small bowel (Figure 13.2B).

Several variants of the so-called gastric bypass operations exist, varying in length as well as in location of the bypassed intestinal segments. The oldest and best studied of these is the roux-en-Y gastric bypass, which also is the most common diversionary operation currently in use.

The most effective, technically difficult operation, biliopancreatic diversion (BPD), today combines a two-thirds gastric sleeve resection, retains the pylorus, which is sutured to the ileum, and achieves a bypass of the duodenum and

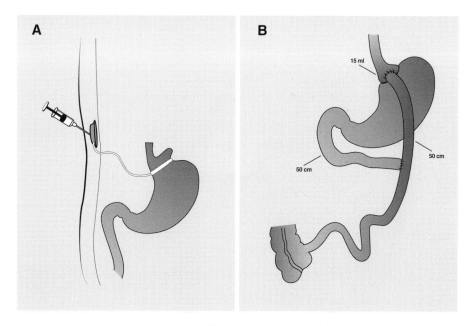

FIGURE 13.2 (A) Laparoscopic adjustable gastric banding, which creates a 15-ml gastric pouch, causing delayed emptying of solid food through the narrowed passage. Adjustments are done by injecting or removing saline from the subcutaneous port. (B) Gastric bypass (roux-en-Y gastric bypass) divides the stomach, leaving a 15-ml pouch connected to a limb of jejunum varying in length.

jejunum, which are reanastomosed into the distal 75–100 cm of ileum (Figure 13.3). This hybrid procedure functions by limiting intake and digestion and causing malabsorption of macronutrients (fat > protein> carbohydrate).[31] BPD

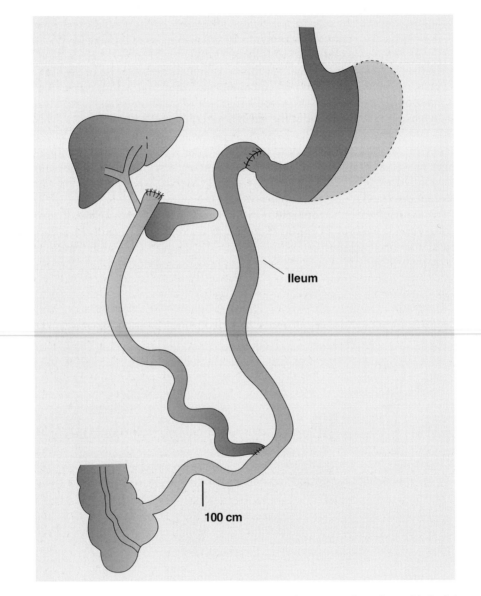

FIGURE 13.3 Biliopancreatic bypass (BPD) consists of sleeve resection of one-third of the stomach and post-pyloric diversion of the duodenum, creating a biliopancreatic duodenojejunal limb that empties into the distal ileum. The proximal duodenoileal anastomosis creates an alimentary limb transporting food to the distal ileum, where it encounters bile and digestive pancreatic enzymes.

requires the greatest attention to supplementation of essential nutrients to avoid deficiencies, a postoperative consideration germane to all obesity operations, whether purely restrictive (banding) or diversionary (gastric and biliopancreatic bypass). *The cost of the increased efficacy of a bariatric operation is the requirement assiduously to supplement and monitor blood levels of vitamins and minerals* (Table 13.2) *indefinitely.*

Complications and side effects of surgery

Surgical morbidity is increased in obese patients, a phenomenon recognized early by gynecologists and obstetricians (see Chapter 15).[32] It was the major concern of surgeons involved in developing the field of obesity surgery and the specific concern that led to major advances in perioperative management of obese patients through routine antibiotic prophylaxis, antithrombotic measures, prevention of atelectasis, and improvement in abdominal wound closure. Laparoscopic approaches have especially benefited severely obese patients, and the various bariatric operations have all been adapted for laparoscopy. Indeed, at centers of excellence, it is the standard of care to perform all primary obesity operations laparoscopically. As is the case with most complex surgery, the hospital's and the individual surgeon's case volume is a key determinant of outcome. At the same time, the long-term therapeutic effects of bariatric surgery are less dependent on technical performance than on patient education preoperatively *and* during frequent follow-up visits with knowledgeable and committed staff.[33]

Predictably, early complications of obesity surgery are related to the complexity and difficulty of the operation, whereas long-term side effects are related to the efficacy in safely maintaining 'controlled undernutrition'.[34] Overall complication rates in centers specializing in bariatric surgery are in the order of 15%, and are usually higher for diversionary operations and lower for purely restrictive ones.

Procedure related
Laparoscopic adjustable banding is the simplest and safest operation; it involves minimal suturing and no anastomoses. As a result, the lack of incisions or staple lines in the gastrointestinal tract obviates any risk of contamination, leaks, or hemorrhage. Complications are related to the device itself, such as fluid extravasation from the tubing, infection around the subcutaneous injectable port, and slippage of the band, with or without herniation of stomach tissue. Gastric bypass and BPD are complicated by bleeding, ulcers, leaks, strictures, and bowel obstruction from internal hernias (Table 13.2).

Side effects
It is in the nature of the procedures to cause vomiting or diarrhea, as should be obvious from their construction. However, these side effects can have behavioral as well as technical causes, emphasizing the need for preoperative education and diligent

TABLE 13.2 Adverse effects of bariatric surgery (approximate prevalence).[35]

Operative (approx prevalence 10%)	Long term (approx prevalence 20–30%)
Thromboembolism	Deficiencies:
Bleeding	Iron
Small bowel obstruction	Calcium
Internal hernia	Vitamins A, D
Pneumonia	Vitamin B$_{12}$
Stenosis	Vitamin B$_1$ (vomiting)
Ulcers	Protein (diarrhea)
Peritonitis (leaks)	Gallstones
Death (< 0.5%)	Weight regain

follow-up. When vomiting or diarrhea does not respond to behavioral adjustments, one must consider surgical–technical causes such as strictures, ulcers, or fistulas.

Deficiencies
These also relate to the nature of the operations. Excessive vomiting, to be suspected when weight loss is rapid and unusually great, can have dire consequences including vitamin B complex deficiency leading to irreversible neuropathy (Wernicke's encephalopathy), dehydration with hypochloremic acidosis and shock, or protein deficiency. Diarrhea after diversionary operations may be related to short bowel syndrome or bacterial overgrowth, but may also have dietary causes. Nevertheless, the deficiencies are preventable and significantly easier to treat than obesity itself.

Weight-loss failure
Long-term follow-up studies after obesity surgery demonstrate differences in median weight loss: generally speaking, BPD is superior to gastric bypass, which is superior to banding. Population differences exist and are attributable to cultural factors. As yet, no consensus addresses a strategy for managing patients with inadequate results entailing recurrence of preoperative, obesity-related morbidity.[35] Reoperative surgery is always associated with higher complication rates, and should be performed only at centers experienced in performing open bariatric surgery. Gastric restrictive operations, with failure percentages as high as 30%, are more prone to fail than diversionary ones, and should be converted to a bypass procedure.

Eating disorders
Few reports describe the development of eating disorders after bariatric surgery. As eating disorders such as anorexia nervosa and bulimia in the general population

are most prevalent in young women, one must consider these among differential diagnoses when refractory vomiting or diarrhea occurs in young women after obesity surgery. Binge-eating disorder (BED) is the most common eating disorder among the obese, with frequencies increasing with increasing BMI. Patients with diagnosed BED preoperatively have increased postoperative complication rates.[36] This potential eventuality should not, however, disqualify such individuals from surgery; rather, preoperative referral for expert treatment is advisable.

Benefits of surgery

Most patients measure 'success' in terms of magnitude and duration of maintained weight loss. Quality of life is subjective, although highly correlated with health-related quality of life. Recently published studies convincingly demonstrate that anti-obesity surgery not only diminishes the severity of the majority of comorbidities[18] and improves the quality of life,[19] but also reduces the increased mortality of severe obesity.[16,17] Of greatest relevance to young obese women planning pregnancy are the dramatic improvements and even cure of infertility, glucose intolerance and type 2 diabetes mellitus, hypertension, and lipid disorders that follow bariatric surgery (see Chapters 5 and 6).[35]

Pregnancies after obesity surgery

During the 45 years that anti-obesity surgery has been practiced, case reports and observational studies describe pregnancy outcomes with fairly consistent findings across different procedures and settings. The lessons learned are applicable to today's practice, although the quality of the evidence has improved with the wider adoption of obesity surgery. It is essential to keep in mind, however, that *major differences in long-term efficacy* have been found *between operations*. Specifically, *clear 'dose–response' relationships exist between amount of sustained weight loss and primary and secondary efficacy variables*.

Gestational complications and side effects

Deficiencies

Women of reproductive age are always cautioned that surgical weight loss increases their risk of unintended pregnancy mainly due to reversal of obesity-related anovulation. Although it is not clear whether obesity itself increases the risk of contraceptive failure,[35] diversionary operations *do* reduce the bioavailability of low-dose oral contraceptives, a fact that needs to be considered post-operatively.[37–39] Nevertheless, after all forms of bariatric surgery, women are strongly advised to avoid becoming pregnant during the period of rapid postoperative weight loss (usually 18–24 months), because of the potential for developing deficiencies. All candidates for weight-loss surgery should have a comprehensive preoperative assessment of blood vitamins and minerals because deficiencies are common among all obese patients,[40] ostensibly in the face of chronic 'overnutrition'. Like all patients having bariatric surgery, women and their physicians are advised of the mandate for the patient routinely to take vitamin and mineral supplements and the need to monitor blood levels regularly to detect and prevent deficiencies. These same recommendations are emphasized to women planning pregnancy. Regardless of these mandates, the most common complication of bariatric operations is deficiency of nutrients and vitamins, as specified in Table 13.2; indeed, the majority of case reports on adverse pregnancy outcomes exhibit deficiencies.[41–45]

Severe complications

Although rare, internal herniation after laparoscopic gastric bypass has been described, with increased prevalence during pregnancy. As with all causes of abdominal pain in the obese, it is especially difficult to diagnose during pregnancy. Unrecognized small bowel obstruction in this setting can easily progress to strangulation, sometimes with fatal outcome.[46] This possibility emphasizes the *need for the experienced bariatric surgical team to continue their involvement with their patients during pregnancy*.

Fetal outcomes

No reliable statistics quantitate early spontaneous abortions after obesity surgery. Fecundity is increased with weight loss, but, as previously mentioned, women are strongly advised to avoid pregnancies during the rapid weight loss phase, making it difficult to validate abortion data regardless of the inherent ability to assess whether pregnancies are unwanted. The early abortion rate after bariatric surgery appears to be lower than in obese women, but similar to that of the general population, but more data are required.[47]

Reports on malformations vary; by most accounts, the prevalence is unchanged. The most significant factor contributing to an increased rate is folate deficiency, but diligent supplementation (and monitoring) should effectively prevent this. The normalization of glucose metabolism postoperatively would be expected to reduce the risks of malformations from hyperglycemia,[48–51] leading to a net decrease of abnormalities following obesity surgery.

Although there is an increase in SGA births compared with before maternal surgery, with a prevalence higher than that of the general population, mean birth weights increase (to population levels) at the same time as the high rate of macrosomia and large-for-gestational-age (LGA) fetuses in obese mothers declines to general population levels after maternal surgery. Owing to the decrease in macrosomia, reductions occur in fetal complications referable to this condition, bringing the prevalences down to community levels. *The reduced prevalence of LGA offspring is probably the most important benefit of preconception obesity surgery*, as the discussion below elucidates.

Maternal outcomes

Evaluating the literature on postsurgical pregnancy complications is complex, as any such evaluation must consider the wide ranges of weight loss and, concomitantly, the interval between surgery and conception, the specific type of operation, and the quality and quantity of postoperative monitoring and care. Case series may achieve equivalent or better results than series having 'better' operations (that is, more effective with respect to sustained weight loss) owing to population differences. In general, US populations, compared with European or Asian, have inferior results with purely restrictive procedures. Recent papers demonstrate the difficulty in understanding the literature, keeping in mind that the criteria for evaluating evidence concerning treatment of obesity need to be redefined.[13,52]

Sheiner and associates analyzed 298 deliveries to patients after unspecified 'bariatric operations' among a total of 159 210 deliveries during the years 1988–2002 in the only hospital in the Negev region of Israel.[53] Unfortunately, this paper did not stratify for obesity by comparing the 10.7% of obese postsurgery patients with the remarkably low 1.2% of obese nonsurgery patients; stratification was also lacking for type of operation. Furthermore, these authors gave no indication of the women's preoperative weight. The paper shows a 9.4% prevalence of macrosomia among operated women versus 4.6% in the larger population ($P <$ 0.001), and higher prevalences of labor induction, failed induction, cesarean delivery, premature rupture of membranes, and fertility treatments (all $P \leq$ 0.001), with no significant differences in placental abruption, placenta previa, dystocia, meconium-stained amniotic fluid, low Apgar scores, or perinatal mortality rates. Despite the deficiencies just mentioned, it is interesting that the perinatal death rate was 0.3% among postoperative pregnancies versus 1.5% in the nonoperated patients ($P = 0.102$).

Outcomes with different techniques

A study from Australia describes 79 consecutive first pregnancies in women following *laparoscopic adjustable gastric banding*, comparing them to the same patients' presurgical penultimate pregnancies ($n = 40$) and to obstetric outcomes in matched, unoperated, obese women ($n = 79$) and community outcomes.[54] The authors found incidences of pregnancy-induced hypertension (10%), gestational diabetes mellitus (GDM) (6.3%), and neonatal outcomes, including stillbirths, preterm deliveries, SGA, and LGA, similar to community levels and significantly lower than their preoperative outcomes or those of the obese controls. It is important to note that these births were a median of 20 months postoperative after a mean weight loss of 23%. Mean gestational weight gain was 9.6 ± 9.0 kg (SD), significantly less ($P < 0.001$) than preoperative (14.4 ± 9.7 kg) or in obese controls (15.5 ± 9.0 kg). In 20 of the 79 pregnancies, conception occurred less than 1 year after operation. Maternal weight gain was 2.3 ± 9.5 kg compared with 11.7 ± 8.4 kg in the remaining 59 patients ($P < 0.001$). Birth weights were similar and there were no differences in outcomes. These results contrast with an Austrian case series of seven unexpected pregnancies occurring a median of 12 months (range 1–22) postoperatively with bad outcomes.[55]

A US study of 34 patients among 2433 having *gastric bypass*, a diversionary operation, during 2001–4 describes outcomes comparing 21 patients who became pregnant within 1 year of surgery (early) with 13 conceiving after 1 year (late).[56] The mean BMI in the early group was 35 and was associated with a mean pregnancy weight gain of 1.8 kg. The late group had mean BMI of 28 ($P = 0.002$), with mean gestational weight gain of 15.5 kg ($P = 0.002$). Although the authors conclude that there were 'no significant episodes of malnutrition, adverse fetal outcomes, or pregnancy complications' in pregnancies occurring within 1 year, it is noteworthy that 23.8% of the early group had 'major complications' (pre-eclampsia and miscarriages) versus 7.7% in the late group, and 25% 'minor complications' (preterm labor, hypertension, cholelithiasis, and iron deficiency) compared with 21% in the late group. Among the 21 early pregnancies there were 5 miscarriages (24%) and 1 ectopic pregnancy versus 1 miscarriage and no ectopics in the late group . The average birth weight among the 15 carried to term was 2868 g, compared with 2727 g among the late pregnancies.

Outcomes of pregnancies after open BPD for severe obesity have been studied since 1984 at Laval University in Quebec City.[57] These outcomes are of special interest because BPD has the greatest potential for causing undernutrition with protein deficiency and various hypovitaminoses. In this analysis, postoperative pregnancies in 132 women resulted in 166 infants delivered by 109 mothers. Comparisons were made with data collected from 568 severely obese women with pregnancies prior to BPD. The miscarriage rates were similar (21.6% before and 26% after surgery), as were the rates of premature deliveries (16.7 vs 13.6%). After the surgery, 90 of the 109 women had a mean gestational weight gain of 9.1 ± 5.9 kg (SD), while 8 women lost a mean of 11.3 ± 8.9 kg. Significantly, mean birth weight was 3.2 ± 0.5 kg among those who gained. Eleven mothers maintained a stable weight and delivered babies weighing 2.8 ± 0.5 kg. Length of time between surgery and pregnancy did not affect gestational weight gain or birth weight, with intervals of means of 3.8 ± 2.3 years in gainers, 3.0 ± 1.7 in losers, and 4.3 ± 3.1 years among weight-stable mothers.

GDM and gestational weight gain

These two topics have come under intense scrutiny with the advent of the obesity epidemic. As recently as within the last 5 years, it was considered necessary and ethical to perform a randomized trial to determine the efficacy of managing gestational diabetes, and it was acceptable to withhold knowledge of the diagnosis because screening was not part of routine pregnancy care! The current standards for gestational weight gain were published in 1990 by the US Institute of Medicine (IOM) (Table 13.3),[58] and are not expected to be revised before 2009 even though maternal mortality is increasing. Perhaps evidence from pregnancy outcomes after anti-obesity surgery can provide valuable information on these two topics.

It is only recently that evidence for beneficial effects of treatment of GDM has been published.[59] Recognition of the association between obesity and impaired glucose tolerance progressing to type 2 diabetes mellitus, and the adverse

TABLE 13.3 Institute of Medicine gestational weight gain recommendations (1990)[58]

| BMI | Weight gain in | | Weekly in 2nd trimester, 3rd trimester |
	kg	lb	
19.8–25.9	11.5–16.0	25–35	~0.5 kg (1 lb)
26.0–29.9	7.0–11.5	15–25	~0.3 kg (0.66 lb)
≥30.0	≥7.0	≥15	~0.3 kg (0.66 lb)

outcomes of the mounting numbers of obese pregnancies, has heightened the awareness of the importance of treating obesity-related GDM.

A 15-year Israeli review of 8014 deliveries of patients with GDM identified a subset of 28 patients with prior obesity surgery (26 restrictive).[60] Remarkably, only 120 (1.5%) of the 7986 nonoperated women were obese in this population. One woman among the 28 bariatric surgery patients (3.6%) was obese. Although the study is too small to draw meaningful conclusions, the authors anticlimactically concluded that previous maternal surgery was not associated with adverse perinatal outcome.

The case series of BPD from Quebec City described above included 1200 obese women (BMI = 48 ± 9 [SD]) over a period of 20 years.[57] Thirty-four had delivered children both before and after surgery, whereas 113 had given birth to 172 children after surgery. The children were assessed when they were 2 years or older. Before surgery 18% of women had type 2 diabetes and 16% had GDM, with both levels significantly above community standards. After surgery, BMI was 32 ± 6.3 at the time of pregnancy. There were no cases of type 2 diabetes and no case of GDM ($P < 0.01$). The prevalence of macrosomia among 638 pregnancies before surgery was 34.8%, dropping to 7.7% among 156 pregnancies after surgery, comparable to community standards. These results are important to compare with the outcomes after the purely gastric-restrictive, adjustable-banding procedures, with less surgical weight loss and shorter postoperative intervals accounting for a relatively low mean gestational weight gain. With longer postoperative intervals after adjustable banding, gestational weight gain increases, leading to higher prevalences of GDM and macrosomia/LGA than after BPD.

Offspring outcomes

The overall experience across operations demonstrates that mean length of gestation is similar, yielding slightly higher birth weights, and dramatically lower rates of LGA, macrosomic babies, and preterm births, with no changes in early Apgar scores, jaundice, or neonatal nursery days.

The ultimate judgment of the advisability of anti-obesity surgery, potentially affecting the unborn or the young, lies with its effects on adult health or longevity. It is in this context that post-BPD pregnancy is a test of the putative adverse effects of limiting nutrient availability during development. Much hesitancy and, indeed, controversy over pediatric anti-obesity surgery[61–63] with its potential to cause undernutrition are predicated on the premise that growth and development might be adversely affected, hypothetically leading to adult disease. Operations with the greatest potential to cause undernutrition during the most vulnerable period of growth and development (gestation) might provide evidence to settle the controversy. Although obesity surgery has been practiced regularly for more than four decades, only one report describes development of offspring conceived after maternal surgery and followed into adolescence. The Quebec report presents outcomes of maternal BPD among offspring born after maternal surgery, comparing them with their siblings born before their mothers' operations.[64] The mean pregestational BMI of the unoperated women was 48 ± 8, compared with mean BMI of 31 ± 9 in postoperative mothers. The study compared 45 children aged 2–18 years with 172 same-age siblings born after maternal biliopancreatic bypass. The prevalence of offspring obesity was 52% lower and severe obesity 45% lower than among siblings ($P = 0.006$). These latter prevalences were similar to Quebec population standards. There were no increases in underweight or SGA infants. Children born after maternal surgery performed scholastically at the same levels as their peers in the community at large.

Summary of gestational outcomes after anti-obesity surgery

In women with BMI of at least 35, surgical weight loss is associated with numerous changes in outcome compared with unoperated women. Although fecundity increases, the postoperative interval affects abortion rates, stillbirths, gestational weight gain, malformation, and IUGR. On the whole, lower prevalences of macrosomia/LGA, dystocia, nerve damage (Erb's palsy), fractures, and hemorrhage are seen, along with lower incidences of labor induction, failed induction, cesarean delivery in primiparas, premature rupture of the membranes (PROM), and infections. Mean birth weight increases, but there are fewer obese infants, no increases in SGA (remains higher than general population), and no increases in preterm birth (remains higher than general population).

Degree of sustained weight loss determines amelioration versus cure/prevention of maternal complications, including GDM, pregnancy-induced hypertension (PIH), pre-eclampsia, eclampsia cesarean delivery, and perineal trauma. To summarize, the preponderance of outcomes after maternal obesity surgery is better than before surgery and better than in unoperated equally obese women. Most but not all postsurgical outcomes reach prevalence rates similar to the general population.

Implications

The experience from pregnancies after biliopancreatic bypass surgery, the operations achieving the greatest sustained weight loss while entailing the greatest risk of gestational undernutrition, supports the need to change substantially the commonly practiced intrapregnancy weight-gain recommendations for obese women with BMI of 35 or greater, which give no consideration to limiting or advising against gain in these women.[58] This proposal is at odds with the premise that women at high levels of 'prepregnancy BMI are likely to benefit the most from gaining within the IOM guidelines', as articulated in a recent study of women's target gestational weight gain.[65] However, what is even more alarming is the recognition that this study additionally found that providers were recommending gains *above* IOM guidelines for obese women.

In comparing BPD outcomes with those after purely restrictive operations, which achieve significantly lower maintained weight loss (and undernutrition), it appears that outcomes, especially GDM and LGA/macrosomia, are superior, with the greater weight loss of BPD operations. Thus, the common practice of routinely deflating adjustable bands when pregnancy has been ascertained after laparoscopic adjustable banding should not continue, except in those cases where there are obvious complications or excessive and rapid weight loss.

The 'fetal overnutrition hypothesis'[66] has been effectively proven through studies of outcomes after anti-obesity surgery.[64] The mechanisms are abrogation of insulin resistance through normalization of glucose and lipid metabolism, and correction of the various factors involved in the pathogenesis of chronic overnutrition manifested as obesity and type 2 diabetes mellitus (see Figure 13.1). In this context, it is likely that obesity surgery reduces maternal stress, an important element of the diathesis, although human data on postoperative stress are not yet available. Dieting, on the other hand, is stressful and increases urinary cortisol in pre- and postmenopausal women.[67,68]

The largely beneficial outcomes of offspring followed into adolescence, compared with siblings born before their mothers' operation, indicate that any undernutrition suffered in the womb does not seem to have similar detrimental effects to those documented in the large epidemiologic studies following catastrophes, such as the Dutch 'Hunger Winter' or the siege of Leningrad during World War II. It is important, however, to note that, although obesity was diagnosed in adolescence in the famine studies, several of the adverse outcomes manifested later in adulthood.[69]

The critical differences between experimental undernutrition in laboratory animals and catastrophic human famine and the putative undernutrition imposed by anti-obesity surgery is that the last is *voluntary* and thus *not perceived by the mothers as threatening or stressful*. However, the postnatal influences of catch-up growth and other maternally controlled influences (bottle-feeding, diet choices, and sedentary behavior), which have been implicated in the pathogenesis of postfamine nutritional 'programming', are still present whether or not obese mothers have been operated on. Mothers who have suffered from obesity sufficiently to undergo surgical treatment are, however, more receptive to education about the hazards of bottle-feeding, catch-up growth, and obesiogenic behaviors.

A small, detailed, metabolic ward study of energy balance in women after biliopancreatic bypass surgery compared with matched controls demonstrated equivalent net energy balance.[31] This means that the operated women absorb enough energy to support pregnancy.[29] *It is this 'eumetabolic' state that accounts for the improvements in fetal–maternal outcomes.* Their only 'undernutrition' might pertain to specific essential nutrients, especially if these are not supplemented. The implication is that anti-obesity surgery, if monitored and supplemented meticulously, might be an option in growing children (especially girls) if all other nonsurgical treatments have failed to return the child to an age-appropriate growth trajectory.[30]

A final implication of the favorable outcomes of offspring after 'successful' maternal bariatric surgery is that the intrauterine environment is of exceptional importance, as it has the capacity to override long-term effects of susceptibility genes *and* a 'toxic' postnatal environment.

Recommendations

1. Prevent obese pregnancies from occurring at any age! An important problem with hormonal contraception is the greatly increased prevalence of thromboembolism associated with combined oral contraceptives in obese women. Any use of such preparations should be accompanied by some form of anticoagulation, although there is no evidence as yet of an increased prevalence of thromboembolism associated with the lower systemic exposure to ethinyl estradiol delivered via the vaginal ring.[70]
2. Defer pregnancy until weight has stabilized regardless of treatment! This is especially important to keep in mind in view of the 'controversy' over fertility treatments.[71] With anti-obesity surgery, it is not hazardous to conceive before weight stability, but it is more prudent to conceive during periods of homeostasis. A side effect of weight-loss surgery in young couples is increased risk of divorce.[72]
3. As part of the treatment plan for fat, albeit fecund, females, include a well-designed monitoring and supplementation schedule (folic acid)!
4. Although effective operations are available, employ a step-care strategy in treating and preventing chronic overnutrition, especially in growing individuals! An important proviso of any step-care strategy is prompt implementation of more aggressive therapy when any method fails (rescue treatment).
5. Prevent excessive and rapid gestational weight gain! Although preconception BMI is the most significant risk factor for gestational weight gain and can be modified, extraordinary educational efforts are needed regarding the hazards of excessive weight gain during pregnancy.

Conclusions

All *treatment* of chronic overnutrition, regardless of mechanism of action, is based on creating a durable negative energy balance, taking care to supplement essential nutrients. Dieting in and of itself is stressful, as exhibited by elevated cortisol levels in both pre- and postmenopausal women who exert high dietary restraint.[67,68] *Prevention*, on the other hand, need only provide protection against periods of positive energy balance, which can mostly be achieved by regular physical activity.[73] An important step in preventing chronic overnutrition in the population would be to provide effective contraception to all obese women with reproductive capacity. Those expressing intent to become pregnant, on the other hand, should effectively and durably reduce weight while taking contraceptive measures prior to conception. The most effective current means of achieving prolonged and sustained weight loss is anti-obesity surgery.

References

1. Catalano PM. Management of obesity in pregnancy. *Obstet Gynecol* 2007;**109**:419–33.
2. Lewis G, ed. *The Confidential Enquiry into Maternal and Child Health (CEMACH). Saving Mothers' Lives: Reviewing Maternal Deaths to Make Motherhood Safer – 2003–2005*. The Seventh Report on Confidential Enquiries into Maternal Deaths in the United Kingdom. London: CEMACH, 2007.
3. Office of the Surgeon General. *The Surgeon General's Call to Action to Prevent and Decrease Overweight and Obesity*. Rockville, MD: Office of the Surgeon General, 2001. Available at: www.surgeongeneral.gov/topics/obesity/calltoaction/CalltoAction.pdf.
4. Chang J, Elam-Evans LD, Berg CJ, et al. Pregnancy-related mortality surveillance – United States, 1991–1999. *MMWR Surveill Summ* 2003;**52**;(SSO2):1–8.
5. Sweeney NM, Glaser D, Tedeschi C. The eating and physical activity habits of inner-city adolescents. *J Pediatr Health Care* 2007;**21**:13–21.
6. Li L, Li K, Ushijima H. Moderate–vigorous physical activity and body fatness in Chinese urban schoolchildren. *Pediatr Int* 2007;**49**:280–5.
7. Olson CM. Food insecurity in women: a recipe for unhealthy trade-offs. *Topics Clin Nutr* 2005;**20**:321–8.
8. Ludwig DS. Childhood obesity – the shape of things to come. *N Engl J Med* 2007;**357**:2325–7.
9. Villamor E, Cnattingius S. Interpregnancy weight change and risk of adverse pregnancy outcomes: a population-based study. *Lancet* 2006;**368**:1164–70.
10. Hillier TA, Pedula KL, Schmidt MM, et al. Childhood obesity and metabolic imprinting. *Diabetes Care* 2007;**30**:2287–92.
11. Ozanne SE, Constância M. Mechanisms of disease: the developmental origins of disease and the role of the epigenotype. *Nat Clin Pract Endocrinol Metab* 2007;**3**:539–46.
12. Reece EA. Perspectives on obesity, pregnancy and birth outcomes in the United States: the scope of the problem. *Am J Obstet Gynecol* 2008;**198**:23–7.
13. Jain A. Treating obesity in individuals and populations. *BMJ* 2005;**33**:1387–90.
14. Angrisani L, Favretti F, Furbetta F, et al. Italian Group for Lap-Band System: results of multicenter study on patients with BMI < or 35 kg/m². *Obes Surg* 2004;**14**:415–18.

15. O'Brien P, Dixon J, Laurie C, et al. Treatment of mild to moderate obesity with laparoscopic adjustable gastric banding or an intensive medical program: a randomized trial. *Ann Intern Med* 2006;**144**:625–33.

16. Sjöström L, Narbro K, Sjöström CD, et al. Effects of bariatric surgery on mortality in Swedish obese subjects. *N Engl J Med* 2007;**357**:741–52.

17. Adams TD, Gress R, Smith SC, et al. Long-term mortality after bypass surgery. *N Engl J Med* 2007;**357**:753–61.

18. Sjöström L, Lindroos AK, Peltonen M, et al. Lifestyle, diabetes, and cardiovascular risk factors 10 years after bariatric surgery. *N Engl J Med* 2004;**351**:2683–93.

19. Karlsson J, Taft C, Rydén A, et al. Ten-year trends in health-related quality of life after surgical and conventional treatment for severe obesity: the SOS intervention study. *Int J Obes* 2007;**31**:1248–61.

20. ACOG Committee on Adolescent Health Care. The overweight adolescent: prevention, treatment, and obstetric-gynecologic implications. *Obstet Gynecol* 2006;**108**:1337–48.

21. Schilling PL, Davis MM, Albanese CT, et al. National trends in adolescent bariatric surgical procedures and implications for surgical centers for excellence. *J Am Coll Surg* 2008;**206**:1–12.

22. van Dam RM, Willett WC, Manson JE, Hu FB. The relationship between overweight in adolescence and premature death in women. *Ann Intern Med* 2006;**145**:91–7.

23. Ford ES, Mokdad AH, Ajani UA. Trends in risk factors for cardiovascular disease among children and adolescents in the United States. *Pediatrics* 2004;**114**:1534–44.

24. Weiss R, Dziura J, Burgert T, et al. Obesity and the metabolic syndrome in children and adolescents. *N Engl J Med* 2004;**350**:2362–74.

25. Geier AB, Foster GD, Womble LG, et al. The relationship between relative weight and school attendance among elementary schoolchildren. *Obesity* 2007;**15**:2157–61.

26. Andersson SE, Dallal GE, Must A. Relative weight and race influence average age at menarche: results from two nationally representative surveys of US girls studied 25 years apart. *Pediatrics* 2003;**111**:844–50.

27. Gigante DP, Rasmussen KM, Victora CG. Pregnancy increases BMI in adolescents of a population-based birth cohort. *J Nutr* 2005;**135**:74–80.

28. Besculides M, Laraque F. Unintended pregnancy among the urban poor. *J Urban Health* 2004;**81**:340–8.

29. Butte NF, Wong WW, Treuth MS, et al. Energy requirements during pregnancy based on total energy expenditure and energy deposition. *Am J Clin Nutr* 2004;**79**:1078–87.

30. Kral JG. Preventing and treating obesity in girls and young women to curb the epidemic. *Obes Res* 2004;**12**:1539–46.

31. Tataranni P, Mingrone G, Raguso C, et al. Twenty-four energy and nutrient balances in weight stable postobese patients after biliopancreatic diversion. *Nutrition* 1996;**12**:239–44.

32. Pitkin RM. Abdominal hysterectomy in obese women. *Surg Gynecol Obstet* 1976;**142**:532–6.

33. Harper J, Madan AK, Ternovits CA, Tichansky DS. What happens to patients who do not follow-up after bariatric surgery? *Am Surg* 2007;**73**:181–4.

34. Cannizzo F Jr, Kral JG. Obesity surgery: a model of programmed undernutrition. *Curr Opin Clin Nutr Metab Care* 1998;**1**:363–8.

35. Kral JG, Näslund E. Surgical treatment of obesity. *Nat Clin Pract Endocrinol Metab* 2007;**3**:574–83.

36. Potoczna N, Branson R, Piec G, et al. Gene variants and binge eating as predictors of comorbidity and outcome of treatment in severe obesity. *J Gastrointest Surg* 2004;**8**:971–82.

37. Brunner Huber LR, Toth JL. Obesity and oral contraceptive failure: findings from the 2002 National Survey of Family Growth. *Am J Epidemiol* 2007;**166**:1306–11.

38. Victor A, Odlind V, Kral JG. Oral contraceptive absorption and sex hormone binding globulins in obese women: effects of jejunoileal bypass. *Gastroenterol Clin North Am* 1987;**16**:483–91.

39. Merhi ZO. Challenging oral contraception after weight loss by bariatric surgery. *Gynecol Obstet Invest* 2007;**64**:100–2.

40. Flancbaum L, Belsley S, Drake V, et al. Preoperative nutritional status of patients undergoing Roux-en-Y gastric bypass for morbid obesity. *J Gastrointest Surg* 2006;**10**:1033–7.

41. Grange D, Finlay J. Nutritional vitamin B_{12} deficiency in a breastfed infant following maternal gastric bypass. *J Pediatr Hematol Oncol* 1994;**11**:311–18.

42. Weissman A, Schachter M, Dreazen E. Severe maternal and fetal electrolyte imbalance in pregnancy after gastric surgery for morbid obesity. *J Reprod Med* 1995;**40**:813–16.

43. Gurewitsch ED, Smith-Levitin M, Mack J. Pregnancy following gastric bypass surgery for morbid obesity. *J Obstet Gynaecol* 1996;**88**:658–61.

44. Huerta S, Li Z, Heber D, Liu C, Livingston EH. Vitamin A deficiency in a newborn resulting from maternal hypovitaminosis A after biliopancreatic diversion for the treatment of morbid obesity. *Am J Clin Nutr* 2002;**76**:426–9.

45. Cools M, Duval EL, Jespers A. Adverse neonatal outcome after maternal biliopancreatic diversion operation: report of 9 cases. *Eur J Pediatr* 2006;**165**:199–202.

46. Moore KA, Ouyang DW, Whang EE. Maternal and fetal deaths after gastric bypass surgery for morbid obesity. *N Engl J Med* 2004;**351**:721–2.

47. Merhi ZO, Pal L. Effect of weight loss by bariatric surgery on the risk of miscarriage. *Gynecol Obstet Invest* 2007;**64**:224–7.

48. Hockett PK, Emery SC, Hansen L, Masliah E. Evidence of oxidative stress in the brains of fetuses with CNS anomalies and islet cell hyperplasia. *Pediatr Dev Pathol* 2004;**7**:370–9.

49. Moley KH, Chi MM, Knudson CM, et al. Hyperglycemia induces apoptosis in pre-implantation embryos through cell death effector pathways. *Nat Med* 1998;**4**:1421–4.

50. García-Patterson A, Erdozain L, Ginovart G, et al. In human gestational diabetes mellitus congenital malformations are related to pre-pregnancy body mass index and to severity of diabetes. *Diabetologia* 2004;**47**:509–14.

51. Moore L, Bradlee L, Singer M, et al. Chromosomal anomalies among the offspring of women with gestational diabetes. *Am J Epidemiol* 2002;**155**:719–24.

52. Kral JG, Dixon JB, Horber FF, et al. Flaws in evidence-based medicine methodologies may adversely affect public health directives. *Surgery* 2005;**137**:279 84.

53. Sheiner E, Levy A, Silverberg D, et al. Pregnancy after bariatric surgery is not associated with adverse perinatal outcome. *Am J Obstet Gynecol* 2004;**190**: 1335–40.

54. Dixon JB, Dixon ME, O'Brien PE. Birth outcomes in obese women after laparoscopic adjustable gastric banding. *Obstet Gynecol* 2005;**106**:965–72.

55. Weiss HG, Nehoda H, Labeck B, et al. Pregnancies after adjustable gastric banding. *Obes Surg* 2001;**11**:303–6.

56. Dao T, Kuhn J, Ehmer D, et al. Pregnancy outcomes after gastric-bypass surgery. *Am J Surg* 2006;**192**:762–6.

57. Marceau P, Kaufman D, Biron S, et al. Outcome of pregnancies after biliopancreatic diversion. *Obes Surg* 2004;**14**:318–24.

58. Institute of Medicine (Subcommittees on Nutritional Status and Weight Gain During Pregnancy, Committee on Nutritional Status During Pregnancy and Lactation, Food and Nutrition Board). *Nutrition During Pregnancy. Part I, Weight Gain*. Washington, DC: National Academy Press, 1990.

59. Crowther A, Hiller JE, Moss JR, et al. Effect of treatment of gestational diabetes mellitus on pregnancy outcomes. *N Engl J Med* 2005;**352**:2477–86.

60. Sheiner E, Menes TS, Silverberg D, et al. Pregnancy outcome of patients with gestational diabetes mellitus following bariatric surgery. *Am J Obstet Gynecol* 2006;**194**:431–5.

61. Kral JG. A stitch in time versus a life in misery. *Surg Obes Relat Dis* 2007;**3**:2–5.

62. Apovian CM, Baker C, Ludwig DS. Best practice guidelines in pediatric/ adolescent weight loss surgery. *Obes Res* 2005;**13**:274–82.

63. Garcia VF, DeMaria EJ. Adolescent bariatric surgery: treatment delayed, treatment denied, a crisis invited. *Obes Surg* 2006;**16**:1–4.

64. Kral JG, Biron S, Hould F, et al. Large maternal weight loss from obesity surgery prevents transmission of obesity to children 2–18 years. *Pediatrics* 2006;**118**:e1644–9.

65. Stotland NE, Haas JS, Brawarsky P, et al. Body mass index, provider advice, and target gestational weight gain. *Obstet Gynecol* 2005;**105**:633–8.

66. Lawlor D, Smith G, O'Callaghan M, et al. Epidemiologic evidence for the fetal overnutrition hypothesis: findings from the Mater University study of pregnancy and its outcomes. *Am J Epidemiol* 2007;**165**:418–24.

67. McLean J, Barr S, Prior J. Cognitive dietary restraint is associated with higher urinary cortisol excretion in healthy premenopausal women. *Am J Clin Nutr* 2001;**73**:7–12.

68. Rideout CA, Linden W, Barr SI. High cognitive dietary restraint is associated with increased cortisol excretion in postmenopausal women. *J Gerontol A Biol Sci Med Sci* 2006;**61**:628–33.

69. Ravelli ACJ, van der Meulen JHP, Osmond C, et al. Obesity at the age of 50 y in men and women exposed to famine prenatally. *Am J Clin Nutr* 1999;**70**: 811–16.

70. Roumen FJME. The contraceptive vaginal ring compared with the combined oral contraceptive pill: a comprehensive review of randomized controlled trials. *Contraception* 2007;**75**:420–9.

71. Nelson SM, Fleming RF. The preconceptual contraception paradigm: obesity and infertility. *Hum Reprod* 2007;**22**:912–15.

72. Hafner R, Rogers J. Husbands' adjustment to wives' weight loss after gastric restriction for morbid obesity. *Int J Obes* 1990;**14**:1069–78.

73. Claesson IM, Sydsjö G, Brynhildsen J. Weight gain restriction for obese pregnant women: a case-control intervention study. *Br J Obstet Gynaecol* 2008;**115**:44–50.

14 Diabetes and obesity

Orli Most and Oded Langer

Introduction

Established diabetes mellitus, either type 1 or 2, is the most common pre-existing medical condition in pregnant women. According to the US Centers for Disease Control and Prevention (CDC), its frequency is 2–5/1000 pregnancies.[1] This calculation was published in 1990 and has in all probability increased by 40% in view of the present epidemic of obesity in the USA. This means that a unit delivering 4000 babies per year will see approximately 8–20 cases by the 1990 CDC calculation and possibly as many as 30 or 40 considering the increased numbers of individuals diagnosed with diabetes in the past decade. A more recent CDC publication shows (Figure 14.1) a marked increase in women of reproductive age (18–44 years) diagnosed with diabetes (from 2.2 in 1997 to 3.5 per 1000). The data cited above reinforce the need for diabetic mothers to be managed in clinics run conjointly by an obstetrician and a physician with expertise in diabetes using standardized protocols. In addition, such clinics should be staffed by a dietitian/nutritionist and a nurse or a midwife trained specifically in managing diabetic mothers. This same team should provide all antenatal care until the completion of the postpartum period.

The value of such coordinated efforts in the UK can be inferred from the latest 'Confidential Enquiries into Maternal and Child Health' (CEMACH in 2007), which noted that the number of maternal deaths related to diabetes mellitus declined continually in each preceding triennia.[2] Whereas four deaths were recorded in 1997–9, only one was listed for 2002–5.[2]

The complications of diabetes affecting the mother and fetus are well known. Maternal complications include preterm labor, pre-eclampsia, nephropathy, birth trauma, cesarean section, and postoperative wound complications, among others. Fetal complications include fetal wastage from early pregnancy loss or congenital anomalies, macrosomia, shoulder dystocia, stillbirth, growth restriction, and hypoglycemia, among others. The presence of obesity among diabetics compounds these complications.[1-3] The nature and type of diabetes-related pregnancy complications were such that the international medical community (World Health Organization and International Diabetes Federation) set forth the St Vincent's declaration of 1989, with one of its aims to achieve similar pregnancy outcomes in diabetic and nondiabetic women.[3]

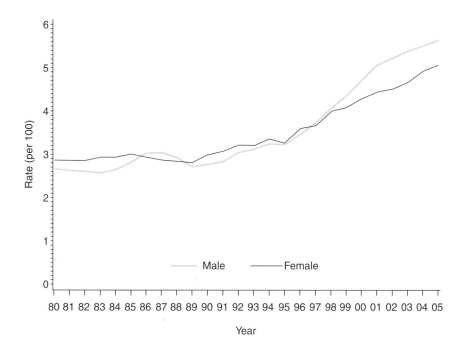

FIGURE 14.1   Age-adjusted prevalence of diagnosed diabetes per 100 population by sex, USA, 1980–2005. From 1980 to 1998, the age-adjusted prevalence of diagnosed diabetes for men and women was similar. However, in 1999, the prevalence for males began to increase at a faster rate than that of females. From 1980 to 2005, the age-adjusted prevalence of diagnosed diabetes increased 111% for men and 76% for women. Data are from Centers for Disease Control and Prevention. Available at: www.cdc.gov/diabetes/statistics/prev/national/figbysex.htm.

Table 14.1 shows important reductions in the stillbirth rate (SBR), early neonatal deaths (ENND), and perinatal mortality rate (PMR) achieved at a tertiary care hospital in Birmingham, UK, as a result of provision of obstetric care to diabetic women who adhered to the guidelines mentioned above.

Diabetes is either present before pregnancy in the form of type 1 or type 2, or detected for the first time during pregnancy. In the latter circumstance, the condition is termed gestational diabetes mellitus (GDM). GDM is also associated with adverse maternal and fetal outcomes, the nature of which does not differ significantly from that associated with diabetes that had been present before pregnancy. However, obesity represents a major risk factor for the onset of diabetes during pregnancy. In general, pregnancy is characterized by decreased insulin sensitivity (increase in resistance of 40–50%) compared with the nonpregnant state.[4] In addition, obesity alone, like GDM, is associated with hyperinsulinemia and increased insulin resistance.[5] This association may explain, at least in part, why obese patients are at greater risk of developing GDM. Both leptin and insulin levels in the fasting state are significantly higher

TABLE 14.1 Changes in stillbirth (SBR), early neonatal mortality (ENND), and perinatal mortality (PMR) before and after St Vincent's declaration of 1989 in a tertiary-care center (modified from Dunne et al[3]).

	Overall diabetes population	Pregestational diabetes
SBR/1000	16 → 6 $P < 0.05$	17 → 11 ns
ENND/1000	23 → 14 ns	28 → 23 ns
PMR/1000	38 → 20 $P < 0.05$	44 → 34 ns

ns, nonsignificant; ENND, early neonatal deaths; PMR, perimortal rate; SBR, stillbirth rate.

(150% and 123%, respectively) in obese than nonobese women.[6] Sebire et al[7] found a twofold increase in the rate of GDM (odds ratio [OR] 1.68, 95% confidence interval [CI] 1.53–1.84). Comparing obese and nonobese patients, Kumari[8] found a rate of GDM of 24.5% for the morbidly obese and 2.2% for the nonobese. Our group studied 6857 women, the majority of whom were Mexican–American; a direct association was found for glucose-screening categories, obesity, and the rate of GDM. For patients with screening results of 130–189 mg/dl, the rate of obesity was approximately 24–30%. Above 189 mg/dl, however, the rate of obesity increased twofold. For nonobese women, the rate of GDM increased for each 10 mg increment in glucose screening, demonstrating that the rates of obesity and glucose tolerance are both associated with the development of GDM.[9]

Diabetes before pregnancy

Prepregnancy

Preparing the diabetic woman for pregnancy represents an ideal, because at least 60% of pregnancies are unplanned in the USA. Even so, healthcare professionals who deal with nonpregnant diabetic women would be remiss not to discuss this eventuality on a regular basis. Preconceptual counseling is a key element in avoiding or reducing the known maternal and fetal risks of diabetes. Counseling should include a thorough discussion of known risks, the importance of good glycemic control, and the necessity to take folic acid supplementation prior to becoming pregnant as well as during the first 12 weeks of pregnancy. Counseling must also emphasize that the dose of folic acid for diabetic mothers is higher than the dose suggested for nondiabetic mothers (5 mg vs 400 μg). Additional topics for counseling sessions include the importance of smoking cessation, avoidance of teratogenic drugs, appropriate contraception, the need for regular screening for nephropathy and retinopathy, proper control of blood pressure, limitation of alcohol consumption, and management of hypoglycemia.

Glycemic control should be assessed by regular determination of HbA1c (glycated hemoglobin) in addition to regular self-monitoring of blood glucose levels. In the UK, the National Service Framework for diabetes recommends that the HbA1c level be less than 7% at the time of conception. Women who achieve tight control preconceptually and maintain control throughout pregnancy significantly reduce their risk of maternal, fetal, and obstetric complications.[10]

An important aspect of the prepregnancy care of any diabetic woman is the avoidance of obesity, or weight reduction if obesity is present. Should weight reduction be advised, the goal should be 5–10% of existing body weight. Behavior modification is the usual first-line management strategy in the form of diet and exercise. If this intervention fails, however, medical management with pharmaceutical agents may be considered, especially for patients with BMI ≥ 35 or those with BMI ≥ 30 who have concurrent medical conditions (see Chapter 12). The two main prescription medications currently used to achieve medically induced weight loss are sibutramine and orlistat. Sibutramine acts on the central satiety centers. Studies have shown that weight lost after 1 year of sibutramine use is on average 10 lb (4.5 kg) more than with diet or placebo alone. The side effects of sibutramine, however, make it a difficult drug for many patients to tolerate (see Chapter 12). Orlistat blocks lipase, a digestive enzyme that breaks down dietary fat to a form that can be absorbed by the body; therefore, it inhibits the absorption of dietary fat by up to 30%. The remainder of the unabsorbed dietary fat is eliminated in the stool, causing an unpleasant side effect to the patients. It is important to note that pharmacotherapy does not work with all patients and often the effect of the drug is diminished after 6 months of use. It is also important to note that these two drugs are not considered appropriate for use during pregnancy, and either patients who are using them should also use effective contraceptives, or these medications should be stopped as soon as pregnancy is suspected.

Patients with BMI ≥ 35 and a failed pharmacotherapy trial may be candidates for bariatric surgery (see Chapter 13). Weight-loss surgery may result in diminution of as much as 50% of the excess weight within the first 2 postoperative years. Complications of bariatric surgery include infection, thrombotic events, gallstones due to the rapid weight loss, hernia at the surgical incision sight, nutritional deficiencies, and the dumping syndrome.

Pregnancy: antenatal care

Ideally, the diabetic patient should continue care with the same multidisciplinary team that provided her care preconceptually. If this is not possible, the physician in charge should arrange a referral to a similar team. The goals of antenatal care include maintenance of glycemic control to reduce the risk of known complications, monitoring for the appearance of pre-eclampsia, avoidance of excess weight gain, and regular monitoring of fetal growth.

Weight gain in pregnancy is defined as the weight at delivery minus the pregravid weight. The recommendations for weight gain in pregnancy in the

1990 US Institute of Medicine report are as follows: 11.2–15.9 kg (25–35 lb) for normal-weight women, 6.8–11.2 kg (15–25 lb) for overweight women, and 6.8 kg (15 lb) for obese women.[11] These guidelines were initially intended to help decrease the risk of fetal growth restriction. However, no established guidelines exist for weight gain in the pregnant patient when fetal macrosomia is the reference. Similarly, no established guidelines are known for weight gain in diabetic pregnancies, regardless of whether the mother was obese or not. Contributors to fetal growth and macrosomia include maternal obesity, excessive weight gain, and poor glycemic control in diabetic pregnancy.[12]

It is axiomatic that the goal of treatment of both pregnant and nonpregnant diabetic patients is to optimize the glycemic profile. In pregnant patients, this is customarily performed with a trial of diet therapy and addition of insulin or oral antidiabetic drugs.[13] Both agents were designed to reduce the level of glycemia. Insulin has been available since 1923 and is without question the reference standard therapy for a disease causing the premature death of countless people and untold morbidity worldwide.

In Europe and South Africa, the first-generation sulphonylureas, glyburide and metformin, have been used for years. The fierce resistance to the use of these agents in pregnancy stems from the lack of data from appropriately powered and well-designed studies. In general, outcome-based research has not been available. In the USA, until the year 2000, the use of oral antidiabetic drugs (hypoglycemic or antihyperglycemic) was contraindicated, and they played a limited role in the management of diabetes in pregnancy. The main objection to their use was the risk of congenital anomalies, fetal compromise, and fetal hypoglycemic episodes through direct stimulation of the fetal pancreas. As so often happens, the ban on the use of oral hypoglycemic agents in pregnancy was based on the scant evidence provided in this instance by case reports and one study of fetal anomalies in 50 poorly controlled diabetic women before pregnancy that failed to address the question: Is it the drug or is it the glucose?[14] Until recently, the American College of Obstetricians and Gynecologists (ACOG) and the American Diabetes Association (ADA) did not recommend the use of oral hypoglycemic agents in pregnancy.[15,16] It is only lately that of the use of oral hypoglycemic agents was considered and then became an accepted practice by scientific forums (North American Diabetes in Pregnancy Study Group and the 5th International Workshop on Gestational Diabetes in 2004).

The concerns regarding the use of oral hypoglycemic agents in the treatment of GDM were recently studied in a systematic format with adequate sample size and a randomized design. This study demonstrated that glyburide is comparable to insulin in achieving maternal levels of glycemia that result in a perinatal outcome similar to that in the general population.[17]

As suggested above, adequate glycemic control is crucial throughout pregnancy and is assessed by serial measurements of HbAlc and daily home glucose monitoring (Table 14.2). Adequate glycemic control cannot be achieved unless the patient has a home monitoring kit. The HbA1c level reflects the mean glucose concentration over the preceding 8 weeks, except in pregnancy when it reflects control over the preceding 6–8 weeks. The management goal is to achieve an HbA1c level as close to normal as possible without inducing hypoglycemia. Awareness of hypoglycemia can be significantly diminished in pregnancy, and patients should be educated appropriately. In a national Dutch study in which 72% of patients had good glycemic control before conception (HbA1c < 7%), a two- to three-fold increase in hypoglycemic episodes was observed in 41% of patients, with 19% experiencing hypoglycemic coma in the first trimester.[18] Table 14.2 also shows the other types of parameters that need frequent monitoring and the frequency of this monitoring to be carried out.

Published guidelines on glycemic control during pregnancy vary, and differences are also noted between the targets of the USA and those of the UK and Europe. Regardless of which guideline is selected by the management team, it is crucial that both short- and long-term targets be communicated to patients, documented in the record at every visit, and revised when necessary. It is unrealistic to expect that the hypoglycemic agents selected and used in the prenatal period will need no revision or addition as pregnancy progresses. Failure to change therapy when necessary may have devastating consequences, especially if accompanied by poor communication between the team and the patient. Table 14.3 shows the recommended glycemic targets of the ADA, the ACOG, and the Guy's and St Thomas' NHS Foundation Trust of the UK.[10] Some units in the USA suggest lower fasting glucose concentration (3.1–3.6 mmol/l) with 1-h postprandial values of < 6.7 mmol/l. (To convert millimoles/liter of glucose to milligrams/deciliter, multiply by 18. To convert milligrams/deciliter of glucose to millimoles/liter, divide by 18 or multiply by 0.055.)

TABLE 14.2   Frequency of testing in pregnancy[10]

Test	Frequency
HbA1c	Every 4–6 weeks
Blood glucose	7 times a day (at least 4 times) and when hypoglycemia is suspected
Urinary ketones	Blood glucose > 11.1 mmol/l, unwell, vomiting, or not eating
Serum creatinine	Every trimester in women with known nephropathy
Thyroid function	Baseline serum-free T_4 and TSH
Blood pressure	Every visit with health team
Proteinuria	Every visit with health team; 24-h urinary collection advised each trimester in women with nephropathy
Retinal screening	Baseline and every trimester in both type 1 and type 2 diabetes

T_4, thyroxine; TSH, thyroid-stimulating hormone.

TABLE 14.3 Recommended glycemic targets[10]

	American Diabetes Association	American College of Obstetricians and Gynecologists	Guy's and St Thomas' NHS Foundation Trust
Fasting glucose concentration (mmol/l)	4.4–6.1	≤5.3	4–5.5
2-h postprandial glucose concentration (mmol/l)	≤8.6	≤6.7	≤7.0

Such values are supported by studies showing improved outcome with particular reference to rates of macrosomia and shoulder dystocia. Regardless of the targets selected, they should be realistic, achievable, and adapted to the needs of the individual patients to avoid severe and recurrent hypoglycemic episodes.

The overriding goals of monitoring for fetal well-being are prevention of stillbirth, reduction in the incidence of macrosomia, and avoidance of fetal growth restriction. Current recommendations suggest that all women should be counseled regarding the regular use of fetal kick counts, although the data to show that this measure conclusively reduces the risk of stillbirth in diabetic women is scant. It is, however, noninvasive and inexpensive, and it may improve maternal bonding. A mainstay of antenatal fetal surveillance is nonstress testing (NST), with or without determination of amniotic fluid volume (AFV) and/or biophysical profile. Kjos and coworkers[19] described obstetric outcomes in 3134 women with all types of diabetes who had twice-weekly NST with AFV determination. No stillbirths occurred within 4 days of the last antepartum testing, but 85 women required cesarean delivery for nonreassuring heart-rate pattern. More recently, Brecher et al[20] reported a retrospective, case–control study in which 1935 women with all types of diabetes were assessed in a similar fashion. Women who experienced stillbirths were more likely to have had suboptimal glucose control and a greater interval from their last fetal surveillance testing.[19,20]

Another type of fetal monitoring is Doppler velocimetry of fetal and maternal vessels. Abnormal fetal blood velocity is associated with increased risk of fetal acidemia. As placental resistance increases, umbilical blood flow becomes increasingly retrograde so that reversed end-diastolic blood flow is a strong predictor of fetal death.[21]

The detection of fetal macrosomia is facilitated by frequent ultrasound examination using modern, high-resolution equipment with built-in biometry. Prior to the advent of ultrasound, assessment of macrosomia was limited to palpation, a method that is inaccurate in the best of hands. This is not to say that ultrasound is error free; it is associated with a recognized over-underestimation rate of 10% on each side. No consensus definition of fetal macrosomia exists. Some authorities cite 4000, others 4500, and still others 5000 g. Nevertheless, the danger of the macrosomic child relates to the possibility of serious fetal morbidity and increased risk of shoulder dystocia. The most accurate ultrasound determinant of fetal size in the third trimester is abdominal circumference. More than 60 formulas assist in the estimation of fetal weight from ultrasound readings. None is perfect or stands out as being most accurate in nondiabetic or diabetic pregnancies. The sensitivity of detecting fetal macrosomia is 50–60% with an 8% margin of error. Serial measurements increase accuracy, but accuracy decreases with increasing fetal size.[21,22]

Intrapartum care

Women with diabetes should be delivered in maternity units with access to senior medical, obstetric, and neonatal staff. In the USA, this generally means a level 3 hospital. In the UK and Europe, such care is delivered in centers of excellence and university teaching hospitals for the most part.[10]

Timing of delivery is determined to avoid risk of stillbirth, and the intentional delivery of women with insulin-treated diabetes at 38 weeks is common. This practice undoubtedly increases cesarean section rates and has prompted some healthcare providers to expectantly manage women under good glycemic control until 40 completed weeks' gestation. Delivery at 38 weeks may impart an additional benefit of reduction of infant size and a lower incidence of shoulder dystocia.[23] Progress of labor should be followed closely by continuous electronic fetal monitoring and regular glycemic checks. The target range for blood glucose during labor and delivery recommended by Diabetes UK is 4–6 mmol/l. In contrast, the ACOG suggests hourly glucose levels be kept at less than 110 mg/dl.[23,24] Tight regulation of maternal glucose levels during labor can reduce the incidence of neonatal hypoglycemia even among women with poor antepartum glycemic control.[25]

At the start of active labor, insulin requirements fall rapidly, and glucose must be given along with insulin to prevent maternal hypoglycemia (2.55 mg dextrose/kg per min). Capillary blood glucose must be checked hourly and the rate of insulin adjusted as needed. Insulin requirements fall once again after delivery of the placenta, with some women not requiring insulin for 24–48 h, at which times insulin requirements must be recalculated.[10,25]

Cesarean delivery rates in women with either pre-existing diabetes or GDM are uniformly increased.[26] At the Parkland Hospital, Dallas, Texas, the cesarean delivery rate in women with overt diabetes has remained around 80% for the past 25 years. Contributing factors include fetal macrosomia, labor induction for maternal and fetal complications of failed labor, and scheduled induction at 38–39 weeks' gestation.

Prophylactic cesarean delivery has been proposed, although such a practice is controversial among diabetic women. Recommendations for fetal weight threshold vary from 4000g to 4250 g and even 4500 g, as proposed by the

ACOG.[26,27] Such a practice is made more difficult by limitations in accurately estimating fetal weight, and the obvious consequence of this inaccuracy is an increase in unnecessary operative deliveries in women with diabetes, concomitant with an increase in cesarean section-associated morbidity and healthcare costs.

Special precautions may be warranted in the case of diabetic patients who are severely or morbidly obese. These precautions pertain to having appropriate equipment, such as blood-pressure cuffs, wheelchairs, trolleys, operating tables, and special laryngoscopes, and healthcare professionals trained to deal with such circumstances. The last CEMACH report of 2007[2] cited the death of a woman who had been operated on on two beds pushed together because she was too heavy for an operating table.

Postpartum care

With placental delivery, insulin requirements diminish greatly in all types of diabetes. Women with type 1 diabetes often require very little insulin during the first 24–72 h after delivery. When regular eating patterns resume, women with multiple-dose therapy or continuous insulin infusion generally require a one-third to one-half reduction of pregnancy insulin doses. Women with type 1 diabetes on fixed split doses can generally be restarted at about 0.6 total daily units of insulin per kilogram of postpartum weight, receiving two-thirds of the total dose before breakfast (one-third short-acting and two-thirds intermediate-acting isophane insulin (NPH)) and one-third of total dose in the evening. The evening dose of short- and intermediate-acting NPH can be given together or further split into a before-dinner dose of short-acting (one-half of evening dose) and a before-bedtime dose of intermediate-acting NPH (one-half of evening dose). Postpartum glycemic targets can be relaxed to fasting and postprandial targets of 100 and 150 mg/dl, respectively. Women with type 2 diabetes often have adequate glycemic control immediately after delivery and may not require any medical therapy during hospitalization. These women can be followed with daily fasting capillary glucose levels during hospitalization and after discharge. If resumption of oral antihypoglycemic agents is necessary, glyburide, glipizide, and metformin have been shown to have little or no transfer into human milk and can be prescribed for breastfeeding women.[28]

Medical nutritional consultation should be obtained and total daily caloric needs recalculated based on the woman's healthy weight target and breastfeeding requirements. Postpartum caloric intake should be about 25 kcal/kg per day and 27–30 kcal/kg per day in nonbreastfeeding and breastfeeding women, respectively.[29] Breastfeeding may be problematic in obese or morbidly obese diabetic mothers because of breast size and difficulty of latching on on the part of the fetus. Despite this, the American Academy of Pediatrics and the US Surgeon General strongly recommend exclusive breastfeeding for the first 6 months of life and preferably the first 12 months. Neither pre-existing diabetes nor GDM presents a contraindication to breastfeeding. In-hospital consultation with a lactation specialist is useful to encourage the mother and to ensure that early attempts at feeding are not traumatic for the mother or her child.

Gestational diabetes mellitus

Definition

Since the obstetric community has been managing diabetic women in pregnancy for almost a century, it is somewhat surprising that there is still no international consensus on the appropriate terminology for diabetes that manifests itself for the first time in pregnancy. It can be defined as carbohydrate intolerance first diagnosed during pregnancy, noting that this definition is problematic because it embraces untold numbers of type 2 diabetic women who remain undiagnosed until the disease is first recognized during pregnancy and classified as GDM.[30,31] It is further noted that different studies report varying rates of population prevalence, as well as short- and long-term complications, with prevalence rates of 1–14% in the USA.

One of the major long-debated issues is whether or not intensive treatment can influence birth weight and reduce prenatal morbidity. As recently as 2003, the UK National Institute for Health and Clinical Excellence (NICE) antenatal care guidelines stated: 'There is an absence of evidence to support routine screening for GDM and therefore it is not recommended.' This issue has been clarified once and for all by the publication of the Australian Carbohydrate Intolerance study (ACHOIS). This double-blind trial randomized 1000 women with GDM to routine antenatal care or treatment. The composite measure of serious perinatal complications declined by 75% from 4% in the routine care to 1% in the treated group. The number of macrosomic babies similarly declined by almost 50% from 22% in the routine care group to 13% in the treated group.[32]

Screening

The detection of GDM is plagued by different approaches to screening with different timings of blood-glucose measurements and blood-glucose loads. Table 14.4 shows three of the current, widely used criteria to detect GDM. These differences compound the calculation of prevalence and accentuate the differences noted between populations. The presence of GDM is a risk factor for the subsequent development of type 2 diabetes, and this risk is modified by ethnic origin. Accordingly, GDM may affect as many as 15% of south Asian women, whereas for white women, whose overall risk of type 2 diabetes is lower, the risk may be as low as 3%.

The question often arises as to how to screen and when to screen. Here again there is no universal consensus. If prevalence rates of GDM are 2–4%, the two-stage screening protocol using the glucose challenge test originally described by Mary O'Sullivan is reasonable. Here, 50 g glucose in 150 ml water is administered to an unprepared woman at 24–28 weeks' gestation. A positive test is a plasma glucose measurement 1 h after ingestion of the glucose of ≥ 7.8 mmol/l. By this test, the sensitivity for a subsequent positive glucose tolerance test (GTT) is 79%, the specificity is 87%, and the positive predictive value is 15%.

TABLE 14.4 Criteria currently used to define gestational diabetes. (Adapted from Fraser and Heller.[30])

WHO	One or more values following a 75-g glucose load; fasting plasma glucose $\geq$ 7 mmol/l, 2-h glucose $\geq$ 7.8 mmol/l
EASD	One or more values following a 75-g glucose load; fasting plasma glucose $\geq$ 6 mmol/l, 2-h glucose $\geq$ 9 mmol/l
ADA	Two or more values following a 100-g glucose load; fasting plasma glucose $\geq$ 5.3 mmol/l, 1-h glucose $\geq$ 10 mmol/l, 2-h glucose $\geq$ 8.6 mmol/l, 3-h glucose $\geq$ 7.7 mmol/l

ADA: American Diabetes Association; EASD: European Association for the Study of Diabetes; WHO: World Health Organization.

On the other hand, in populations where the prevalence is expected to be over 4%, screening should be replaced by a diagnostic test as well as the 2-h GTT applied to the whole population. A modified version of this test using the 2-h value only has been described by Åberg et al[33] as being successful in a Swedish community, and this version might be useful. A means to reduce the cost and inconvenience of large-scale screening in any of the above scenarios would be to use the ADA's low-risk criteria for GDM to exclude women from screening who are aged less than 25 years, of normal weight for height, and from a low-prevalence ethnic group. It has been calculated that, by applying these exclusions, only 3% of positive diagnoses would be missed.[30] Other, albeit less specific, means of identifying GDM include the following: persistent urinary glycosuria, unexplained polyhydramnios, and the classic triad of polydypsia, polyphagia, and polyuria. All require intensive follow-up, as none is specific.

Pregnancy: antenatal care

Antenatal care for women diagnosed with GDM differs in one important aspect from that provided to women with established diabetes. Although most of the routine interventions for pregnancy surveillance are similar if not identical, the patient with established diabetes is already medicated, whereas the patient with newly diagnosed GDM is confronted with two possibilities. The first is dietary modification with input based on the nutritionist's recommendations, accompanied by self-monitoring of glucose on a routine basis and close follow-up and surveillance. Patient education plays a key role at this point. Such patients should be informed that, if this intervention is not successful, medication will be required. Here, gaining the patient's trust and cooperation is crucial so that she becomes aware of the serious nature of GDM and its potential consequences to herself and her fetus.

The second possibility is the immediate institution of pharmacologic therapy. There are two thresholds for the initiation of pharmacologic therapy.[31] The traditional threshold requires fasting plasma glucose of at least 105 mg/dl, whereas the more intense approach uses fasting plasma glucose of at least

95 mg/dl in conjunction with postprandial levels of at least 120 mg/dl for 2 h or 140 mg/dl for 1 h. By these criteria, for a given population, approximately 30–50% of women who have GDM will require pharmacologic therapy when diet alone fails to reduce glycemic levels.[34] However, it has recently been suggested that to obtain improved perinatal outcome in obese women who have GDM, pharmacologic (insulin) treatment will be required, even in the presence of good glycemic control with diet alone.[35] Accordingly, the rate of GDM patients who require pharmacologic therapy may be even higher than previously suggested. Although there is a paucity of information regarding the length of time that diet should be maintained before initiation of pharmacologic therapy, caregivers need to note that the time from diagnosis to delivery in GDM is short. Most patients who have GDM are diagnosed at 28–32 weeks and deliver at 37–39 weeks' gestation. Any delay in initiation of pharmacologic therapy with its potential to achieve the established levels of glycemic control will result in irreversible adverse outcome (macrosomia, metabolic complications, and so forth). Among patients who have threshold fasting plasma of less than 95 mg/dl and therefore qualify for the trial of diet therapy, a 2-week, diet-alone period will identify most patients who can achieve the desired level of glycemic control. Therefore, obese GDM patients (BMI > 29) and patients who have fasting plasma of over 95 mg/dl, or those who have fasting plasma glucose of under 95 mg/dl who fail to achieve the desired level of glycemic control within 2 weeks, all require pharmacologic therapy. Still, for every valid recommendation, there is a valid exception; in these cases, the practitioner's clinical wisdom supersedes this recommendation. For example, when GDM is diagnosed after 28–30 weeks' gestation and there is less time to influence the desired level of control, the care provider needs to be more liberal in the early initiation of pharmacologic therapy. In contrast, there will be more flexibility when GDM is diagnosed during the second trimester, when the growth stimulation to the fetus is not yet prominent.[31]

Oral antihypoglycemic agents in GDM

Earlier in this discussion, it was noted that there previously had been some concern regarding the value of continued treatment with oral antihypoglycemics during pregnancy. Table 14.5 is a recent amalgamation of published data reporting successful treatment with oral antidiabetic agents during pregnancy.[31]

Postpartum care and future risks

Women with GDM differ from overt diabetics in their immediate postpartum needs for glycemic control. No medication is needed in the majority of cases. If, on the other hand, the woman diagnosed with GDM is really an undiagnosed overt diabetic, medication will be needed on a regular basis. Moreover, such patients require referral to and follow-up with a diabetologist.

Women with GDM have a 50–60% lifetime risk of developing diabetes, most commonly type 2. This risk is modulated by obesity, the extent of weight gain during pregnancy, and the percentage of gained weight that is retained post

TABLE 14.5 Studies reporting successful treatment of oral antidiabetic agents in pregnancy

| Study | Study design | Type of diabetes | No. of patients | | Achievement of good control |
			Glyburide	Regular insulin	
Langer, 2000[31]	RCT	GDM	201	203	82% and 88%
Lim, 1997[44]	Prosp, observ	GDM	33	21	No significant difference
Conway, 2004[45]	Prosp, observ	GDM	75	—	84%
Kremer, 2004[46]	Prosp, observ	GDM	73	—	81%
Chmait, 2004[47]	Prosp, observ	GDM	69	—	82%
Gilson, 2002[48]	Prosp, observ	GDM	22	22	82%
Fines, 2003[49]	Retro (case–control)	GDM	40	44	NA
Velazques, 2003[50]	Case series	GDM	31	7	Glyburide 82%
Pendsey, 2002[51]	RCT	Type 2	—	23	Improved level of glycemic control
Coetzee, 1979[52]	Prosp, observ	GDM and type 2		GDM: 81.4%	
Hellmuth, 2000[53]	Prosp, observ	GDM	Sulfonylurea: 68	42	Type 2 diabetes 46.2%
Notelowitz, 1971[54]	RCT	GDM and type 2	Tolbutamide chlorpropamine: 2 × 52	52	Using oral hypoglycemic: 80%
Yogev, 2004[55]	Prosp	GDM	25	30	Mean blood glucose similar in all groups
Moore, 2005[56]	RCT	GDM	Metformin: 32	31	Blood glucose similar
Jacobson, 2005[57]	Retro	GDM	236	316	Blood glucose similar

Observ, observational; Props, prospective; RCT, randomized controlled trial; Retro, retrospective.
GDM, gestational diabetes mellitus; RCT, randomized control trial.

partum. If any fasting pregnancy glucose is over 121 mg/dl, the risk of diabetes is 21 greater than if fasting levels remain below 95 mg/dl.[36] The Fifth Workshop Conference on GDM recommended that the postpartum glycemic status of women with recent GDM be established 6 weeks later with a 75-g, 2-h oral glucose test repeated in 1 year and then at least every 3 years after.[36,37] Women with prior GDM and postpartum impaired glucose tolerance (IGT) test have a 16% annual incidence rate of developing diabetes.[38] The onset of type 2 diabetes can be delayed or prevented in women with IGT. Two controlled trials found that intensive lifestyle interventions over 4–6 years reduced the risk of diabetes by 58% compared with nonintervention.[39] Metformin, acarbose, and Orlistat reduce the risk by 31%, 25%, and 37%, respectively.[40–42]

A systematic review of recurrence of GDM in 2007 noted marked variation across studies. The most consistent predictor of future recurrence was nonwhite ethnicity, even granting that racial breakdowns within a study were not always explicit. Minority populations had markedly higher recurrence rates of GDM than non-Hispanic whites. Risk factors such as maternal age, parity, BMI, oral glucose tolerance test levels, and insulin use were inconsistently useful in prediction of recurrent GDM.[43]

References

1. Centers for Disease Control. Perinatal mortality and congenital malformations in infants born to women with insulin-dependent diabetes mellitus – United States, Canada, and Europe, 1940–1988. *JAMA* 1990;**264**:437–41.
2. Lewis G, ed. *The Confidential Enquiry into Maternal and Child Health (CEMACH): Saving Mothers' Lives: Reviewing Maternal Deaths to Make Motherhood Safer – 2003–2005.* The Seventh Report on Confidential Enquiries into Maternal Deaths in the United Kingdom. London: CEMACH, 2007.
3. Dunne F, Brydon P, Proffitt M, et al. Approaching St Vincent. Working toward the St Vincent targets. *Diabetic Med* 2001;**18**:333–4.
4. Catalano PM, Tyzbir ED, Roman NM, et al. Longitudinal changes in insulin release and insulin resistance in nonobese pregnant women. *Am J Obstet Gynecol* 1991;**165**(6 Pt 1):1667–72.
5. Ramsay JE, Ferrell WR, Crawford L, et al. Maternal obesity is associated with dysregulation of metabolic, vascular, and inflammatory pathways. *J Clin Endocrinol Metab* 2002;**87**:4231–7.
6. Sattar N, Gaw A, Packard CJ, Greer IA. Potential pathogenic roles of aberrant lipoprotein and fatty acid metabolism in pre-eclampsia. *Br J Obstet Gynaecol* 1996;**103**:614–20.
7. Sebire NJ, Jolly M, Harris JP, et al. Maternal obesity and pregnancy outcome: a study of 287,213 pregnancies in London. *Int J Obes Relat Metab Disord* 2001;**25**:1175–82.
8. Kumari AS. Pregnancy outcome in women with morbid obesity. *Int J Gynaecol Obstet* 2001;**73**:101–7.

9. Yogev Y, Langer O, Xenakis EM, Rosenn B. Glucose screening in Mexican-American women. *Obstet Gynecol* 2004;**103**:1241–5.

10. Chaudry R, Gilby P, Carroll PV. Pre-existing (type 1 and type 2) diabetes in pregnancy. *Obstet Gynaecol Reprod Med* 2007;**17**:339–44.

11. US Institute of Medicine. Nutritional status and weight gain. In: *Nutrition During Pregnancy*.Washington, DC: National Academy Press, 1990: 227–33.

12. Sunehag A, Berne C, Lindmark G, Ewald U. Gestational diabetes-perinatal outcome with a policy of liberal and intensive insulin therapy. *Ups J Med Sci* 1991;**96**:185–98.

13. Langer O. Maternal glycemic criteria for insulin therapy in gestational diabetes mellitus. *Diabetes Care* 1998;**21**(Suppl 2):B91–B8.

14. Piacquadio K, Hollingsworth DR, Murphy H. Effects of in-utero exposure to oral hypoglycaemic drugs. *Lancet* 1991;**338**:866–9.

15. American College of Obstetricians and Gynecologists. *Technical Bulletin 92*. Washington, DC: ACOG, 1996: 1–2.

16. Metzger BE, Coustan DR. Summary and recommendations of the Fourth International Workshop-Conference on Gestational Diabetes Mellitus. *Proceedings of the Fourth International Workshop-Conference on Gestational Diabetes Mellitus*, 1998;**21**:B161–7.

17. Langer O, Conway DL, Berkus MD, et al. A comparison of glyburide and insulin in women with gestational diabetes mellitus. *N Engl J Med* 2000;**343**:1134–8.

18. Visser GHA. How to improve outcome of pregnancy of women with type 1 diabetes: the Dutch experience. National Dutch Audit. Oral Presentation at Diabetes UK Annual Professional Conference, 14–16 March 2007, Glasgow.

19. Kjos SL, Leung A, Henry OA, et al. Antepartum surveillance in diabetic pregnancies: predictors of fetal distress in labor. *Am J Obstet Gynecol* 1995;**173**:1532–9.

20. Brecher A, Tharakan T, Williams A, Baxi L. Perinatal mortality in diabetic patients undergoing antepartum fetal evaluation: a case-control study. *J Matern Fetal Neonatal Med* 2002;**12**:423–7.

21. Dudley DJ. Diabetic-associated stillbirth: incidence, pathophysiology, and prevention. *Clin Perinatol* 2007;**34**:611–26, vii.

22. Wallace S, McEwan A. Fetal macrosomia. *Obstet Gynaecol Reprod Med* 2007;**17**:58–61.

23. Lurie S, Insler V, Hagay ZJ. Induction of labor at 38 to 39 weeks of gestation reduces the incidence of shoulder dystocia in gestational diabetic patients class A2. *Am J Perinatol* 1996;**13**:293–6.

24. American College of Obstetricians and Gynecologists. *Pregestational Diabetes*. ACOG Practice Bulletin no. 60. Washington, DC: ACOG, 2005.

25. Curet LB, Izquierdo LA, Gilson GJ, et al. Relative effects of antepartum and intrapartum maternal blood glucose levels on incidence of neonatal hypoglycemia. *J Perinatol* 1997;**17**:113–15.

26. Casey BM, Lucas MJ, Mcintire DD, Leveno KJ. Pregnancy outcomes in women with gestational diabetes compared with the general obstetric population. *Obstet Gynecol* 1997;**90**:869–73.

27. American College of Obstetricians and Gynecologists. Clinical management guidelines for obstetrician–gynecologists. ACOG Practice Bulletin no. 40, 2002. *Obstet Gynecol* 2002;**100**.

28. Kjos SL. After pregnancy complicated by diabetes: postpartum care and education. *Obstet Gynecol Clin North Am* 2007;**34**:335–49, x.

29. Jovanovic L, Nakai Y. Successful pregnancy in women with type 1 diabetes: from preconception through postpartum care. *Endocrinol Metab Clin North Am* 2006;**35**:79–97, vi.

30. Fraser R, Heller SR. Gestational diabetes: aetiology and management. *Obstet Gynaecol Reprod Med* 2007;**17**:345–8.

31. Langer O. Oral anti-hyperglycemic agents for the management of gestational diabetes mellitus. *Obstet Gynecol Clin North Am* 2007;**34**:255–74, ix.

32. Fraser R. Gestational diabetes: after the ACHOIS trial. *Diabetic Med* 2006;**23**(Suppl 1):8–11.

33. Åberg A, Rydhstroem H, Frid A. Impaired glucose tolerance associated with adverse pregnancy outcome: a population-based study in southern Sweden. *Am J Obstet Gynecol* 2001;**184**:77–83.

34. Zhu S, Wang Z, Heshka S, et al. Waist circumference and obesity-associated risk factors among whites in the third National Health and Nutrition Examination Survey: clinical action thresholds. *Am J Clin Nutr* 2002;**76**:743–9.

35. Langer O, Yogev Y, Xenakis MJ, et al. Overweight and obese in gestational diabetes: the impact on pregnancy outcome. *Am J Obstet Gynecol* 2005;**192**: 1768–76.

36. Schaefer-Graf UM, Buchanan TA, Xiang AH, et al. Clinical predictors for a high risk for the development of diabetes mellitus in the early puerperium in women with recent gestational diabetes mellitus. *Am J Obstet Gynecol* 2002;**186**:751–6.

37. Metzger BE, Buchanan TA, Coustan DR, et al. Summary and recommendations of the Fifth International Workshop Conference on Gestational Diabetes Mellitus. *Diabetes Care* 2007;**30**(Suppl 2):251–60.

38. Kjos SL, Peters RK, Xiang A, et al. Predicting future diabetes in Latino women with gestational diabetes. Utility of early postpartum glucose tolerance testing. *Diabetes* 1995;**44**:586–91.

39. Tuomilehto J, Lindstrom J, Eriksson JG, et al. Prevention of type 2 diabetes mellitus by changes in lifestyle among subjects with impaired glucose tolerance. *N Engl J Med* 2001;**344**:1343–50.

40. Chiasson JL, Josse RG, Gomis R, et al. Acarbose treatment and the risk of cardiovascular disease and hypertension in patients with impaired glucose tolerance: the STOP–NIDDM trial. *JAMA* 2003;**290**:486–94.

41. Knowler WC, Barrett-Connor E, Fowler SE, et al. Reduction in the incidence of type 2 diabetes with lifestyle intervention or metformin. *N Engl J Med* 2002;**346**:393–403.

42. Torgerson JS, Hauptman J, Boldrin MN, Sjostrom L. XENical in the prevention of diabetes in obese subjects (XENDOS) study: a randomized study of orlistat as an adjunct to lifestyle changes for the prevention of type 2 diabetes in obese patients. *Diabetes Care* 2004;**27**:155–61.

43. Kim C, Berger DK, Chamany S. Recurrence of gestational diabetes mellitus: a systematic review. *Diabetes Care* 2007;**30**:1314–19.

44. Lim JM, Tayob Y, O'Brien PM, Shaw RW. A comparison between the pregnancy outcome of women with gestation diabetes treated with glibenclamide and those treated with insulin. *Med J Malaysia* 1997;**52**:377–81.

45. Conway DL, Gonzales O, Skiver D. Use of glyburide for the treatment of gestational diabetes: the San Antonio experience. *J Matern Fetal Neonatal Med* 2004;**15**:51–5.

46. Kremer CJ, Duff P. Glyburide for the treatment of gestational diabetes. *Am J Obstet Gynecol* 2004;**190**:1438–9.

47. Chmait R, Dinise T, Moore T. Prospective observational study to establish predictors of glyburide success in women with gestational diabetes mellitus. *J Perinatol* 2004;**24**:617–22.

48. Gilson G, Murphy N. Comparison of oral glyburide with insulin for the management of gestational diabetes mellitus in Alaskan native women. *Am J Obstet Gynecol* 2002;**187**:S152.

49. Fines V, Moore T, Castle S. A comparison of glyburide and insulin treatment in gestational diabetes mellitus on infant birth weight and adiposity. *Am J Obstet Gynecol* 2003;**189** (Suppl 108):161.

50. Velazquez MD, Bolnick J, Cloakey JL, et al. The use of glyburide in the management of gestational diabetes. *Obstet Gynecol* 2003;**101**:88S.

51. Pendsey SP, Sharma RR, Chalkhore SS. Repaglinde: a feasible alternative to insulin in management of gestational diabetes mellitus. *Diabetes Res Clin Pract* 2002;**56**(Suppl 1):S44–S5.

52. Coetzee EJ, Jackson WP. Metformin in management of pregnant insulin-independent diabetics. *Diabetologia* 1979;**16**:241–5.

53. Hellmuth E, Damm P, Molsted-Pedersen L. Oral hypoglycaemic agents in 118 diabetic pregnancies. *Diabetic Med* 2000;**17**:507–11.

54. Notelowitz M. Sulfonylurea therapy in the treatment of the pregnant diabetic. *S Afr Med J* 1971;**45**:226–9.

55. Yogev Y, Ben-Haroush A, Chen R, et al. Undiagnosed asymptomatic hypoglycemia: diet, insulin, and glyburide for gestational diabetic pregnancy. *Obstet Gynecol* 2004;**104**:88–93.

56. Moore CX, Cooper GJ. Co-secretion of amylin and insulin from cultured islet beta-cells: modulation by nutrient secretagogues, islet hormones and hypoglycemic agents. *Biochem Biophys Res Commun* 1991;**179**:1–9.

57. Jacobson GF, Ramos GA, Ching JY, et al. Comparison of glyburide and insulin for the management of gestational diabetes in a large managed care organization. *Am J Obstet Gynecol* 2005;**193**:118–24.

SECTION 4
Surgery and Anaesthesia

15 Operative delivery

LaTasha Nelson and Alan M Peaceman

Background

The growing obesity epidemic has resulted in increasing numbers of obese women requiring obstetric care and presenting unique challenges for their medical care providers.[1-5] Of particular concern is the increased rate of cesarean delivery in obese compared with nonobese patients.[6] The presence of obesity may help explain a portion of the rising rates of cesarean deliveries observed in industrialized societies.

Crane et al studied a population of 20 130 women with live births stratified by maternal prepregnancy body mass index (BMI), to compare route of delivery. In the population of women designated as nonobese, defined by a maternal BMI less than 29, the rate of cesarean delivery was 20.2%, whereas women with BMI between 29 and 34.9 had a rate of 30.1%, those with BMI between 35 and 39.9 had a rate of 38.6%, and when BMI exceeded 39.9, a rate of 45.9%.[7] In the preterm prediction study published by Brost et al, the authors were able to show a linear relationship between increasing prepregnancy BMI and increasing rate of cesarean delivery[8] (Figure 15.1). Studies in low-risk populations mirror the trend of increased rates of cesarean delivery among obese women. Kaiser et al demonstrated an odds ratio of 3.99 for the risk of cesarean delivery in a low-risk obese population of women managed by midwives. The authors defined the low-risk population as healthy women without chronic conditions (diabetes, hypertension, and unstable asthma), prenatal complications (multiple gestations, fetal malformations, and gestational diabetes), and those who chose repeat cesarean delivery.[9]

This increase in cesarean deliveries is of great concern because of the potential for increased morbidity that is so common, especially when compared with that associated with vaginal delivery. In addition, obese women undergoing cesarean delivery experience more complications than nonobese women, including increased blood loss, operative time, and rates of thromboembolic events. Complications occur during the procedures as well as in the postpartum period.[7,10,11] Postoperatively, obese women are also at increased risk of wound complications, admission to an intensive care unit (ICU) for postoperative recovery, and prolonged hospital stays.[12] This increase in morbid events leads to

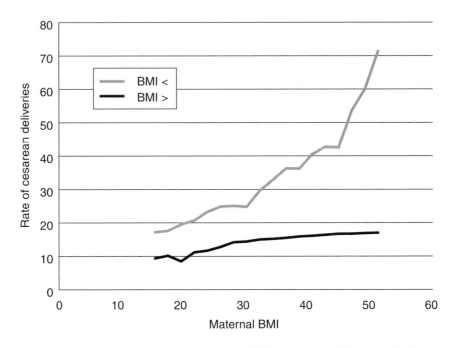

FIGURE 15.1 Cesarean delivery rate by maternal BMI (constructed from data in Crane et al[7])

increased personal and financial burdens that affect the individual, the hospital, and the healthcare system as a whole.

This chapter discusses preoperative planning and evaluation, operative concerns, and the prevention and management of postoperative complications in the care of obese patients. Counseling for future pregnancies is addressed at the end.

Preoperative planning

Any facility caring for obese and severely obese patient should have equipment designed for obese patients in order to provide adequate care (Table 15.1). These include appropriate-size dressing gowns, extra-large BP monitors, and automated beds able to support the weight and width of obese patients. Specialized surgical supplies include extra-long abdominal instrument sets with appropriate retractors and automated extra-wide beds with appropriate weight capacity. Medical and surgical teams must be aware of the potential need for the ICU after surgical procedures.[13]

Preparation for surgical procedures involves consideration of the special needs of this population. The obstetric literature is fairly limited with regard to the discussion of technical aspects of surgical preparation in obese and morbidly obese patients. However, the literature pertaining to patients who desire weight-loss surgery provides excellent descriptions of planning algorithms that improve surgical management[13] (Table 15.1).

TABLE 15.1   Patient care algorithm

Preoperative

1. Recommended equipment

   a. Surgical beds with appropriate weight capacity

   b. Equipment for patient lifting and transfer

   c. Wheelchairs and stretchers with appropriate weight capacity

   d. Extra-long abdominal instrument sets

   e. Extra-long abdominal retractors

2. Preoperative evaluation

   a. Consultation of medical services for surgical clearance if necessary

   b. Consider pulmonary function tests to evaluate respiratory status and risk of sleep apnea

   c. Baseline electrocardiogram for patients with chronic hypertension or cardiac conditions

   d. Anesthesia consultation for planning of optimal anesthesia/analgesia

3. Assemble obstetric team

   a. Physicians experienced in the care of obese patients

   b. Additional support staff to assist with surgical visualization

   c. Consider scheduling the case during times when additional physicians are available to provide assistance if necessary

4. Laboratory evaluation

   a. Complete blood count

   b. Screening for blood products

Operative

1. Operating room organization

   a. Physician and support staff placement should provide access both during the procedure and for emergent situations

   b. Patient placement should promote easy ventilation without hindering the surgical team

2. Pneumatic compression devices should be used for prophylactic thromboprophylaxis

3. Surgical approach

   a. Decide on the appropriate abdominal skin incision

   b. Consideration of impaired exposure secondary to redundant soft tissue

   c. Forceps and vacuum instruments should be available in the event that soft tissue dystocia hinders delivery of the fetus

TABLE 15.1 (continued)

4. Antibiotics

a. Additional antibiotics should be available in the event of blood loss > 1500 ml

b. Additional antibiotics should be available in the event that operative time exceeds 3 h

5. Closure of surgical incision

a. Use of delayed absorbable suture should be considered for closure of the fascia layer

b. Mass closure should be considered for midline incisions

c. Layered closure is appropriate for transverse incisions

d. Suture closure of subcutaneous tissue should be considered when this layer exceeds a depth of 3 cm

e. Consider use of surgical staples for closure of the skin incision

Postoperative

1. Considerations should be made for optimal postoperative recovery

a. Patients with respiratory disorder may be better served in intensive care units

b. Many patients can be managed in standard postpartum recovery units

2. Thromboprophylaxis should be continued until the patient is ambulatory

3. Patients should be encouraged to attempt early assisted ambulation

4. Wound care

a. Patients should be counseled on the importance of good wound hygiene

b. Patients should be given close follow-up after discharge for removal of staples and evaluation of wound complications

Caring for obese and morbidity obese patients is very much a multidisciplinary effort. The team should include obstetric physicians experienced in the care of obese patients. The same may be said for the anesthetic and nursing teams. The general approach should be geared to ensuring patient safety while, at the same time, optimizing the surgical environment for the surgical team. Soft tissue dystocia is a common concern during vaginal delivery of obese patients, but this problem is even more pressing at cesarean delivery.[13] Maneuvers usually relied upon to assist in the delivery may be difficult if not impossible due to increased maternal girth; therefore, it is helpful to employ the assistance of persons experienced with the use of forceps and/or vacuum to facilitate safe and timely delivery. Ideally, these often complicated deliveries would be performed only on an elective basis when preoperative planning is possible. However, the reality is that emergencies occur when least expected, and mechanisms for mobilizing additional support staff should be available in institutions with a patient population that includes numerous obese and morbidly obese patients.

Preoperative laboratory evaluation should include at a minimum blood bank screening, with type and cross-match being performed prior to need due to the increased risk of blood loss during surgical cases. Evaluation of hemoglobin and/ or hematocrit is essential upon admission to labor and delivery. It is inappropriate to rely on clinic records, which may be out of date for this crucial information. Cardiac and respiratory evaluation may also be appropriate in instances where additional comorbid conditions, such as hypertension or diabetes, exist (see Chapter 16).

Pregnancy-related respiratory changes are exaggerated in obese obstetric patients; vital capacity, respiratory rate, and tidal volume are all compromised.[14] At the time of cesarean delivery, respiratory changes (specifically in vital capacity and tidal volume), are of particular importance; obstetricians therefore must rely heavily on experienced anesthesia staff (see Chapter 16). The planning for elective cases should include anesthesia consultations to evaluate respiratory and cardiac issues prior to the time of surgery. At the time of cesarean delivery, positioning of the patient is an important consideration. A delicate balance must be struck between optimizing surgical exposure and accessibility, and respiratory management in a potentially compromised patient.

Antibiotic therapy

Infectious complications are the leading cause of operative and postoperative morbidity in patients undergoing cesarean delivery.[12] Infectious morbidity includes wound infections and endometrial infections, both of which diagnoses are usually made during the immediate postpartum period and prior to discharge. Both also lead to increased length of hospital stay and patient dissatisfaction. This trend occurs in both low-risk and high-risk populations. Cesarean delivery is associated with an eightfold increase in infectious morbidity compared with vaginal delivery.[15] The obese patient is at increased risk, most likely due to increased operation times, increased blood loss, and increased difficulty of procedure. Tran et al studied a cohort of 969 women delivered by cesarean section and described risk factors for post-cesarean surgical site infections.[16] Every 5-unit increase of maternal BMI doubled the risk of postoperative infection.

Prevention of postsurgical infections has been well studied, and the administration of prophylactic antibiotics to patients undergoing elective and in-labor cesarean delivery results in as much as a 75% decrease in infectious morbidity. Current recommendations of the American College of Obstetricians and Gynecology include the use of narrow-spectrum antibiotics with adequate coverage for common skin pathogens.[1] First-generation cephalosporins, such as cefazolin, are generally used in patients without documented penicillin allergy.[17] Cefazolin is just as effective as newer cephalosporins at a lower cost. Dosing recommendations range between 1 and 2 g depending on the weight of the patient, duration of the case, and estimated amount of blood loss. Patients with penicillin allergies may be treated with second-line agents such as clindamycin or metronidazole,[1] which provide adequate coverage for skin pathogens. The use of broad-spectrum antibiotics is discouraged, as they are unnecessary and potentially increase the development of antibiotic-resistant organisms.

Standard dosing is successful in achieving adequate tissue levels of antibiotics in the majority of patients. However, in morbidly obese patients, dosing should be individualized.[18,19] In cases that are prolonged and with blood loss exceeding 1500 ml, additional doses of antibiotics may be necessary.[19,20] It is important to address the timing of antibiotic administration. There has been much debate as to whether prophylactic antibiotics should be administered prior to skin incision or at the time of umbilical cord clamping. Proponents of the administration of antibiotics prior to skin incision cite findings from classic animal studies by Burke,[21] who showed that adequate antibiotic levels achieved prior to bacterial inoculation with a susceptible pathogen resulted in a significant decrease in infection. Proponents of awaiting umbilical cord clamping before administering antibiotics believe that placental transport of antibiotics results in suboptimal therapy for the neonate, thus increasing the risk of sepsis with antibiotic-resistant pathogens. Moreover, the presence of antibiotic therapy could potentially complicate the evaluation of infectious morbidity in the nursery.[22,23]

Sullivan et al published a prospective, randomized, placebo-controlled trial to determine when prophylactic antibiotics should be administered during cesarean deliveries.[24] One group was given antibiotic therapy 15–60 min prior to skin incision, whereas the second group was given antibiotics at the time of umbilical cord clamp. The authors found that the group of women given antibiotics prior to skin incision had decreased rates of endometritis (1% vs 5%), as well as decreased rates of skin infections (3% vs 5%). Furthermore, this benefit was achieved without increasing rates of neonatal sepsis, neonatal ICU admission, or length of hospital stay. There were significantly fewer neonatal ICU admissions in the preoperative administration group. In the population of neonates with documented sepsis, the group found no difference in the types of pathogens or antibiotic resistance between the two groups.[24]

Thrombosis prophylaxis

While in developing countries the leading cause of maternal mortality is maternal hemorrhage, in developed countries it is thromboembolic conditions, including venous thrombosis, arterial thrombosis, and pulmonary embolism. The increased rate of thrombotic events is due to pregnancy-related enhancement of all aspects of Virchow's triad: hypercoagulability, venous stasis, and endothelial damage. During the ante- and postpartum periods, the number of thrombotic events increases 5–10-fold, accounting for 0.5–3 maternal deaths per 1000 deliveries. Cesarean delivery increases this risk above that experienced with vaginal parturition by 3–10-fold.[25–28]

The impact of obesity as an independent risk factor for thrombotic events is well documented. Stein et al conducted a retrospective cohort study, using the database of the National Hospital Discharge Survey (NHDS) to compare

12 015 000 obese patients and 691 000 000 normal-weight patients.[29] These patients represented a nonobstetric, nonsurgical, hospital-based population. For obese women, the relative risk (RR) of deep venous thrombosis was 2.50, and the RR of pulmonary embolism was 2.21. Obese women ran a greater risk than obese men (RR = 2.2). The impact of obesity on thrombotic disease was greatest in women less than 40 years of age when the RR of deep venous thrombosis was 6.1 compared with 3.7 in age-matched men.[29]

Obese pregnant women requiring cesarean delivery have three risk factors for thrombosis: obesity, female gender, and surgical procedure. Current recommendations advocate prophylactic therapy for high-risk women undergoing cesarean delivery.[28,30,31] A number of investigators have looked at optimal regimens of thromboprophylaxis that can be used at the time of cesarean delivery.

A retrospective cohort study conducted by Lindqvist et al in 1999 put to rest the notion that the prevalence of thromboembolic events is greater in the postpartum period than in the antepartum period. The incidence of thromboembolic events (13 per 10 000 deliveries) was evenly distributed between antepartum and postpartum events.[30]

Quinones et al conducted a decision analysis comparing four strategies for managing patients after cesarean delivery: universal subcutaneous heparin prophylaxis, heparin prophylaxis for patients with documented genetic thrombophilia, use of pneumatic compression stockings, and no prophylaxis.[31] The decision analysis showed that pneumatic compression stockings were the intervention associated with the lowest incidence of adverse events while decreasing the risk of thrombotic events. Their recommendation was to use universal pneumatic compression devices (PCDs), especially in high-risk patients undergoing cesarean delivery.[31]

Casele and Grobman performed a decision analysis evaluating the cost-effectiveness of thromboprophylaxis during cesarean delivery utilizing intermittent pneumatic compression. The final analysis demonstrated that the use of intermittent PCDs reduced the incidence of deep venous thrombosis by at least 50% at a cost of less than US$180 in most institutions.[32]

Operative incisions

An effective abdominal incision is one that can be made quickly, provides adequate exposure, allows for easy extension when necessary, and is associated with few postoperative complications. In terms of the satisfaction of patients, the cosmetic result is perhaps even more important, as this is often the only sign that remains evident to them. The appropriate placement of abdominal incisions is of particular concern in obese patients. One must weigh the benefit of improved access against the complications associated with wound closure and wound disruption.

The rationale behind different incisions is based on a thorough understanding of the anatomy of the abdominal wall. What follows is written from a practical point of view.[33]

Skin

The outermost layer of the abdominal incision has little to do with wound integrity but much to do with esthetics. Considerable care should be taken to consider the appearance of the final scar. Langer's lines are lines of tension or cleavage within the skin that are characteristic for each part of the body. Incisions made parallel to these lines heal well and produce fine, linear scars. Incisions made perpendicular to these lines produce irregular points of tension, and thus create a more pronounced scar and a poorer cosmetic finish. Langer's lines traverse the abdomen wall; thus, incisions that are transverse produce the best cosmetic effect.[33]

Fascia

The anterior abdominal wall possesses two superficial layers of fascia: a superficial fatty layer, Camper's fascia, and a deep and more fibrous layer, Scarpa's fascia. In addition to these superficial layers, a even deeper and more fibrous layer, the rectus sheath, originates from the aponeuroses of the transverse abdominal and oblique muscles as they meet in the abdominal midline. This layer, along with the muscles of the abdominal wall, holds the abdominal viscera in place.

Fascial fibers are oriented in a transverse fashion, a fact that is increasingly important at the time of incision closure. Transverse incisions are along the direction of the fibers, and repair of these incisions places suture around the fibers, thus producing a more secure closure. Vertical incisions are perpendicular to the fibers. Repair of this incision separates the fibers, reducing the strength of the fascia along the line of the incision.[33]

Muscle fibers

The anterior abdominal wall is made up of two groups of muscles. The flat muscles course diagonally and transversely and comprise the external obliques, the internal obliques, and the transversalis muscles. The second and more anterior group of muscles runs vertically and includes the rectus and pyramidalis muscles. These muscle fibers possess a healthy blood supply, as evident by the way in which they heal following trauma. Incisions that require sectioning of these muscles are generally well tolerated, healing well and without functional compromise.[33]

Abdominal incisions

Gaining and maintaining surgical access during abdominal cases is a major concern in the obese and morbidly obese patient. Operative time is extended and blood loss is increased, both issues increasing the risk of infectious morbidity and potentially prolonging operative recovery. Vertical and transverse incisions are used in the majority of cesarean deliveries; both are associated with potential benefits as well as potential morbidity. A number of studies have compared the use of vertical and transverse incisions in obese patients in an effort to determine which is best (see below).[34,35]

Transverse incisions

Transverse incisions are often favored in surgical procedures, as they present the best cosmetic results. Moreover, the strength of the closed transverse incision is superior to that of the vertical incision, leading to less wound breakdown. Furthermore, postoperative pain issues are decreased, and these incisions tend to interfere less with postoperative respiratory efforts.

Of the transverse incisions, the Pfannenstiel is most commonly used in obstetric and gynecologic surgical procedures.[33] This incision provides an excellent cosmetic result as well as a strong secure wound closure. Pfannenstiel incisions are described as slightly curved transverse incisions that are generally 10–15 cm in length. This incision requires dissection of the rectus fascia and separation of the rectus muscles in order to gain access to the abdominal viscera.

Maylard incisions are also used in obese patients to provide better access to the pelvic/abdominal cavity. These incisions are transverse and transect the rectus muscles. Identification of the inferior epigastric vessels is required prior to cutting the muscles in order to reduce blood loss. These vessels may be preserved or ligated at the discretion of the surgeon. With this incision, the rectus muscles are not dissected from the overlying fascia, thus facilitating better reapproximation at the time of incision closure.[33]

Disadvantages of both transverse incisions include awkward exposure, particularly in the obese and morbidly obese and in cases where the upper abdomen must be visualized. In addition, transverse incisions necessitate the division of fascial and muscle layers, which may increase hemorrhage and the risk of postoperative hematoma. Of great importance, in obese or morbidly obese patients, this incision is often placed in the skin folds of the panniculus, where it might increase infectious morbidity. Transverse incisions take longer (6–15 min) to perform than vertical incisions.[33–35] Closure of transverse incisions is generally layered with or without closure of the subcutaneous tissue. Another disadvantage of transverse incisions is that retraction of the large pannus, in order to gain good access, can compromise the maternal cardiopulmonary system and cause anesthetic problems (see Chapter 16).[36]

Vertical incisions

Vertical incisions provide the best exposure of the abdominal cavity during surgical procedures. They allow rapid entry in emergent situations, thus decreasing overall operative time. This partly results from the fact that entry does not require division of the rectus muscles from the associated fascia and is therefore less likely to lead to hemorrhage and hematoma formation.[33,35,37] Disadvantages of vertical incisions include the appearance of a scar that is very visible, greater postoperative pain than with transverse incisions, and higher likelihood of respiratory complications, possibly due to splinting and decreased motion secondary to pain.

Many surgical techniques are utilized in the closure of vertical incisions, including layered and mass closure. Two meta-analyses have shown that mass closures are superior to layered closures for midline incisions in terms of decreased rates of postoperative wound hernia, wound dehiscence, suture sinuses, infection, and wound pain.[38,39]

The question remains of which incision is optimal. Wall conducted a retrospective cohort study of 239 women with BMI greater than 35 undergoing primary cesarean delivery. The primary outcome measure was a wound complication requiring reopening of the incisions. The overall incidence of wound complications was 12%, which is comparable to that experienced in similar studies. The incidence of wound complications in patients with vertical compared with transverse incisions was significantly higher (35% vs 9%).[37] Although the data from this study are impressive, it is hampered by the fact that patients receiving vertical incisions tended to have higher BMI. Thus, it is unclear whether the significant difference in wound complications was due to confounding or to characteristics of the incision. In the final analysis, it is important to make individualized decisions pertaining to incision techniques. One must always take into account prior incisions (if any), maternal body habitus, the urgency of the procedure, and the number and competency of available surgical assistants.

Postoperative considerations

Postoperative complications are increased in obese and morbidly obese patients undergoing cesarean delivery compared with those delivering vaginally. The most common cause of postoperative morbidity is postoperative wound complications, including wound infections, seromas, and hematomas. Wound complications occur in 2.5–29.7% of all cesarean deliveries. This percentage far exceeds that of other, nonobstetric, abdominal procedures, most likely due to contamination from organisms found in infected amniotic fluid. The most common cause of wound disruption is from infectious etiologies.[40,41] Abdominal adiposity is a strong risk factor for postoperative wound complications, especially when subcutaneous tissue thickness exceeds 2–3 cm.[42,43] The reason for this increased morbidity is related to the poor vascular supply of fatty tissue and the fact that suboptimal blood flow increases the susceptibility to infection following contamination.[44]

Vermillion et al conducted a prospective study of 140 obstetric patients undergoing cesarean delivery of varying BMI which attempted to estimate the effect of subcutaneous wound thickness as a risk factor for wound complications.[45] These women had an average BMI greater than 44.5. The only single independent risk factor related to wound complications was maximum subcutaneous tissue thickness greater than 3 cm (RR = 2.8). The authors showed no relationship between absolute body weight or BMI, only body habitus and the distribution of adiposity.[45]

Del Valle et al conducted a study to evaluate risk factors that increase postoperative wound complications in obese populations.[46] They considered 438 women with average BMI greater than 30 undergoing cesarean delivery. Of the total of 22 wound complications, 6 were in the group of patients with subcutaneous closure and 16 in the group without closure. The addition of subcutaneous closure decreased wound complications from 7.4% to 2.7% ($P = 0.03$). These authors postulated that this benefit was due to a decrease in the functional dead space between skin and fascia, as well as increased tensile strength provided by the addition suture. In addition, it was determined that the benefit of subcutaneous wound closure diminished as BMI increased.[46]

Naumann et al also demonstrated that a significant decrease in postoperative wound complications could be achieved by closuring subcutaneous tissue at the time of cesarean delivery.[47] They randomized 245 women with at least 2 cm of subcutaneous fat to either subcutaneous closure or no closure at the time of cesarean delivery. Prophylactic antibiotics were given at the time of umbilical cord clamping in all women. The overall rate of wound complications was 20.8%, subclassified into 14.5% in the closure group and 26.6% in the no-closure group ($P = 0.02$). These authors concluded that closure of subcutaneous tissue can significantly reduce postoperative wound complications in women possessing greater than 2 cm of subcutaneous fat.[47]

The prevailing recommendation is for placement of absorbable sutures for subcutaneous tissue approximation in patients with greater than 2 cm of subcutaneous tissue, as a means to decrease the rate of postoperative wound disruption.

The subject of use of drain placement in obese patients remains a matter of discussion. A number of studies report no difference in wound morbidity with use of subcutaneous drain placement versus suture alone without drain. Magann et al published a randomized controlled trial comparing no-closure, subcutaneous stitch closure and subcutaneous drain placement in women with 2 cm or more subcutaneous tissue.[48] The no-suture-closure group comprised 205 women with average BMI of 39.8 ± 7.2, the suture closure group comprised 191 women with average BMI of 39.4 ± 8.6, and the drain placement group comprised 194 women with average BMI of 40.7 ± 12.7. They found no significant difference in wound morbidity among the three groups.[48]

The Cochrane Collaboration published a review of wound drainage for cesarean section.[49] Seven randomized controlled trials were included, representing a total of 1993 women. The authors of this study found that there was no evidence to support the routine placement of drains after cesarean delivery. They also found no difference in the risk of wound infections, other wound complications, febrile morbidity, or endometritis in women with wound drains compared with women without drains. A trend toward longer operative time and increased blood loss was present in patients with drains compared to women without wound drains.[49]

Finally, Ramsey et al looked at whether drains could be used in addition to subcutaneous sutures to improve outcome.[50] This group found that the addition of a wound drain was ineffective in reducing wound complications. In fact, the women with both interventions had higher rates of wound complications than the women with suture alone, though this number did not reach statistical significance.[50]

Delivery after cesarean section in obese women

The management of future deliveries and appropriate patient counseling deserves mention. It is not always clear whether these patients should be advised to undergo elective repeat cesarean delivery or be encouraged to consider a vaginal trial of labor. A study published in 2006 by the National Institute of Child Health and Human Development Maternal-Fetal Medicine Units Network addressed this question.[51] This study evaluated 14 142 women with singleton pregnancies undergoing a trial of labor after cesarean delivery compared with 14 304 women with singleton pregnancies undergoing elective cesarean delivery over a 4-year period. The failure rate increased in a dose-related manner with increasing BMI. In women with BMI of 18.5–24.9 (normal), the rate of vaginal trial failure was 15.2%. The rate of failure in women with BMI of 25.0–29.9 (overweight) was 22.3%, and for women with BMI of 30.0–39.9 (obese) it was 29.9%. Finally, the rate of failure in women with BMI greater than 40 (morbidly obese) was 39.9% (Figure 15.2). The morbidly obese women failing a trial of vaginal delivery experienced a sixfold higher maternal morbidity, and increased rates of hospital stay greater than 4 days, endometritis, and neonatal ICU admissions. Morbidly obese women undergoing elective repeat cesarean delivery experienced a rate of uterine rupture/dehiscence fivefold greater than women with lower BMI.[51]

Obese and morbidly obese women considering a trial of labor after cesarean delivery should be counseled on the potential maternal and neonatal risks.

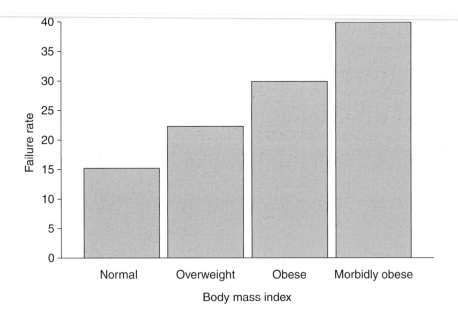

FIGURE 15.2 Percentage of women failing vaginal trial of labor. (Adapted from Hibbard et al.[51])

Clinicians should individualize patients, always taking into account the indication for the initial operative delivery as well as prior obstetric history when counseling patients about delivery options.[51]

References

1. ACOG Committee Opinion 315: Obesity in pregnancy. *Obstet Gynecol* 2005;**106**:671–5.
2. Kumari AS. Pregnancy outcome in women with morbid obesity. *Int J Obstet Gynaecol* 2001;**73**:101–7.
3. Wolfe HM, Gross TL, Sokol RJ, et al. Determinants of morbidity in obese women delivered by cesarean. *Obstet Gynecol* 1988;**71**:691–6.
4. Kliegman RM, Gross T. Perinatal problems of the obese mother and her infant. *Obstet Gynecol* 1985;**66**:299–305.
5. Robinson HE, O'Connell CM, Joseph KS, et al. Maternal outcomes in pregnancies complicated by obesity. *Obstet Gynecol* 2005;**106**:1357–64.
6. Young TK, Woodmansee B. Factors that are associated with cesarean delivery in a large private practice: the importance of prepregnancy body mass index and weight gain. *Am J Obstet Gynecol* 2002;**187**:312–20.
7. Crane SS, Wojtowycz MA, Dye TD, et al. Association between pre-pregnancy obesity and the risk of cesarean delivery. *Obstet Gynecol* 1997;**89**:213–16.
8. Brost BC, Goldenberg RL, Mercer BM, et al. The preterm prediction study: association of cesarean delivery with increases in maternal weight and body mass index. *Am J Obstet Gynecol* 1997;**177**:333–41.
9. Kaiser PS, Kirby RS. Obesity as a risk factor for cesarean in a low-risk population. *Obstet Gynecol* 2001;**97**:39–43.
10. Perlow JH, Morgan MA. Massive maternal obesity and perioperative cesarean morbidity. *Am J Obstet Gynecol* 1994;**170**:560–5.
11. Perlow JH, Morgan MA, Montgomery D, et al. Perinatal outcomes in pregnancy complicated by massive obesity. *Am J Obstet Gynecol* 1992;**167**:958–62.
12. Houston MC, Raynor BD. Postoperative morbidity in the morbidly obese parturient woman: supraumbilical and low transverse abdominal approaches. *Am J Obstet Gynecol* 2000;**182**:1033–5.
13. Whittemore AD, Kelly J, Shikora S, et al. Specialized staff and equipment for weight loss surgery patients: best practice guidelines. *Obes Res* 2005;**13**:283–9.
14. Ungern-Sternberg BS, Regli A, Bucher E, et al. Impact of spinal anesthesia and obesity on maternal respiratory function during elective Cesarean section. *Anesthesia* 2004;**59**:743–9.
15. Lang CT, King JC. Maternal mortality in the United States. *Best Pract Res Clin Obstet Gynaecol* 2008 [Epub ahead of print].
16. Tran TS, Jamulitrat S, Chongsuvivatwong V, et al. Risk factors for postcesarean surgical site infection. *Obstet Gynecol* 2000;**95**:367–71.
17. Chelmow D, Hennesy M, Evantash EG. Prophylactic antibiotics for non-laboring patients with intact membranes undergoing cesarean delivery: an economic analysis. *Am J Obstet Gynecol* 2004;**191**:1661–5.

18. Forse RA, Karam B, Maclean LD, et al. Antibiotic prophylaxis for surgery in morbidly obese patients. *Surgery* 1989;**106**:750–6.

19. Ohge H, Takesue Y, Yokoyama Y, et al. An additional dose of cefazolin for intraoperative prophylaxis. *Surg Today* 1999;**29**:1233–6.

20. Swoboda SM, Merz C, Kostnik T, et al. Does intraoperative blood loss affect antibiotic serum and tissue concentrations. *Arch Surg* 1996;**131**:1165–71.

21. Burke JF. The effective period of preventive antibiotic action in experimental incision and dermal lesions. *Surgery* 1961;**50**:161–8.

22. Chelmow D, Ruehli MS, Huang E. Prophylactic use of antibiotics for nonlaboring patients undergoing cesarean delivery with intact membranes: a meta-analysis. *Am J Obstet Gynecol* 2001;**184**:656–61.

23. Thigpen BD, Hood WA, Chauhan S, et al. Timing of prophylactic antibiotic administration in the uninfected laboring gravida: a randomized clinical trial. *Am J Obstet Gynecol* 2005;**192**:1864–71.

24. Sullivan SA, Smith T, Chang E, et al. Administration of cefazolin prior to skin incision is superior to cefazolin at cord clamping in preventing postcesarean infectious morbidity: a randomized controlled trial. *Am J Obstet Gynecol* 2007;**455**:e1–5.

25. James AH, Grotegut CA, Brancazio LR, et al. Thromboembolism in pregnancy: recurrence and its prevention. *Semin Perinatol* 2007;**31**:167–75.

26. Krivak TC, Zorn KK. Venous thromboembolism in obstetrics and gynecology. *Obstet Gynecol* 2007;**109**:761–77.

27. Myles TD, Gooch J, Santolaya J. Obesity as an independent risk factor for infectious morbidity in patients who undergo cesarean delivery. *Obstet Gynecol* 2002;**100**:959–64.

28. Jacobsen AF, Drolsum A, Klow NE, et al. Deep vein thrombosis after elective cesarean section. *Thromb Res* 2004;**113**:283–8.

29. Stein PD, Beemath A, Olson RE. Obesity as a risk factor in venous thromboembolism. *Am J Med* 2005;**118**:978–80.

30. Lindqvist P, Dahlback B, Marsal K, et al. Thrombotic risk during pregnancy: a population study. *Obstet Gynecol* 1999;**94**:595–9.

31. Quinones JN, James DN, Stamilio DM, et al. Thromboprophylaxis after cesarean delivery. *Obstet Gynecol* 2005;**106**:733–40.

32. Casele H, Grobman WA. Cost-effectiveness of thromboprophylaxis with intermittent pneumatic compression at cesarean delivery. *Obstet Gynecol* 2006;**108**:535–40.

33. Burke JJ, Gallup DG. Incisions for gynecologic surgery. In: *Operative Gynecology*, 9th edn. Philadelphia: Lippincott Williams and Wilkins, 2003: 256–90.

34. Houston MC, Raynor BD. Postoperative morbidity in the morbidly obese parturient woman: supraumbilical and low transverse abdominal approaches. *Am J Obstet Gynecol* 2000;**182**:1033–5.

35. Grantcharov TP, Rosenberg J. Vertical compared with transverse incisions in abdominal surgery. *Eur J Surg* 2001;**167**:260–7.

36. Perlow JH. Obesity in the obstetric intensive care patient. In: Foley M, Strong T, eds. *Obstetric Intensive Care: A practical manual*. Philadelphia: WB Saunders, 1997: 77–90.

37. Wall PD, Deucy EE, Glantz JC, et al. Vertical skin incisions and wound complications in the obese parturient. *Obstet Gynecol* 2003;**102**:952–6.

38. Richards PC, Balch CM, Aldrete J. Abdominal wound closure. *Ann Surg* 1983;**197**:238–43.

39. Cardosi RJ, Drake J, Holmes S, et al. Subcutaneous management of vertical incisions with 3 or more centimeters of subcutaneous fat. *Am J Obstet Gynecol* 2006;**196**:607–16.

40. Chelmow D, Huang E, Strohbehn K. Closure of the subcutaneous dead space and wound disruption after Cesarean delivery. *J Matern Fetal Neonatal Med* 2002;**11**:403–8.

41. Martens MG, Kolrud BL, Faro S, et al. Development of wound infection or separation after cesarean delivery. *J Reprod Med* 1995;**40**:171–5.

42. Emmons SL, Krohn M, Jackson M, et al. Development of wound infections among women undergoing cesarean section. *Obstet Gynecol* 1988;**72**:559–64.

43. Cetin A, Cetin M. Superficial wound disruption after cesarean delivery: effect of the depth and closure of subcutaneous tissue. *Int J Gynaecol Obstet* 1997;**57**:17–21.

44. Chelmow D, Rodriguez EJ, Sabatini MM. Suture closure of subcutaneous fat and wound disruption after cesarean delivery: a meta-analysis. *Obstet Gynecol* 2004;**103**:974–80.

45. Vermillion ST, Lamoutte C, Soper DE, et al. Wound infection after cesarean: effect of subcutaneous tissue thickness. *Obstet Gynecol* 2000;**95**:923–6.

46. Del Valle GO, Combs P, Qualls C, et al. Does closure of camper fascia reduce the incidence of post-cesarean superficial wound disruption? *Obstet Gynecol* 1992;**80**:1013–16.

47. Naumann RW, Hauth JC, Owen J, et al. Subcutaneous tissue approximation in relation to wound disruption after cesarean delivery in obese women. *Obstet Gynecol* 1995;**85**:412–16.

48. Magann EF, Chauhan SP, Rodts-Palenik S, et al. Subcutaneous stitch closure versus subcutaneous drain to prevent wound disruption after cesarean delivery: a randomized clinical trial. *Am J Obstet Gynecol* 2002;**186**:1119–23.

49. Gates S, Anderson ER. Wound drainage for caesarean section. *Cochrane Database Syst Rev* 2005; (1):CD004549.

50. Ramsey PS, White AM, Guinn DA, et al. Subcutaneous tissue reapproximation, alone or in combination with drain, in obese women undergoing cesarean delivery. *Obstet Gynecol* 2005;**105**:967–73.

51. Hibbard JU, Gilbert S, Landon MB, et al. Trial of labor or repeat cesarean delivery in women with morbid obesity and previous cesarean delivery. *Obstet Gynecol* 2006;**108**:125–33.

16 Anaesthetic techniques

Melanie J Woolnough and Steven M Yentis

Introduction

Pregnancy is well known to pose particular risks to women undergoing anaesthesia, and attention to these risks is thought to be one of the major factors resulting in the decline of maternal deaths directly due to anaesthesia over the last 20–30 years. Obesity is also associated with increased risks of anaesthesia, and the combination of obesity and pregnancy presents the obstetric anaesthetist with an exceptional challenge; it also puts the obese parturient into a high-risk group (Table 16.1),[1] irrespective of any obstetric complication that she may also be more likely to suffer (see previous chapters).

Antenatal assessment

The last triennial report of the UK 'Confidential Enquiries into Maternal Death' found that, of those who died, 52% had a body mass index (BMI) greater than 25, and of the deaths due directly to anaesthesia 4 out of 6 women were obese.[2] It recommended that obstetric units develop protocols for the management of morbidly obese women, including early referral for anaesthetic assessment. However, the practical problems posed by antenatal anaesthetic assessment of all such women, ideally by an experienced obstetric anaesthetist, are enormous – at least in the UK, where pregnant women are not routinely seen antenatally by anaesthetists. A recent national survey found that 67% of units did not routinely refer parturients with BMI > 35, and many leading obstetric anaesthetists felt that a threshold of > 40 would be more clinically relevant.[3] Even the latter cut-off carries the risk that anaesthetic resources may become overloaded, especially if the prevalence of obesity continues to increase.

The assessment should include a detailed history and examination, including an evaluation of the respiratory and cardiovascular system, airway, peripheral veins, and lower back. Blood pressure should be measured with an appropriate size cuff to ensure accurate readings depending on the circumference of the woman's arm: < 33 cm (13 inches) = regular cuff; 33–41 cm (13–16 inches) = large cuff; and > 41 cm (> 16 inches) = thigh cuff.[4]

Investigations at this time should be directed by the findings of the history and physical examination, but may include further blood tests, including arterial

TABLE 16.1 Increased anesthetic-related risks associated with obesity.

Respiratory	o Difficult airway and intubation*
	o Decreased functional residual capacity, vital capacity and oxygen reserve;* increased incidence of hypoxaemia*
	o High airway pressures during controlled ventilation*
	o Chronic respiratory insufficiency
	o Obstructive sleep apnoea or obesity hypoventilation syndrome
	o Pulmonary hypertension
Cardiovascular	o Hypertension
	o Difficulty monitoring blood pressure
	o Ischaemic heart disease
	o Increased risk of deep vein thrombosis*
Gastrointestinal	o Hiatus hernia; increased gastric volume/acidity and intra-abdominal pressure,* i.e., increased risk of aspiration *
Metabolic/endocrine	o Diabetes*
	o Hypercholesterolaemia
	o Gallbladder and biliary disease; fatty liver*
Pharmacological	o Altered pharmacokinetics*
	o Difficulty calculating appropriate dosage*
Technical aspects	o Difficult monitoring
	o Difficult regional anaesthesia
	o Difficult venous access
	o Difficult positioning and moving; need for specialized equipment, e.g., operating tables, lifting equipment

Those marked * indicated risks that are also conferred by pregnancy

blood gas analysis, electrocardiography, echocardiography, and pulmonary function tests.

With the results of these evaluations available, and in communication with the obstetricians, midwives, and the woman herself, a joint management plan for the intra- and postpartum periods should be formulated and documented clearly in the antenatal case notes. Any comorbidity should be treated aggressively at this time with referral to the appropriate clinicians. A third-trimester weight should ideally be available in the notes, though units may find measuring very large women's weight difficult. At this time, it would be useful to consider the need for any extra equipment. It is imperative that appropriate labour ward beds, theatre tables, and hoists are available, not to mention scales to obtain the patient's weight when she is ambulatory. Many older manual operating tables have a maximum weight limit of 135 kg, whereas the joint guidelines from the Obstetric Anaesthetists' Association (OAA) and Association of Anaesthetists of Great Britain and Ireland (AAGBI) recommend that operating tables should withstand at least 165 kg.[5] Many commercially available mechanical operating tables will sustain weights of 250–300 kg, and these tables have the added advantage of not needing manual adjustment, which may require intense effort.

Intrapartum care – anaesthetic techniques

When the woman arrives on the labour ward she should be assessed early by the anaesthetist and obstetrician. Senior members of both teams must be informed and stand ready to give a hand if required. In extreme cases, extra staff should be allocated to the team (this would include obstetric, anaesthetic, anaesthetic assistant, and midwifery), since most procedures will be more difficult. Details of general intrapartum care are described in Chapter 9. Of particular relevance to anaesthesia is the need for intravenous cannulation (which may be difficult and should be done early), appropriate blood pressure monitoring (with an appropriate size cuff), and anti-aspiration prophylaxis (e.g., nil by mouth, regular doses of ranitidine), as obese women are more at risk of intervention, including general anaesthesia. Women should also wear graduated pressure stockings throughout their admission to help prevent thromboembolism, though care should be taken to ensure that stockings are of adequate size so that they themselves do not cause restriction of blood flow.

Analgesia for labour

Analgesia may be broadly classified into non-drug, systemic drug, and regional techniques. The implications of non-drug methods and systemic drugs (typically Entonox and pethidine or other opioids) in obesity are broadly similar to those for women of lower BMI. Although side effects, such as sedation and respiratory depression, can be especially detrimental in obese women, no evidence suggests that the latter are more at risk from them – though drug regimens based on weight may cause difficulty, as it is not clear whether to estimate drug doses according to ideal weight, lean body weight, or actual weight.[6] Conversely, giving fixed doses irrespective of weight (e.g., 100 mg pethidine) may result in inadequate dosage, whereas intramuscular injections may be unreliable, with the drug being unintentionally placed in the subcutaneous tissues instead of the muscle.

Regional anaesthesia/analgesia describes the loss of sensation artificially produced by the administration of one or more agents at some point along the course of a nerve, blocking the passage of impulses along that nerve pathway to the brain. In the context of obstetrics, it usually refers to an epidural, spinal, or combined spinal–epidural (CSE) technique (Figure 16.1). All of these techniques are commonly used in obstetric practice; *analgesia* refers to relief of pain during labour while *anaesthesia* refers to insensitivity to surgical interventions, though the distinction is sometimes blurred (e.g., low-dose techniques that provide pain

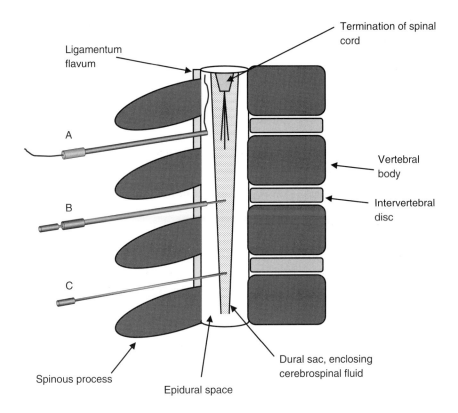

FIGURE 16.1 Diagram of vertebral canal, showing different regional anaesthetic/analgesic techniques. (A) Epidural showing insertion of catheter; (B) combined spinal–epidural showing placement of spinal needle through epidural needle; (C) spinal. Reprinted with permission from Richards NA, Yentis SM. Anaesthesia, analgesia and peripartum management in women with pre-existing cardiac and respiratory disease. *Fetal Matern Med Rev* 2006;**17**:327–47.

relief in labour can also allow certain procedures, such as perineal suturing, to be painless). Other regional techniques include paracervical and pudendal blocks, though these are rarely, if ever, performed by the anaesthetist. The advantages and disadvantages of the different regional techniques over each other are similar to those in non-obese parturients. In general, epidurals confer flexibility, i.e., they may be extended for several hours and/or topped up for delivery, spinals offer more rapid, dense anaesthesia suitable for surgical procedures, and CSEs are technically more complex but offer the advantages of both techniques. In obese women, the choice of technique mainly depends on the personal preference of the anaesthetist, the nature of the indication (labour, delivery, etc.), and the technical aspects of achieving regional anaesthesia in obese patients (see below).

Regional analgesia in labour has many advantages for the obese woman. It usually offers excellent analgesia and, in doing so, decreases maternal cardiovascular and respiratory work by decreasing oxygen consumption.[7] Good analgesia may also facilitate vaginal examination/placement of a fetal scalp electrode, if these are made more difficult by the mother's obesity. Since obese women are more at risk of obstetric interventions, the ability to top up the epidural as required reduces the need for urgent new anaesthesia that may be difficult and/or hazardous in this patient group. Establishing regional analgesia early in labour is particularly beneficial, as it will be technically easier if the woman can sit or lie still, and the anaesthetist can be sure that it is working before the contractions become too intense.

Difficulties with regional blockade

Regional techniques can be extremely challenging in very obese patients. The bony landmarks used to identify the position of the lumbar interspaces are more difficult or even impossible to palpate and, in some individuals, even locating the midline is difficult. The latter is usually easier with the patient in the sitting position, but this may require several helpers to assist the woman into position. The distance from the skin to the epidural space exhibits considerable individual variation depending on the distribution of adipose tissue,[8] but does show some correlation with BMI.[9] Standard epidural and spinal needles (8–10 cm) may be too short, so most manufacturers now market longer needles (13–15 cm) for use in obese individuals (Figure 16.2), though even these may not be long enough in extreme cases. In recent years, ultrasonography imaging has been used to aid the placement of regional blocks, and several studies describe its use in the obese obstetric population, either as an indirect measurement before epidural placement or used directly during the procedure.[10–12] Many departments now have access to portable ultrasound machines, as they are routinely used for the placement of central venous catheters, and, of course, there are ultrasound scanners available in the maternity unit. However, these devices are not designed for this purpose and may be less suitable for epidural/spinal techniques, especially in extreme obesity. Clearly, their optimal use requires operator training and practice.

Once the epidural space has been located and cannulated, obese women are at greater risk of the catheter migrating out of the epidural space during labour.[13,14] For example, Hood and Dewan found that 42% of morbidly obese women had their initial epidural catheter fail, compared with 6% of controls.[15] This could be related to increased mobility of the skin and subcutaneous tissues overlying the vertebral column, so that, even if the catheter is well fixed to the skin, movement of the patient during labour could pull the tip out of the epidural space.[16,17] However, leaving a greater length of catheter in the epidural space to counteract this is more likely to result in a partially effective block, as the catheter is more likely to lie laterally.

Apart from failure, the increased difficulty in placing regional blocks in obese women is likely to result in more accidental dural punctures. Furthermore, the risk of extensive block, with unintended motor block (adding to difficulty in moving the patient and possibly increasing the risk of deep vein thrombosis) and cardiorespiratory embarrassment, may also be increased. Several studies indicate

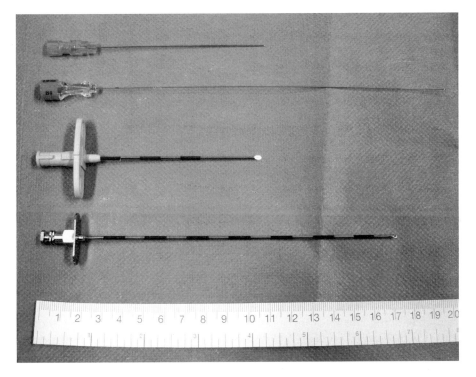

FIGURE 16.2 Examples of standard and extra-length spinal (upper) and epidural (lower) needles. Even the extra-long needles may be too short in extreme obesity

that in obesity there is increased cephalad spread of spinal solutions and that a higher sensory block is achieved than in normal individuals.[18-22] Furthermore, a study to estimate the minimum analgesic concentration of bupivacaine required for effective analgesia found that obese women required significantly less than women with normal BMI.[23] This circumstance is probably due to a decreased volume of spinal cerebrospinal fluid (CSF) in obesity and pregnancy, so that any local anaesthetic injected into the CSF is therefore less dilute.[24,25] Similarly, epidural solutions may spread more than in non-obese women, because the space available in the epidural compartment is reduced as a result of epidural fat and engorgement of epidural veins consequent to abdominal compression. One possible beneficial consequence of the increased epidural pressure is the observation that, should accidental dural puncture occur, the incidence of postdural puncture headache may be reduced in obesity.[26]

Anaesthesia for surgery

Obese parturients have an increased incidence of instrumental and operative delivery (see Chapters 9 and 15), so anaesthesia will be required more often. Most of the anaesthetic concerns can be considered under anaesthesia for caesarean section. Realistically, there are but two options for caesarean section: general and regional anaesthesia. Although the operation can be performed under local infiltration,[27] this is extremely rare in developed countries and would be a particular challenge for all concerned.

Caesarean sections can be subdivided by the degree of urgency to the mother and fetus;[28] this determines how quickly the fetus is to be delivered. However, preparing for and performing caesarean section on an obese woman invariably is more difficult and takes longer, for all the reasons previously mentioned[29,30] (see also previous chapters). It is imperative, therefore, that the obstetricians and midwives keep the anaesthetist appraised of the woman's status and any change in her condition or management plan. Apart from urgency of the case, other factors to consider include the experience and skill of the individual anaesthetist, whether the woman already has a working epidural in situ, any underlying medical or obstetric complications, and the preferences of the woman herself. Further considerations include the experience and skill of the obstetrician and the need to call for senior members of either or both parts of the team in advance rather than waiting for problems to become evident.

Potential difficulties with intravenous access and monitoring have already been mentioned. If these prove impossible with standard methods, central venous cannulation and invasive arterial monitoring may need to be considered, though these too may be difficult and time-consuming. As a last resort, surgical cut-down may be necessary. Pneumatic calf compression should be added to the graduated pressure stockings that should already be worn throughout admission. Positioning is a particular problem as previously mentioned. Uterine displacement to avoid aortocaval compression with a wedge and/or lateral table tilt may be difficult and of questionable efficacy with a grossly increased abdominal bulk. Arm boards are often useful, as they add width to the operating table, and may improve the accuracy of the monitoring. For procedures that require the lithotomy position, the standard operating table fittings may be inadequate and staff should be assigned to hold the woman's legs. The resultant effect on respiratory and cardiovascular function may limit the amount of hip flexion that is possible.

Regional anaesthesia

If there is an epidural catheter in situ, it can usually be topped up, time permitting, to provide anaesthesia for caesarean section, with most studies reporting an onset time of about 8–15 min and a failure rate of about 4% in non-obese parturients.[31,32]

If new anaesthesia must be provided, a 'single-shot' spinal would be a common choice for the non-obese parturient, and this technique may indeed be suitable for the morbidly obese. However, there appears to be an enormous amount of individual variability with regard to anaesthetic spread in obese patients, and particular caution is required. First, an inadequate block without the ability to extend it (i.e., without a catheter) has significant implications. Conversion to general anaesthesia mid-operation in the obese pregnant population carries an especially high risk, and any operative delay may be detrimental to the mother, fetus, or both. Surgical time is often prolonged in the obese, so a single-shot spinal may not provide adequate duration of anaesthesia, even if an opioid is added to the injectate. Therefore, continuous methods of regional anaesthesia are often preferred, such as CSE, using standard or low doses with the ability to extend the block.[33–35] If time allows, a deliberately low, initial spinal dose can be followed by extension of the block via the epidural, in order to avoid sudden onset of an excessively high block. An alternative is a continuous spinal (in which a microcatheter is placed *intrathecally*). The latter is less commonly used because of technical difficulties (the catheters are very fine and may easily kink, block, or fall out) and because of a spate of neurological complications in the USA 10–15 years ago, originally thought to be related to the technique itself but subsequently shown to be due to the high concentrations of lidocaine in common use at the time. However, continuous spinal anaesthesia has been advocated for caesarean section for the morbidly obese because of its ability to provide rapid and particularly controllable anaesthesia,[36,37] and the technique can also be used to provide analgesia in labour, allowing faster extension than epidural analgesia should caesarean section be required.

A second potential problem with regional anaesthesia in the obese is that as the block level rises it can contribute to respiratory embarrassment – even if the ultimate level of block is not considered excessive. This is thought to be due to block of the intercostal nerves, causing temporary paralysis of the intercostal muscles, combined with the reduction in functional residual capacity seen in obesity and exacerbated in both pregnancy and the supine position. A study of spirometry in obstetric patients receiving spinal anaesthesia for caesarean section found that respiratory function worsened after the spinal and that patients with BMI > 30 had the most significant deterioration.[38] The authors advocated early mobilization as the best method to restore respiratory function. Functional residual capacity and respiratory excursion can be improved in the supine position by tilting the patient head-up, but in the morbidly obese this may further impede surgery, already difficult, by increasing the impingement of adipose tissue on to the surgical site.

General anaesthesia

General anaesthesia is more hazardous than regional for obstetric procedures, and, in the UK, the large decline in its use over the last 20–30 years is thought to be the main factor contributing to the reduced anaesthetic maternal mortality over this time.[2] Currently, only 6–9% of caesarean sections in the UK are performed under general anaesthesia,[39] with most of these listed as emergencies. In such situations, the risks are higher, first because of whatever underlying condition necessitates urgent delivery, and second because of the haste that is often required. Obesity is an independent factor that also increases the risks involved (Table 16.1).

Before contemplating any general anaesthesia, an assessment of the woman's airway is mandatory. A short neck, increased fat deposition within the soft tissues, and large breasts increase the likelihood that airway management and tracheal intubation will be difficult.[40,41] This difficulty may be compounded by the naturally increased oedema of the soft tissues associated with pregnancy. Failed intubation in the obstetric population may be as high as 1 in 250 compared with 1 in 2000 in the general population,[42,43] and this risk is correspondingly higher in the morbidly obese. Standard assessment of the airway includes a Mallampati score (view of the pharynx during maximal mouth opening and tongue protrusion), assessment of neck mobility (e.g., measurement of thyromental and thyrosternal distances and neck circumference), and assessment of whether the mandible can be protruded or is receding, and whether there are prominent or missing upper incisors.[44,45] Because these indicators are relatively poor in their predictive power, a high index of suspicion is required even if they appear normal. A history of obstructive sleep apnoea is informative, as it may suggest the presence of increased pharyngeal soft tissue. Due to the anatomical differences in obese parturients the standard intubating position (neck flexed on the body and head extended on the neck) may be difficult to achieve. A 'ramped' position may provide an improved view at laryngoscopy;[46] this is accomplished by placing blankets under the individual's upper body until the external auditory meatus is in line with the sternal notch. If the airway is determined to be very difficult and there is time, awake fibreoptic intubation can be considered, although training and expertise in this technique is often limited in many centres.

By the second half of pregnancy, anatomical and physiological changes place women at increased risk of aspiration of stomach contents.[47] The obese parturient's risk is increased further as a result of increased intra-abdominal pressure, especially if hiatus hernia (common in obesity) is present. Obese parturients should therefore be premedicated with a histamine H_2-receptor antagonist (e.g., ranitidine) and metoclopramide as well as receive an antacid (sodium citrate; the particulate antacids traditionally used have been shown to be themselves irritant if inhaled) immediately before induction of anaesthesia. Anaesthesia is initiated by a rapid sequence induction (preoxygenation, rapidly acting drugs, and cricoid pressure), which provides optimal conditions for intubation and allows the airway to be secured quickly, while preventing passive reflux of gastric contents.

The mother's functional residual capacity must be denitrogenated before induction to increase the store of oxygen in the lungs to allow for a period of apnoea. Both obesity and pregnancy reduce functional residual capacity due to cephalad movement of the diaphragm and increased intra-abdominal pressure, so that the period of apnoea before which oxygen saturation begins to decrease is shorter in the obese parturient.[48,49] Preoxygenation usually consists of 3 min of tidal breathing with 100% inspired oxygen; if time is particularly short, 4–6 maximal inspired breaths may achieve considerable denitrogenation. Carrying out preoxygenation with the woman positioned head-up or semi-sitting may increase the efficacy of pre-oxygenation and prolong the time before arterial desaturation occurs.[50,51] Most obese women feel more comfortable sitting up than lying completely flat.

Standard drugs are used to induce anaesthesia, typically thiopental with suxamethonium, to cause neuromuscular blockade. The doses of these drugs are based on the patient's actual body weight rather than estimated lean body weight to avoid underdosing, though this may require more drug to be prepared than is usual (e.g., two syringes of each), and this must be accounted for when preparing emergency drugs in advance, as is commonly done. A risk of relative overdosing is present with this dose estimation, and this may contribute to prolonged action (notably sedation), though it is generally considered preferable to underdosing.

Controlled ventilation requires high positive airway pressures to achieve adequate tidal volumes, because of the weight of chest wall in addition to the tissue pushed up from the abdomen when the patient assumes the supine position. This pressure will be exacerbated if the abdominal panniculus is retracted in a cephalad direction during surgery, and it may be better if the excess tissue is suspended vertically,[52] though the necessary equipment may not always be available. The use of positive end-expiratory pressure may help prevent hypoxaemia due to small airway closure by increasing functional residual capacity, though it should be used with caution as the increased intrathoracic pressure that it produces may combine with any existing aortocaval compression, further reducing venous return and cardiac output.

Blood loss is increased with difficult and prolonged surgery, and it is easy not to appreciate the significance of measured losses, as the calculation of circulating blood volume according to body weight may underestimate the proportional loss. Along with raised intrathoracic pressure during ventilation, aortocaval compression persisting after the baby is delivered, difficulty in measuring blood pressure, and potentially difficult venous access, the anaesthetic team must be vigilant for cardiovascular instability and consider hypovolaemia early. Blood should be cross-matched and available when the surgery starts, and the individual whose job it is to bring it from the blood bank if required should be designated and ready to go with no other duties to leave unattended. Instability may be exacerbated by cardiovascular disease such as hypertension and/or myocardial ischaemia.

At the end of surgery, it is particularly important that neuromuscular blockade is adequately reversed since obese women are at increased risk of postoperative hypoxaemia. Airway problems may occur on emergence from anaesthesia as well as on induction, so the tracheal tube should be removed only when the mother is awake and with full monitoring; while this is true of any obstetric case, it is even more important in morbid obesity. Extubation in the sitting position reduces passive regurgitation, due to the effect of gravity, and functional residual capacity and lung excursion are also better in this position. Obese and morbidly obese women often require systemic opioids for postoperative analgesia. Because dosage may be difficult to estimate and the consequences of respiratory depressant side effects especially serious, such drugs should be carefully titrated against response. Multimodal analgesia with opioid, paracetamol, and non-steroidal anti-inflammatory drugs can be supplemented with local anaesthesia, either infiltrated or given as bilateral ilioinguinal blocks,[53,54] though the latter may be difficult to perform in morbid obesity.

Postpartum care

Obese patients are at increased risk of postoperative complications, and this caution is especially valid in the morbidly obese.[15] A period of high-dependency care is beneficial postpartum, especially if the patient has had an operative procedure, has an arterial or central lines in situ, has suffered any complications, or has pre-existing medical problems. Such individuals should be recovered and nursed in a reclining position and supplemental oxygen given routinely after surgery, even if regional anaesthesia has been used. Hypoxaemia due to hypoventilation and/or atelectasis may be reduced by good analgesia, encouragement, early mobilization, and even physiotherapy and/or repiratory therapy. Anti-thromboembolic prophylaxis is imperative, and all women should wear appropriate-size, graduated compression stockings and receive prophylactic low-molecular-weight heparin. Morbidly obese women are more likely to have postoperative wound infections and wound dehiscence, and also prolonged hospital stays.[30] If any complications require further surgery, the same considerations exist as those described above, in terms of anaesthetic risk.

References

1. Brown DL. *Risk and Outcome in Anesthesia*, 2nd edn. Philadelphia: JB Lippincott, 1992.
2. Cooper GM, McClure JH. Anaesthesia. In: *The Confidential Enquiry into Maternal and Child Health (CEMACH). Saving Mothers' Lives: Reviewing Maternal Deaths to Make Motherhood Safer – 2003–2005.* Seventh Report of the Confidential Enquiries into Maternal Deaths in the United Kingdom. London: CEMACH, 2007: 107–16.
3. Smith H, Varghese B, Gill P, Swales H. National survey of anaesthetic assessment of pregnant women with increased body mass index. *Int J Obstet Anesth* 2007;**16**(Suppl 1):47.
4. O'Brien, E. Review: a century of confusion; which bladder for accurate blood pressure measurement? *J Hum Hypertens* 1996;**10**:565–72.
5. Obstetric Anaesthetists' Association, Association of Anaesthetists of Great Britain and Ireland. *Guidelines for Obstetric Anaesthetic Services.* London: AAGBI, 2005.
6. Cheymol G. Effects of obesity on pharmacokinetics: implications for drug therapy. *Clin Pharmacokinet* 2000;**39**:215–31.
7. Maitra AM, Palmer SK, Bachhuber SR, Abram SE. Continuous epidural analgesia for caesarean section in a patient with morbid obesity. *Anesth Analg* 1979;**58**:348–9.
8. Watts RW. The influence of obesity on the relationship between body mass index and the distance to the epidural space from the skin. *Anaesth Intensive Care* 1993;**21**:309–10.
9. Clinkscales CP, Greenfield MLVH, Vanarase M, Polley LS. An observational study of the relationship between epidural space depth and body mass index in Michigan parturients. *Int J Obstet Anaesth* 2007;**16**:323–7.

10. Wallace DH, Currie JM, Gilstrap LC, Santos R. Indirect sonographic guidance for epidural anesthesia in obese pregnant patients. *Reg Anesth* 1992;**17**:233–6.

11. Grau T, Leipold RW, Horter J, et al. The lumbar epidural space in pregnancy: visualization by ultrasonography. *Br J Anaesth* 2001;**86**:798–804.

12. Grau T, Bartusseck E, Conradi R, et al. Ultrasound imaging improves learning curves in obstetric epidural anesthesia: a preliminary study. *Can J Anaesth* 2003;**50**:1047–50.

13. Wasson C. Failed epidural in an obese patient – blame it on Pythagoras! *Anaesthesia* 2000;**56**:605.

14. Bishton IM, Martin PH, Vernon JM, Liu, WHD. Factors influencing epidural catheter migration. *Anaesthesia* 1992;**47**:610–12.

15. Hood DD, Dewan DM. Anesthetic and obstetric outcome in morbidly obese parturients. *Anesthesiology* 1993;**79**:1210–18.

16. Faheem M, Sarwar N. Sliding of the skin over subcutaneous tissue is another important factor in epidural catheter migration. *Can J Anaesth* 2002;**49**:634.

17. Tackaberry CJT, Wadsworth R. Epidural catheter clamp fixes too firmly? *Anaesthesia* 1999;**54**:914.

18. Hodgkinson R, Husain FJ. Obesity and the cephalad spread of analgesia following epidural administration of bupivacaine for cesarean section. *Anesth Analg* 1980;**59**:89–92.

19. Hodgkinson R, Husain FJ. Obesity, gravity, and the spread of epidural anesthesia. *Anesth Analg* 1981;**60**:421–4.

20. Taivainen T, Tuominen M, Rosenberg PH. Influence of obesity on the spread of spinal analgesia after injection of plain 0.5% bupivacaine at the L3–4 or L4–5 interspace. *Br J Anaesth* 1990;**64**:542–6.

21. McCulloch WJD, Littlewood DG. Influence of obesity on spinal analgesia with isobaric 0.5% bupivacaine. *Br J Anaesth* 1986;**58**:610–14.

22. Pitkänen MT. Body mass and spread of spinal anesthesia with bupivacaine. *Anesth Analg* 1987;**66**:127–31.

23. Panni MK, Columb MO. Obese parturients have lower epidural local anaesthetic requirements for analgesia in labour. *Br J Anaesth* 2006;**96**:106–10.

24. Hogan QH, Prost R, Kulier A, et al. Magnetic resonance imaging of cerebrospinal fluid volume and the influence of body habitus and abdominal pressure. *Anesthesiology* 1986;**84**:1341–9.

25. Carpenter RL, Hogan QH, Liu S, et al. Lumbosacral cerebrospinal fluid volume is the primary determinant of sensory block extent and duration during spinal anesthesia. *Anesthesiology* 1998;**89**:24–9.

26. Faure E, Moreno R, Thisted R. Incidence of postdural puncture headache in morbidly obese parturients. *Reg Anesth Pain Med* 1994;**19**:361–3.

27. Gautam PL, Kathuria S, Kaul TK. Infiltration block for caesarean section in a morbidly obese parturient. *Acta Anaesthesiol Scand* 1999;**43**:580–1.

28. Lucas DN, Yentis SM, Kinsella SM, et al. Urgency of Caesarean section: a new classification. *J R Soc Med* 2000;**93**:346–50.

29. Weiss JL, Malone FD, Emig D, et al. Obesity, obstetric complications and cesarean delivery rate – a population-based screening study. *Am J Obstet Gynecol* 2004;**190**;1091–7.

30. Perlow JH, Morgan MA. Massive maternal obesity and perioperative cesarean morbidity. *Am J Obstet Gynecol* 1994;**170**:560–5.
31. Allam J, Malhotra S, Hemingway C, Yentis S. Epidural lidocaine–bicarbonate–adrenaline vs levobupivacaine for emergency caesarean section: a randomised controlled trial. *Anaesthesia* 2008;**63**:243–9.
32. Malhotra S, Yentis S. Extending low-dose epidural analgesia in labour for emergency Caesarean section – a comparison of levobupivacaine with or without fentanyl. *Anaesthesia* 2007;**62**:667–71.
33. Reyes M, Pan PH. Very low-dose spinal anesthesia for cesarean section in a morbidly obese preeclamptic patient and its potential implications. *Int J Obstet Anaesth* 2003;**13**:99–102.
34. Lim Y, Loo CC, Goh E. Ultra low dose combined spinal and epidural anesthesia for cesarean section. *Int J Obstet Anaesth* 2004;**14**:198–9.
35. Emett A, Gowrie-Mohan S. Standard dose hyperbaric bupivacaine is safe and effective for CSE in morbidly obese patients. *Int J Obstet Anaesth* 2004;**13**:298–9.
36. Milligan KR, Carp H. Continuous spinal anaesthesia for Caesarean section in the morbidly obese. *Int J Obstet Anaesth* 1992;**1**:111–13.
37. Imbelloni LE, Gouveia MA. Continuous spinal anesthesia with Spinocath® for obstetric anesthesia. *Int J Obstet Anaesth* 2006;**15**:171–2 (correspondence).
38. Von Ungern-Sternberg BS, Regli A, Bucher E, et al. Impact of spinal anaesthesia and obesity on maternal respiratory function during elective Caesarean section. *Anaesthesia* 2004;**59**:743–9.
39. Department of Health. *NHS Maternity Statistics, England 2003–2004*. London: Government Statistical Service for the Department of Health, 2005. Available at: www.dh.gov.uk/prod_consum_dh/idcplg?IdcService=GET _FILE&dID= 15265&Rendition=Web.
40. Halpern SH, Douglas JM, eds. *Evidence-based Obstetric Anaesthesia*. Oxford: Blackwell, 2005.
41. Juvin P, Lavaut E, Dupont H, et al. Difficult tracheal intubation is more common in obese than in lean patients. *Anesth Analg* 2003;**97**:595–600.
42. Hawthorne L, Wilson R, Lyons G, Dresner M. Failed intubation revisited: 17-year experience in a teaching maternity unit. *Br J Anaesth* 1996;**76**:680–4.
43. Barnardo PD, Jenkins JG. Failed tracheal intubation in obstetrics: a 6-year review in a UK region. *Anaesthesia* 2000;**55**:685–94.
44. Naguib M, Malabarey T, Alsatli RA, et al. Predictive models for difficult laryngoscopy and intubation. A clinical, radiological and three dimensional computer imaging study. *Can J Anaesth* 1999;**46**:748–59.
45. Rocke DA, Murray WB, Rout CC, Gouws E. Relative risk analysis of factors associated with difficult intubation in obstetric anesthesia. *Anesthesiology* 1992;**77**:67–73.
46. Collins JS, Lemmens HJM, Brodsky JB, et al. Laryngoscopy and morbid obesity: a comparison of the 'sniff' and 'ramped' positions. *Obes Surg* 2004;**14**:1171–5.

47. Miller RD, ed. *Miller's Anesthesia*, 6th edn. Philadelphia: Elsevier Churchill Livingstone, 2005.
48. Berthoud MC, Peacock JE, Reilly CS. Effectiveness of preoxygenation in morbidly obese patients. *Br J Anaesth* 1991;**67**:464–6.
49. Jense HG, Dubin SA, Silverstein PI, O'Leary-Escolas U. Effect of obesity on safe duration of apnea in anesthetized humans. *Anesth Analg* 1991;**72**:89–93.
50. Dixon BJ, Dixon JB, Carden JR, et al. Preoxygenation is more effective in the 25 degrees head-up position than in the supine position in severely obese patients: a randomized controlled study. *Anesthesiology* 2005;**102**:1110–15.
51. Altermatt FR, Muñoz HR, Delfino AE, Cortínez LI. Pre-oxygenation in the obese patient: effects of position on tolerance to apnoea. *Br J Anaesth* 2005;**95**:706–9.
52. Whitty RJ, Maxwell CV, Carvalho JCA. Complications of neuroaxial anesthesia in an extreme morbidly obese patient for cesarean section. *Int J Obstet Anesth* 2006;**16**:139–44.
53. Bunting P, McConachie I. Ilioinguinal nerve blockade for analgesia after Caesarean section. *Br J Anaesth* 1988;**61**:773–5.
54. Ganta R, Samra SK, Maddineni VR, Furness G. Comparison of the effectiveness of bilateral ilioinguinal nerve block and wound infiltration for postoperative analgesia after Caesarean section. *Br J Anaesth* 1994;**72**:229–30.

Index

Page references to *figures, tables and text boxes* are shown in *italics*.
Registries, studies and trials have been grouped together.